PAIN

Clinical Manual
for Nursing Practice

Withdrawn

Margo McCaffery RN, MS, FAAN
Consultant in the Nursing Care of Patients with Pain
Santa Monica, California

Alexandra Beebe RN, MS, OCN
Founder and Director
InControl: Cancer Pain Care Associates
Washington, DC

Adapted from the US edition by
Jane Latham RN, DipDN
Nurse Consultant in Pain Management
Honorary Lecturer, Trinity Hospice
London

with
Dermot Ball MSc, MRPharmS
Senior Clinical Pharmacist
Derbyshire Royal Infirmary
Derby

 Mosby

London Philadelphia St. Louis Sydney Tokyo

Publisher:	Nicola Horton
Developmental Editor:	Amy Salter
Project Manager:	Linda Kull
Production:	Cathy Martin
Index:	Wendy Adamson
Design:	Anne-Marie Woodruff
Cover Design:	Anne-Marie Woodruff

Copyright © 1994 Times Mirror International Publishers Limited

Published in 1994 by Mosby, an imprint of Times Mirror International Publishers Limited

Printed by Grafos SA Arte sobre, Barcelona, Spain

Reprinted in 1997

ISBN 0 7234 1992 2

For full details of all Times Mirror International Publishers Limited titles, please write to Times Mirror International Publishers Limited, Lynton House, 7–12 Tavistock Square, London WC1H 9LB, England.

A CIP catalogue record for this book is available from the British Library.

Preface

What is the purpose of this manual?

Authors Margo McCaffery and Alexandra Beebe, leading authorities in the field of pain management, have developed this manual to assist nurses and their colleagues in increasing their knowledge of pain, thus enhancing their unique contribution to the care of patients with pain. This manual provides a comprehensive selection of basic information, tools and specific techniques nurses and other health professionals may use to assess and effectively manage patients with pain.

Why an adapted edition?

This manual has been edited by a British nurse specialist in pain management to provide additional and/or equivalent information of specific relevance to health-care practitioners outside the USA. These adaptations include adding or changing information, such as drug names and usage, health-care terminology, differences in the health-care systems, and the philosophy and practise of pain management in the United Kingdom. Although such changes will make this manual more useful to readers outside the USA, the integrity of McCaffery and Beebe's original work is maintained throughout.

Who should use this manual?

This manual is designed for use by all nurses who specialize in pain management, including those who care for patients in primary care settings such as hospitals, homes or other care settings. Other health-care professionals, such as physiotherapists, doctors, occupational therapists and psychologists, will also find this information useful in their care of patients with pain.

What are the unique features of the manual?

This manual is designed not only for reading and learning, but also for *using* in clinical practice. The following features and tools are provided throughout the manual to assist you in providing optimal care in pain management:

Patient examples and **Immediate help sections**: use these to help you understand how to use the information provided and how to apply this information to specific patient situations.

Sample assessment sheets, Nursing guidelines and suggested **Nursing care plans**: use these to analyse particular nursing-care problems associated with specific patients, to organize appropriate patient care, and to communicate effectively with other colleagues involved in the patient's care.

Chapter references and **Annotated references**: use these to locate background and research information for further investigation into particular topics of interest, and to exchange ideas and information effectively among your colleagues.

Patient/family teaching points: use these to teach patients and their families about pain and how to manage it. Each teaching point corresponds to topics covered in particular chapters of the manual. You will find cross references to these teaching points at the beginning of their associated chapters and throughout that chapter. The teaching points are located in the Appendix for easy access and so you may photocopy them to distribute to patients.

Resources for health professionals and patients: use the comprehensive list, located at the end of Chapter 1, to locate organizations that may provide further information and services for you and your patients.

Acknowledgements

The editor and publisher gratefully acknowledge those who contributed to this edition: Virginia Dunn, Michele Hiscock, Anne Hunt, Noelle Llewelyn, Tony Nunn, Pam Price, Pat Schofield, Kate Seers, and Janet Walker.

Jane Latham, RN, DipDN
Nurse Consultant in Pain Management
London, 1994

The publishers also wish to acknowledge those who contributed to the original edition of this book: Lucie Ferrell, Craig Colbert, and Dolores Stammer; colleagues of Margo McCaffery and Alexandra Beebe; Judith Beyer, Jo Eland, Shoosh Lettick, Noreen Meinhart, Madelyn Miscally, Judith A. Paice, Susan C. Schafer, Sandy Sentivany, Carol Wenzl, Fran Wiley, Donna Wong, Paul Koren, Linda Duncan, and Susie Baxter; Melissa McCaffery, Mary Katherine Smith, Don Smith, Rick Brewer, Elaine, Lee, Ren, Bill, Carol, Jo, Noreen and Mark; Schuyler Savage, Camilla, Debbie, Dolores S., Connie, Eleanor, Joyce, and Dolores R.

Contents

Perspectives on Pain: History, Current Status, and Developing the Nurse's Role

Unquestionably, pain is extremely prevalent. Pain is a universal human experience, and it is the most frequent reason that people seek health care. However, very few data exist that accurately reveal the incidence of either brief or prolonged pain of any sort. Three studies on the general population state the incidence of chronic pain as 9.4% (Baker and Merskey, 1967), 8.7% (Frolund and Frolund, 1986) and 11% (Cook et al, 1984). Potter (1989) also reviews these studies. This chapter provides a general overview of current perspectives on and knowledge about pain management. Please refer to subsequent chapters for detailed discussions of specific topics.

HISTORICAL PERSPECTIVE ON PAIN CONTROL

Traditionally, pain has been viewed as a symptom for which a cause is diagnosed, and pain is then eliminated by cure or control of the cause. However, during the last 15–20 years, health professionals have looked beyond this approach to see what can be done in the meantime to help the patient with pain. That is, how do we help the patient with pain during the process of diagnosis, and of cure or control of the cause of pain? What can we do for the patient whose pain cannot be cured or controlled? Such a patient might have an end-stage illness, but the person might live for months with pain. The patient might

have a normal life expectancy with a non–life-threatening cause of pain, such as arthritis or peripheral neuropathy. How do we help people with these various sorts of pain? The *palliative*, as well as the *curative* approach is now seen as important.

Relief from pain has probably been a concern of mankind since the beginning of time, but health professionals have not, until relatively recently, devoted much clinical effort or research to pain relief. The study of pain, i.e. *algology*, is in its infancy. Before the introduction of the gate control theory in 1965 by Melzack and Wall, very little appeared in the professional literature about pain. Today there are an increasing number of books on the subject, and professional journals in all the health-care disciplines regularly feature articles on pain.

Not only must information about pain control be disseminated, but also *pain management must be recognized as a priority*. Historically, this has not been the case.

The question of responsibility or accountability for pain relief was studied in the late 1960s and early 1970s, and the conclusion was drawn that health care systems did not hold health-care team members accountable for pain relief (Fagerhaugh, 1974; Fagerhaugh and Strauss, 1977; Strauss et al, 1974; Weiner, 1975). This problem continues today. The nurse may work within the hospital or the community, and the nurse personally may want to relieve the patient's pain; however, the nurse may discover that the system does not actually regard pain relief as a high priority. The importance of assessing and relieving pain may be verbalized, but other forms of communication, such as assessment tools, may be lacking.

Interestingly, most high priorities have fairly predictable indicators, such as standardized "paper work". For example, delivery of medications to the patient is a legitimate high priority and one for which the nurse is held accountable by the hospital. Very predictable paperwork goes into this: the doctor writes and signs prescriptions that are transferred onto various places such as nursing-care plans, and all medications are usually recorded on a standardized medication record, easily located on the patient's chart, so that all health-care team members can quickly access this information.

By contrast, this is not always the case with pain. Many clinical areas where patients with pain are cared for do not have standardized pain-assessment records nor do they have a systematic method of recording all pain-relief measures for the individual patient, and whether those measures have been safe and effective. Thus information about the problem of pain and possible solutions are not easily identified and transmitted quickly to other members of the health-care team. Furthermore, if pain-relief measures are not implemented (e.g. an analgesic is not given when requested by the patient), the nurse is less likely to be questioned about this than if he/she fails to administer scheduled medications, such as penicillin 6 hourly.

Unfortunately, the studies of responsibility for pain management reveal that health-care team members are held accountable for controlling the patient's *expression* of pain, which may include the patient asking for an analgesic, moaning, saying he/she hurts, or splinting the painful area. These expressions of pain can be controlled by relieving the pain; however, since the health-care team are not necessarily held responsible for pain relief, an attempt may be made to control the expression of pain without relieving the pain. This may take the form of statements such as "Try to take control of yourself," "It's not as bad as you think," and "You're going to have to learn to cope with this on your own." In essence, we are saying to the patient "We are not responsible for relieving your pain; you are responsible for your being quiet about it." We are asking the patient to suffer in silence, to learn to live with the pain and leave us alone. Obviously, this is not good-quality patient care; while it is a problem for all health professionals, it is a special problem for nurses. Nurses spend more time with patients with pain than do any other health-care team members. The nursing profession must come to grips with its unique contribution to the care of patients with pain, and must recognize the need to learn how to provide adequate coping mechanisms in addition to good clinical practice.

CURRENT STATUS OF PAIN CONTROL

Overall, some progress has been made in the last 15–20 years. Health professionals have begun to focus on pain control. This progress is reflected in the following six ways:

1. Widespread development of pain-relief units that explicitly state pain control as a high priority. Certainly some clinical areas or hospitals may make an effort to make pain relief a high priority; however, only a few state that pain control is a high priority. That is, if a patient is referred to such a pain-relief unit, pain control will definitely be addressed. Examples of such units are:
The Hospice Movement. St Joseph's Hospice, Hackney, started in 1905, followed by St Christopher's Hospice, Sydenham, in 1967. There are now hundreds of hospices of various types worldwide. Every hospice programme states that pain control is one of its primary goals.
Multidisciplinary pain clinics. Nerve block clinics for pain relief have existed for many years, but today we have many pain clinics, more of which are becoming multidisciplinary. In the early 1960s there were probably only two multidisciplinary pain centres in the United States. In Britain, among the first at that time were Liverpool and Oxford.
Childbirth education programmes. Regardless of the type of preparation for childbirth, almost always one explicit goal is to make labour and delivery a more positive and comfortable experience. Many of these programmes, e.g. Lamaze, Kitzinger, and Bradley, grew rapidly during the 1970s and early 1980s.

2. Founding of professional organizations concerned with pain management. *The Pain Society* (the British and Irish Chapter of the IASP) was founded in 1967. This was followed in 1974 by the *International Association for the Study of Pain* (IASP) and other national Chapters. The IASP and its Chapters have as their goal the promotion of multidisciplinary education and research on pain.

The *International Pain Foundation*, formed in 1986, has as its goal the support of public and professional education about pain disorders and their treatment.

The Royal College of Nursing formed the *Pain Research Group* in 1989 (now known as the Pain Forum).

Help the Hospices is a national resource for hospice care organizations and provides grant aid for capital and educational needs.

The *Information Service at St. Christopher's Hospice* provides a resource and link for members of the public and for health-care professionals seeking information on the work of the hospice movement. This includes a UK and Republic of Ireland Directory of Hospice Services.

Cancer Relief Macmillan Fund and *Marie Curie Cancer Care* are two major organizations involved in giving financial support to hospital and community units and to patients themselves.

3. Publication of professional journals that focus primarily or exclusively on pain management. Such publications include the *Journal of Pain and Symptom Management, The Clinical Journal of Pain, Pain Management*, and *Pain.*

4. National and international meetings with pain as the primary topic. These are fairly common now and include meetings every 3 years for the IASP and yearly for many Pain Societies, such as that in the United Kingdom.

In May 1986, health professionals and lay persons participated in a consensus development conference on pain sponsored by the National Institutes of Health (NIH) in the United States (Engber, 1986a). The following were noted in the consensus statement:

Progress has been made since the last conference in 1979, including new commitment to utilizing a multidisciplinary team approach for chronic pain, advances in pharmacological techniques, and increased research in non-pharmacological methods.

Deficiencies continue in the clinical management of pain, including undermedication of patients with acute pain and those with prolonged pain due to malignancy, especially children; overmedication of people with chronic non-malignant pain; inadequate education of health professionals; and inadequate communication between professionals and patients.

The nurse's role is the key link in facilitating communication between the patient, family, and health-care team. The role of the nurse (in the hospital and community)

includes teaching the patient about pain, administering medications in relation to the individual's needs, and using non-pharmacological pain relief methods.

5. Worldwide concern for cancer pain control. The World Health Organization (WHO) recognizes cancer pain relief as a worldwide priority. Its booklet, *Cancer Pain Relief*, discusses the prevalence of cancer pain, education and training, legislative factors, and specific pharmacological guidelines.

6. National initiatives for improving pain management. These are often facilitated by organizations such as Macmillan Cancer Relief Fund and Marie Curie Cancer Care when considering cancer pain. More recently the National Association of Health Authorities (NAHA) has also become more actively involved through conference and financial commitment.

The Royal College of Surgeons and College of Anaesthetists of England's *Report on Pain after Surgery* (September 1990), has also laid down findings and guidelines for future care in the field of acute postoperative pain control.

Information about some of the above is included at the end of this chapter in the "Resources" section.

In addition, there has been a dramatic increase in books on pain and in articles in journals representing the various health-care disciplines. Considerably more research is being done on assessment and relief of pain by a variety of approaches, both pharmacological and non-pharmacological.

URGENT NEED FOR RE-EDUCATION OF HEALTH PROFESSIONALS

The newness of the science of pain has practical implications regarding professional education. It takes years for a new science to gain acceptance and for the body of knowledge to be disseminated and incorporated in basic education. Hence many health professionals practising today were taught very little about pain relief, and much of what they were taught has now been superseded by new knowledge. It is often disconcerting for these health-care providers to be re-educated about pain control. Many of the current approaches are different from what they were taught originally and sometimes are even the opposite of what they have conscientiously been doing.

Health professionals who have received inadequate or inaccurate education about pain control very often *are unaware of their lack of knowledge about pain control*. They have been doing what they were taught. Because the sensation of pain is subjective, and cannot be measured by anyone except the person who feels it, the health professional may not always realize when their efforts have not been effective. If the health-care provider does not believe what the patient says or if the patient is not carefully assessed, it may appear that efforts to relieve pain are successful when in fact they are not. It is difficult at times to convince health professionals of the need for re-education. Because of misconceptions about how to assess pain and a lack of knowledge about the pharmacology of analgesics, situations that at first seem simple can easily be misunderstood and can lead to faulty conclusions about a patient.

Patient Example

John, 20 years old, was hospitalized 2 days ago for fractures and lacerations following a car accident. Within the last 24 hours he has become a "problem" for the staff. The analgesics prescribed for him are pethidine 75mg IM or orally every 4 hours. He has become a "clock watcher" and "prefers injections to tablets." He jokes with the staff and is often smiling or watching TV. He has many visitors throughout the day and evening. He says he never really gets good pain relief, but about 30 minutes after he receives the injectable narcotics he is usually on the telephone laughing and talking with his friends. The staff are convinced that he does not have as much pain as he says, because he does not act as though he is in pain. The staff also believe his preference for the injection over the pill and his regular requests by the clock are indications that he was or is becoming a drug abuser.

These *inaccurate conclusions* are a result of the staff's failure to understand this patient's effective coping mechanisms for handling pain and stress, in addition to their lack of pharmacological information about the analgesics prescribed. These inaccurate conclusions interfere with effective treatment and evaluation of John's pain. Re-education of all health-care team members is *essential* if adequate pain control is to be achieved. Advances in this area have recently been made by both the IASP and the RCN in the form of guidelines for curriculum and training in pain management for nurses and doctors. Post-registration courses are also being set up in recognition of the need to enable practitioners to develop the knowledge skills and attitudes required in pain management. This need has been highlighted by Cohen (1980) and Watt-Watson (1987). Details of such courses can be obtained from the National Boards listed in the Resources section.

THE NURSE'S UNIQUE ROLE

Many different health-care team members care for the patient with pain. There seems to be much overlap in the functioning of team members, as well there should be if a multidisciplinary approach is being used.

From a practical point of view, the nurse's unique role in the care of people with pain can be distinguished from the roles of other members of the health-care team, simply because the nurse spends more time with people with pain than does any other team member. Although the care of patients with pain ideally is multidisciplinary, in most cases *nursing care is the cornerstone*. In well-developed programmes of pain control, such as in the hospice or the multi-disciplinary pain-relief unit, this role of the nurse is well-recognized.

The nurse's role in the care of people with pain most often includes carrying out pain-relief methods with and for the patient, identifying the need for change or additional methods, implementing them, and assessing the impact on the patient. It is usually through the nurse that many patients can receive the best pain control.

When the nurse is knowledgeable about pharmacological approaches to pain control, along with non-invasive methods such as relaxation and transcutaneous nerve stimulation, there is a unique opportunity to individualize these interventions for the patient.

THE AUTHORS' BELIEFS ABOUT PAIN RELIEF AND THE PATIENT'S RIGHTS

Our beliefs about pain relief and the patient's rights form the foundation of our suggested approaches to the care of people with pain. Some of these beliefs have been presented before (McCaffery, 1979), and we continue to be committed to them. These beliefs are not, however, truths. They are simply an honest statement of what we have become convinced of as we have cared for people with pain. We hope that the statements will enable the reader to understand our underlying philosophy and will provoke thought and discussion among nurses. Above all, we urge others to address the issue of the patient's rights.

We believe that pain control:
1. Is a legitimate therapeutic goal.

2. Contributes significantly to the patient's physical and emotional well-being.

3. Must rank high in the list of priorities in patient care.

4. Is patient-controlled, i.e. the patient is the final authority about assessment of pain and all methods of pain control to the extent that it is safe and that communication, including the non-verbal kind, is possible.

We believe that the patient has a right:

1. To decide the duration and intensity of pain he/she is willing to endure or tolerate.

2. To be informed of all possible methods of pain relief along with the favourable and unfavourable consequences, as well as the controversial aspects.

3. To choose which pain-control method(s) he/she wishes to try.

4. To choose to live with or without pain.*

We also recognize that the health-care provider has a right to refuse to treat a patient with pain by a method that the health-care provider deems harmful.

REFERENCES AND SELECTED READINGS

Baker, JW, Merskey, H: Pain in general practice. *Journal of Psychosomatic Research,* **10**: 383–387, 1967.

Cohen, F Post-surgical pain relief: Patients' status and nurses' medication choices. *Pain* **9**: 265–274, 1980.

Crook, J, Rideout, E, Browne, G: The prevalence of pain complaints in a general population. *Pain,* **18**:299–314, 1984.

Engber, D: Report on the NIH consensus development conference on pain, *J. Pain Sympt. Manag.,* **1**:165-167, Summer 1986a.

Engber, D: Wisconsin initiative for improving cancer pain management: progress report. *J. Pain Sympt. Manag.,* **1**:58–59, Winter 1986b.

Fagerhaugh, SY: Pain expression and control on a burn unit. *Nursing Outlook,* **22**:645–650, Oct 1974.

Fagerhaugh, SY, Strauss, A: *Politics of Pain Management: Staff–Patient Interaction,* Addison-Wesley Publishing Co., Menlo Park, Cal, 1977.

Frolund, F Frolund, C: Pain in general practice. *Scandinavian Journal of Primary Health Care,* **4**: 97–100, 1986.

Liebeskind, JC, Melzack, R: The international pain foundation: meeting a need for education in pain management. *Pain,* **30**:1–2, 1987.

McCaffery, M: *Nursing Management of the Patient with Pain.* JB Lippincott Co., New York, 1979.

Potter, RG: Chronic non-malignant pain: time to take on the challenge. *Journal of the Royal College of General Practitioners,* **39**:486–487, Dec 1989.

Schofield, PA: The role of sensation in the management of chronic pain. In: Rom PA, ed. *Sensory Environments—leisure, education and therapy,* 1992. A collection of ideas and experiences reflecting current activity and possible future developments.

Strauss, A, Fagerhaugh, SY, Glaser, B: An organizational-work-interactional perspective. *Nursing Outlook,* **22**:560–566, Sept 1974.

Watt-Watson, J: Nurses' knowledge of pain issues: a survey. *Journal of Pain and Symptom Management,* **4**:207–211, 1987.

Weiner, CL: Pain assessment on an orthopedic ward. *Nursing Outlook,* **23**:508–516, Aug 1975.

RESOURCES FOR HEALTH PROFESSIONALS AND FOR PATIENTS

Publications

The Journal of Pain and Symptom Management
(expansion of PRN forum)
Quarterly
Elsevier Publishing Co, Inc
Journal Fulfillment Department
PO Box 882, Madison Square Station
New York, NY 10160-0200

The Clinical Journal of Pain
Quarterly
Raven Press Books Ltd
1140 Avenue of the Americas
New York, NY 10036

Pain Management
Bimonthly
CORE Medical Journals
3131 Princeton Pike, Bldg 2A
Lawrenceville, NJ 08648

Cancer Pain Relief, 1986
74-page booklet
WHO Publications Center USA
49 Sheridan Ave
Albany, NY 12210

---

* There may be exception to this right if it endangers another person. For example, the mother's right to take certain medications for the sole purpose of her own comfort during pregnancy or labour and delivery may be questioned if these medications endanger the health or life of the baby. Likewise, there may be questions about an individual's right to take an analgesic that also sedates him/her while he driving a vehicle or operating machinery that could injure other people if operated improperly.

Another ethical dilemma is the person with chronic non-malignant pain who "chooses" to live without pain? What then?

Principles of Analgesic Use in the Treatment of Acute Pain and Chronic Cancer Pain: A Concise Guide to Medical Practice, 1987
9-page booklet
American Pain Society
1615 L Street NW, Suite 925
Washington DC 20036
(202) 296-9200

Textbook of Pain. (Ed. Wall, PD, Melzack, R), Churchill Livingstone. 2nd Edition 1989.

The Royal College of Surgeons of England and The College of Anaesthetists Commission on the Provision of Surgical Services. Report of the Working Party on Pain After Surgery, September 1990.

Organizations

IASP (International Association for the Study of Pain)
Membership includes subscription to the journal *Pain,* monthly.
IASP Secretary
909 NE 43rd St, Suite 306
Seattle, WA 98105-6020
(206) 547-6409

The Pain Society of Great Britain & Ireland
The Association of Anaesthetists
9 Bedford Square
London WC1B 3RA
071-631 1650

Help The Hospices
BMA House
Tavistock Square
London WC1H 9JP
071-388 7807/0649

Hospice Information
St Christopher's Hospice
51 Laurie Park Road
Sydenham
London SE26 6DZ
081-778 9252

Royal College of Nursing Pain Forum
20 Cavendish Square
London W1M 0AB
071-409 3333

Cancer Relief Macmillan Fund
Anchor House
15/19 Britten Street
London SW3 3TZ
071-351 7811

Marie Curie Cancer Care
28 Belgrave Square
London SW1X 8QG
071-235 3325

Companies that manufacture analgesics and equipment used for pain management have a variety of resources available concerning pain control.

The English National Board for Nursing, Midwifery and Health Visiting
Victory House
170 Tottenham Court Road
London W1T 0HA
071-388 3131

The National Board for Nursing and Health Visiting for Northern Ireland
RAC House
79 Chichester Street
Belfast BT1 4JE
0232-238152

The National Board for Nursing, Midwifery and Health Visiting for Scotland
22 Queen Street
Edinburgh EH1 1JX
031-226 7371

The Welsh National Board for Nursing, Midwifery and Health Visiting
13th Floor, Pearl Assurance House
Greyfriars Road
Cardiff CF1 3AG
0222-395535

Self-Help in Pain
33 Kingsdown Road
Whitstable
Kent CT5 2DT

Relaxation for Living
168–170 Oatlands Drive
Weybridge
Surrey KT13 9ET

2

Assessment

If patients could always tell us that they hurt and we could accept this as fact, the assessment and treatment of pain would be a great deal simpler than they are. However, we do not always readily believe and help people who say they hurt. Furthermore, not all people can or will tell us about their pain. Some people who hurt may deny pain or refuse pain relief. These complexities of assessing pain initially and performing on-going assessments that enable us to refine the relief of pain are addressed here along with an overview of simple classifications and treatment approaches to major types of pain problems and of specific assessment tools that may be easily used in the clinical setting.

MISCONCEPTIONS THAT HAMPER ASSESSMENT OF PATIENTS WHO INDICATE THEY HAVE PAIN

Virtually all of us grow up thinking in certain ways that cause us to erroneously doubt others who indicate they have pain. Unfortunately, these misconceptions are sometimes reinforced in our professional education. Since almost everyone is prone at times to discount another's report of pain, it is essential to become aware of the misconceptions that cause us to doubt the patient with pain so that we can accomplish the following goals:

- Prevent ourselves from acting on our misconceptions. Many of our misconceptions are well-entrenched in our thinking from early childhood. They may be emotional reactions that are not possible or easy to eliminate and may creep into our thinking no matter how well we understand them logically. Therefore we simply hope to prevent them from having a detrimental effect on what we actually do for the patient. When we think in these ways, ideally we will recognize it and stop ourselves before we act.
- Help others, e.g. health-care team and family, think through reasons why they may unjustifiably doubt the patient.
- Identify our *professional* responsibility to the patient who claims to have pain.

The misconceptions covered in this chapter apply to all types of pain. Extensions of and additions to them are discussed later in relation to chronic nonmalignant pain, children, and the elderly. The misconceptions overlap to some degree; an understanding of the first one is, however, basic to comprehending the others. Table 2.1 provides a glossary of ten misconceptions and corrections. These ten points will be discussed in more detail below.

Misconception	Correction
1. The health-care team is the authority on the existence and nature of the patient's pain sensation.	The person with pain is the only authority about the existence and nature of that pain, since the sensation of pain can be felt only by the person who has it.
2. Our personal values and intuition about the trustworthiness of others constitute a valuable tool in identifying whether a person is lying about pain.	Personal values and intuition do not constitute a professional approach to the patient with pain. The patient's credibility is not on trial.
3. Pain is largely an emotional or psychological problem, especially in the patient who is highly anxious or depressed.	Having an emotional reaction to pain does not mean that pain is caused by an emotional problem. If anxiety or depression is alleviated, the intensity of pain will not necessarily be any less.
4. Lying about the existence of pain, or malingering, is common.	Very few people who say they have pain are lying about it. Outright fabrication of pain is considered rare.
5. The patient who obtains benefits or preferential treatment because of pain is receiving secondary gain and does not hurt as much as he/she says or may not hurt at all.	The patient who uses pain to his/her advantage is not the same as a malingerer and may still hurt as much as is claimed. Also, secondary gain may be an inaccurate diagnosis.
6. All real pain has an identifiable physical cause.	All pain is real, regardless of its cause. Almost all pain has both physical and mental components. Pure psychogenic pain is rare.
7. Visible signs, either physiological or behavioural, accompany pain and can be used to verify its existence and severity.	Even with severe pain, periods of psychological and behavioural adaptation occur, leading to periods of minimal pain or no signs of pain. Lack of pain expression does not necessarily mean lack of pain. How must the patient act for us to believe pain is being experienced?
8. Comparable physical stimuli produce comparable pain in different people. The severity and duration of pain can be predicted accurately for everyone on the basis of the stimuli for pain.	Comparable stimuli in different people do *not* produce the same intensities of pain; such stimuli will produce different intensities of pain that last different periods. There is no direct and invariant relationship between any stimulus and the perception of pain.
9. People with pain should be taught to have a high tolerance for pain. The more prolonged the pain or the more experience a person has with pain, the better is the tolerance for pain.	Pain tolerance is the individual's unique response, varying between patients and varying in the same patient from one situation to another. People with prolonged pain tend to have an increasingly low pain tolerance. Respect for the patient's pain tolerance is crucial for adequate pain control.
10. When the patient reports pain relief following a placebo, this indicates malingering or that the pain is psychogenic.	There is not a shred of evidence anywhere in the literature to justify using a placebo to diagnose malingering or psychogenic pain.

Table 2.1 Misconceptions about assessment of patients who indicate they have pain.

1. Authority on pain: health-care team vs. patient

Misconception: The health-care team is the authority about the existence and nature of the patient's pain sensation.

Correction: The person with the pain is the only authority on the existence and nature of that pain, since the sensation of pain can be felt only by the person who has it.

The basic question is "Whose pain is it?" The answer, of course, is that it is the patient's pain. The content of this entire book revolves around a thorough understanding of the fact that the patient is the only authority about his/her pain.

Sometimes the issue of who is the authority about pain unfortunately boils down to a battle between the health-care team or family and the patient. Members of the health-care team or the family may erroneously believe that they can determine whether the patient hurts and just how much he/she hurts—regardless of what the patient says about it. This is the most detrimental attitude that one can have if the intention is to help the patient.

The most important and most difficult aspect of helping the patient with pain is to accept and appreciate that only the patient can feel the pain. The sensation of pain is completely subjective. The health-care team would rather deal with a symptom that can be detected and measured objectively. It is reassuring to read a pathology report or get back some numbers from the lab; however, when the symptom is pain, we must ask the patient about it. We have no direct measure of the pain sensation—no pain thermometer. When we treat the patient experiencing pain, we must again ask about the pain to determine if we have succeeded. We do not know about pain or the effect of our treatment of it unless we get this information from the patient. Caring for patients with pain can be a humbling experience.

Remember too that patients do not like the fact that the pain sensation is subjective. Sooner or later, most patients with pain realize that they cannot prove their pain. Their only hope is to find someone who will believe them.

Because the pain sensation is subjective, considerable research has been devoted to developing assessment tools that help the patient communicate information about the sensation of pain. Many tools have been developed for adults and, recently, for children as young as 3 years of age.

Still, some patients, such as a baby, a confused or sedated patient, or a patient who speaks a different language, are not able to verbally communicate the pain experience. With these patients it is necessary to make an educated guess about what pain may be felt. This may be based on our knowledge of the physical pathology and the type of pain other patients have told us they experienced from comparable physical causes. We may also be able to obtain some notion of pain by observing non-verbal behaviour such as crying, restlessness, or rigid posture. However, we must remember that here we are merely guessing about pain and we must be ever-ready to revise our guess based on additional information from the patient, from others who know the patient and from new information on the patient's pathology.

Thus some patients may be unable to effectively communicate verbally about the pain felt, and others with pain may deny it or refuse pain relief (discussed later in this chapter). Whenever the patient is able to indicate he/she has pain, we believe the patient's statements are the most valid measurement of pain.

Because pain is subjective, the definition of pain we propose for use in clinical practice, originally proposed in 1968 (McCaffery, p. 95) is "Pain is whatever the experiencing person says it is, existing whenever the experiencing person says it does." Specifically this definition means that when the patient *indicates* he/she has pain, the health-care team responds positively. The patient's report of pain is either believed or given the benefit of the doubt. This is the professional response. Each health-care team member is entitled to his or her personal opinion about whether the patient is telling the truth about the pain felt. However, the issue is professional responsibility, which is to accept the patient's report of pain and to help the patient in a responsive and positive manner.

This approach to pain is difficult to accept. People look at the definition proposed and its implications and voice the fear that if they believe every person who claims to have pain or if they give every person the benefit of the doubt, they will end up being fooled. Indeed, they *will* be fooled sooner or later. Pain is subjective, and being fooled is simply a reality in dealing with something that can never be proved or disproved. This point must be acknowledged by all members of the health-care team. The risk of being fooled does not justify doubting the patient or withholding pain relief. Furthermore, the incidence of malingering, discussed below, is not as high as we usually think. Nevertheless, caring for the patient with pain is, as said, truly a humbling experience. Here, and in other areas of caring for the patient with pain, the subjectivity of pain affects all who care for patients with pain.

No matter which approach we use in responding to the patient's report of pain, we will eventually make a mistake. If we doubt some patients and withhold treatment, we may avoid being fooled by the minority who are addicts, abusers, or malingerers, but we will eventually fail to help someone who does have pain. On the other hand, if we give everyone the benefit of the doubt and try to relieve pain in all who say they have it, we inevitably will be fooled by some who are addicts, abusers, or malingerers, but we will never fail to help someone who does have pain. Either way, we will make a mistake. Therefore we must address our professional responsibility and consider which mistake we can afford. (Of course, some addicts and abusers do have pain that requires narcotics for relief, see pp. 81–82.)

What may happen if we do not believe or respond positively to a patient's report of pain? Pain specialists are very specific about the issue of believing or accepting the patient's report of pain. For example, the booklet *Cancer Pain Relief* published by the World Health Organization, 1986, which represents the combined efforts of pain specialists from throughout the world, lists simply and clearly as the first of eight steps for assessing cancer pain "Believe the patient's complaint of pain" (p. 14). This statement is not discussed—there are no exceptions. The point is made that to ignore the main steps in clinical assessment of cancer pain is the major cause of misdiagnosis and inappropriate management.

One study of children showed that pain caused by cancer was experienced for as long as 821 days before initiation of cancer therapy (Miser et al, 1987). Obviously, failure to believe or respond to a patient's report of pain may cause us to miss a diagnosis until the disease is too far advanced for treatment or to delay treatment until the prognosis is poor.

An equally disastrous outcome may be seen almost daily in the clinical situation when a patient's report of pain is ignored because it is doubted, an altogether too familiar scene. The patient says he/she hurts, and the health-care team doesn't really believe this. They do little to help, and the patient senses their disbelief and concludes that they will not do much to help; however, the patient still hurts and wants pain relief. He/she reacts to this situation with anger and perhaps some sadness or depression and may become irritable and demanding. Perhaps the patient tries a different approach because the truth did not work, resulting in exaggeration or lying to get others belief and help. The health-care team see this change in behaviour and become frustrated, perhaps believing that the patient is manipulative. Thus evolves the adversarial relationship, with the health-care team and patient disagreeing about whether the patient has pain. Enormous emotion and energy are wasted on the part of both patient and health-care team over something that can never be proved or disproved.

Whenever this occurs, ask why it is difficult to believe that this patient hurts. Many of the more common answers are covered below. Ideally, these can be discussed with other members of the health-care team, and the result will be a positive approach, based either on believing the patient or being willing to give him/her the benefit of the doubt. However, this doesn't always happen. If the health-care team continues in the adversarial relationship, it is essential to remember the following:

- An adversarial relationship is not a therapeutic one. It is doubtful that anything helpful can be done for the patient in the context of an adversarial relationship.
- Every time the patient indicates that he/she hurts and the health-care team indicates that they do not believe this, the team is effectively calling the patient a liar. This is insulting and degrading and is not a professional approach to the patient. It is an unethical and unprofessional response to a client's stated need.
- If we are unable to respond professionally and positively to the patient, it is our responsibility to consult with the patient or refer the patient to those who can respond positively to his/her expressed needs. Referral or consultation is the same approach we use for any health/illness problem presented by a patient when we do not know how to treat it or are not able to do so.

2. Patient credibility: personal values vs. professional responsibility

Misconception: Our personal values and intuition about the trustworthiness of others constitute a valuable tool in identifying whether a person is lying about pain.
Correction: Personal values and intuition may serve us well in our social lives, but they do not constitute a professional approach to the patient with pain. Further, the patient's credibility is not on trial, and the health-care team is not called upon to judge this.

In our daily personal lives, it is not uncommon for us to make tentative judgments about those we meet even briefly. It is almost unavoidable to encounter someone without forming some impression of him or her, including whether the person is honest and dependable. When we are unsure, we may or may not decide to take the risk of depending on the person.

What information we use to make these judgments and decisions may be largely unconscious or at least difficult to specify. On the other hand, sometimes visual impact alone causes us to be cautious of a person. For example, if you are walking alone at dusk in a strange neighbourhood with no one else on the street except some strange-looking person walking toward you, you may decide to avoid any risk associated with this person by crossing to the other side of the street to put distance between the two of you. You may be wrong about the person's character, but in daily life decisions such as this may help us avoid being taken advantage of by others, e.g. being hurt or robbed. Such decisions may cause little or no harm to others. In our professional activities, however, such judgments are a disservice to the patient.

Because the sensation of pain is totally subjective, it is understandable how health-care team members might inadvertently rely on personal biases and judgments about human nature to determine the truthfulness of a patient's report of pain. When the patient reporting pain has an entirely different life-style from ours, it may be tempting to invoke personal judgments. The patient may even engage in activities that are illegal or that we consider immoral. Although we have the right to choose not to socialize with such a person in our personal lives, we have no right as health professionals to be punitive or to withhold appropriate treatment. As professionals we have the responsibility to provide, at the very least, humane care.

Putting aside personal values so that the highest quality of care can be provided for the patient is not always easy. Sometimes it helps a health-care team member if he/she is allowed to acknowledge that the patient is not exactly someone to readily invite home to dinner.

3. Pain and emotion: reaction vs. cause

Misconception: Pain is largely an emotional or psychological problem, especially in the patient who is highly anxious or depressed or who has an unclear physical cause of pain.

Correction: An emotional reaction to pain does not mean that pain is caused by an emotional problem. Pain will not simply disappear or necessarily be any less intense if the patient stops being anxious or depressed. Similarly, if a diagnosis of cancer causes the patient to become upset, this does not mean that cancer is mostly a psychological problem that can be treated with appropriate psychotherapy. Furthermore, inability to diagnose a physical cause for the pain does not mean that there is no physical cause of pain, a misconception further discussed below in relation to known physical causes of pain.

Pain almost always results in some degree of anxiety or depression. To experience pain without any emotional response would be abnormal. However, the relationship between pain and anxiety or depression is complicated and unclear. Although anxiety or depression is rarely the sole cause of pain, it certainly affects how the patient handles pain. For example, anxiety or depression probably makes pain more difficult to bear and adversely affects the patient's outlook and motivation or ability to be involved in his/her own pain control.

Intensity of pain, however, is not nearly as likely to be affected by anxiety or depression as is the patient's ability to handle pain. A study of cancer patients has shown that depressed patients are not more likely to have more intense pain than those who are not depressed. The depression associated with cancer pain did not alter the patients' reports of the intensity of pain. However, depression did affect the patients' perception of life's quality (Cleeland, 1984; see also Chapter 7 on the relationship between depression and chronic nonmalignant pain). Thus the intensity of pain is not likely to subside simply because anxiety and depression are alleviated.

Anxiety is usually associated with brief pain whereas depression tends to accompany prolonged pain; an element of both is usually present with all pain. When anxiety or depression is caused by pain, the preferred treatment is to relieve the pain. In other words, if a patient is anxious because of severe pain, he/she should not be given a tranquilliser or sedative. Rather, every effort should be made to relieve the pain.

An appreciation of the fact that pain is not simply a psychological problem, but rather a physical problem accompanied by emotional responses, is especially important in understanding the difference between narcotic addiction and use of narcotics for pain relief (see discussion of addiction on pp. 76–77). Although it is usually clearly understood that a patient in accident and emergency with bloody lacerations and multiple fractures needs narcotics to relieve pain and not to meet a psychological need, this distinction may be less obvious to the observer after the patient begins the process of recovery. Weeks later when the patient still has musculoskeletal pain from nonunion fractures, the anxiety and depression accompanying this pain and the continued requests for narcotics to relieve the pain may be misunderstood as an example of using narcotics to meet psychological needs. The use of narcotics for psychological (or psychic) reasons rather than for an approved medical reason such as pain relief would fit the definition of narcotic addiction. Such a patient might erroneously be labelled a narcotic addict unless it is understood that pain is primarily a physical problem with psychological effects.

4. Malingering: lies vs. truth

Misconception: Lying about the existence of pain, or malingering, is common.
Correction: Very few people who say they have pain are lying about it. Outright fabrication of pain is rare (Hendler, 1984; Leavitt and Sweet, 1986; Reesor and Craig, 1988). Malingering does exist, but it simply is not as likely as many of us believe.

Regarding pain, the malingerer may be defined as a person who says that pain is present when it is not, i.e. the person fakes pain or pretends to have pain, usually to avoid or gain something. The malingerer does not feel pain but tries to make others believe that he/she does. It is a conscious lie because the malingerer by definition does not imagine pain and does not believe it is present. An example of malingering on a small scale is the person who does not want to accept a dinner invitation and who uses the excuse of having a headache when in fact there is none.

The fear of being duped by the malingerer has bothered practitioners for years. Many attempts have been made to devise a test that would detect malingering, but none has been proved effective. Therefore we must accept the reality that believing the patient with pain could result in our believing someone who is deliberately lying to us about having pain. This vulnerability seems unavoidable. Although by believing a malingerer we may aid the accomplishment of his/her goals, our professional responsibility is to treat patients with respect and believe them or give them the benefit of the doubt.

Great care must be taken to avoid inaccurate labelling of patients as malingerers. Patients with chronic non-malignant pain are especially likely to be inaccurately diagnosed as malingerers (see Chapter 7). Patients may be labelled as malingerers simply because the cause of the pain is unknown or because the patient fails to respond to treatment (i.e. patients with vague or unresponsive symptoms seem likely to be labelled malingerers).

Interestingly, documented cases of malingering usually involve patients with textbook symptoms. The patient may identify expected symptoms on the basis of the way he/she is physically assessed by the physician or he/she may actually go to the library and read about the condition. If the patient's intent is to fool the health-care team, it makes sense that the patient would try to do as good a job as possible.

Sometimes malingering is confused with psychogenic pain or secondary gain. However, malingering, secondary gain, and psychogenic pain are three separate conditions. Further, all of them except malingering involve feeling pain. Psychogenic pain may hurt as much as any type of pain of primarily physical origin. The patient with pain who receives secondary gain may also have a very painful condition.

5. Secondary gain: apparent benefits of pain vs. intensity or existence of pain

Misconception: The patient who obtains benefits or preferential treatment because of pain is receiving secondary gain and does not hurt as much as is claimed or may not hurt at all.
Correction: The patient who uses pain to gain an advantage is not the same as a malingerer and may still hurt as much as is claimed. Secondary gain may be an inaccurate conclusion, since what is secondary gain for one person is not for another.

Secondary gain is defined as any practical or emotional advantages that result from having the symptom of pain, especially financial compensation and preferential treatment at home or work, including special favours or attention from friends or family. By definition, the patient has pain and is not malingering, i.e. is not lying about the presence of pain. It may not always be easy to distinguish between malingering and secondary gain because the sensation of pain is totally subjective, and both malingering and secondary gain result in benefits to the patient. However, it is important to remember that malingering involves lying about the existence of pain and is relatively uncommon. By contrast, with secondary gain pain is assumed to be present, and secondary gain may be a fairly common component of the prolonged pain experience.

Secondary gain need not be negative. The term *secondary gain* usually has negative connotations of involving gains that could be more appropriately achieved by behaviours other than reporting pain. When this is true, secondary gain may be a disability (discussed below). Certain secondary gains, however, are appropriate, such as attention and assistance from others when pain limits activity or financial compensation for a work-related injury resulting from unsafe conditions.

In daily life, secondary gain from pain is not unusual. Just as a person may lie about having a headache to avoid accepting a dinner invitation, so may a person use an already existing headache to decline the dinner invitation. In both cases the person wants to avoid attending the dinner, but in one case the excuse is malingering (lying) and in the other case the excuse is based on fact.

Obviously, if pain is prolonged and if the patient begins to use pain as a means of handling many problems or inconveniences of daily life, secondary gain may become a disability. For example, if the patient has chronic low back pain, he/she may begin to use this to avoid a job or spouse not liked. Rather than find a new job or go to work and find ways to make the job better, the pain may be used as an excuse to stay at home. When the patient has disagreements with either husband or wife, the pain may be used as an excuse to avoid the spouse by taking a nap or resting, rather than finding ways to resolve the conflict. Using pain to handle these significant problems disables the patient to the extent of becoming increasingly isolated and less able to function in life.

Whenever the patient uses pain to deal with many problems, this may result in a disability that requires treatment. The question becomes: How can problems of daily living be handled more constructively? Vocational counselling, family therapy, and assertiveness training may be helpful. Many structured pain-management programmes include these therapies, recognizing that it is not unusual for people with prolonged pain to be accused of using, or to actually use, pain to their advantage.

However, it is extremely important to be sure that secondary gain has been accurately diagnosed. The question is not whether the patient has pain – the patient is given the benefit of the doubt. Even if the patient exaggerates the pain to obtain secondary gain, this still does not mean there is no pain at all. In fact, exaggeration of pain may not be for secondary gain but may reflect ineffective coping mechanisms or may be for the purpose of obtaining appropriate treatment for the pain. Exaggeration may be due to the failure of others to believe a patient when telling the truth about the pain felt or due to the patient lacking effective coping styles and being overwhelmed by the pain (see further discussion in Chapter 7). Possible exaggeration may be prevented or minimized by ensuring that the existence of pain is acknowledged to the patient.

Accurate diagnosis of secondary gain involves not only recognizing that the presence of pain is not in question but also recognizing that certain types of behaviour are not always secondary gain. What is secondary gain for one person is not necessarilysecondary gain for another. The patient's responses to pain may appear to be for secondary gain, but this may or may not be the case. For example, the patient may use pain as a reason to rest. Resting at work may enable avoidance of a disliked task. Thus the patient may be using pain for secondary gain. However, it is also possible that in spite of disliking certain tasks, the patient does have pain and may benefit from pacing him/herself and resting at that time. If the latter is true, pain is not being used for secondary gain. In both instances the behaviour of resting is the same and the disliked task is avoided, but in only one instance is the diagnosis of secondary gain appropriate.

It is often erroneously assumed that patients who are awaiting litigation after an injury or who are receiving workers' compensation are likely to prolong or exaggerate their pain to benefit from financial secondary gain. Numerous studies have failed to support this view (Dworkin et al, 1985; Melzack, Katz and Jeans, 1985; see also Chapter 7). Financial gain from pain may in fact be appropriate financial compensation for an injury.

Accurate assessment of secondary gain is not necessarily simple. Useful assessment guidelines may include observing whether patients *regularly* uses pain to avoid activity that they would not want to engage in even if they did not have pain or to obtain benefits that they could not without the pain. If a patient does this regularly and often, secondary gain may be a disability in need of treatment. In discussing with the health-care team the possibility that the patient receives secondary gain from pain that might be more appropriately obtained in other ways, important points are:

- Secondary gain from pain is not the same as malingering, nor does it mean that pain is psychogenic, i.e. caused solely by mental events.
- Pain with demonstrable physical causes, including severe pathology, may be used for secondary gain.
- What is secondary gain for one person is not for another. Accurate assessment of whether a certain type of behaviour is for the purpose of secondary gain may be difficult to make.
- Secondary gain is not always inappropriate, e.g. financial gain or attention resulting from pain may be necessary or justifiable.
- The occasional use of pain to obtain certain advantages is not unusual and does not necessarily warrant any special treatment.
- Secondary gain from pain becomes a problem for which the patient requires assistance when it leads to disablement, i.e. when the patient uses pain instead of a more constructive method of solving daily problems. The patient should then be approached with suggestions for alternatives to solving specific problems of daily living, e.g. marital conflict or job placement. The patient should not be berated for using pain as a solution nor be accused of faking or exaggerating pain.

6. Cause of pain: known vs. unknown physical cause

Misconception: All "real" pain has an identifiable physical cause.

Correction: All pain is real, regardless of its cause. Almost all pain has both physical and mental components. The absence of an identifiable physical cause of pain does not mean the pain is purely psychogenic.

It is easier to believe a patient's report of pain when he/she has a physical diagnosis that corresponds to what is said. We are mistakenly tempted to rely more on identifiable cellular pathology than the patient's statement of what is felt.

Because the sensation of pain is subjective, our thinking about a physical cause may inadvertently disintegrate into a fallacy. If this happens with the healthcare team, it is helpful to state the problem, saying that

it seems that we are thinking the following misconception: "If there is pain, there is a cause. If there is a cause, we can find it. If we can't find the cause, there is no pain and no pain relief is needed." Such thinking is based on the absurd assumption that our own assessment and the diagnostic tests we use are infallible.

In addition to stating the problem clearly, using an analogy (something similar to the situation but not as threatening) may also help promote more logical thinking. For example, you might say "If a patient came into accident and emergency vomiting blood but our assessment revealed no cause for the vomiting and bleeding, would we then doubt that the patient was vomiting and bleeding and do nothing about it?" The point is that vomiting and bleeding, unlike the pain sensation, are objective and potentially life threatening, so we do not dare indulge in the omnipotent thinking expressed in relation to pain. We must remind ourselves and others that just as patients may bleed or vomit without our knowing why, so may they have pain without our being able to identify a cause. Our failure to identify the cause in no way justifies saying that the problem does not exist or does not deserve treatment. Once again, we find that the subjectivity of pain haunts us and that caring for patients with pain is indeed a humbling experience.

In the absence of a readily identifiable physical cause of pain, another interesting and unjustifiable type of thinking tends to occur. We may begin to speculate about whether the pain is imaginary, "all in the head," or psychogenic.

The matter becomes even more complicated if the patient is very anxious or depressed about his/her pain. In the absence of a diagnosed physical cause for pain, it may be reasoned that these emotions indicate a largely psychological cause of the pain. The patient then faces an almost insoluble problem. Anxiety and depression normally associated with pain become even more intense when the patient realizes that the physical cause cannot be found and that the staff are beginning to doubt his/her pain. The more upset the patient becomes, the more basis the staff seem to have for suspecting that the reported pain is psychological in origin. The vicious cycle continues with the patient becoming more anxious or depressed and the staff becoming more sure that the pain is psychogenic.

To have pain acknowledged and validated, particularly by the diagnosis of a physical cause, is extremely important to both staff and patient. Until this happens the staff may become confused and the patient may fear abandonment by the staff or fear loss of sanity. To help both the patient and the health-care team understand the reality of this situation, it may help to examine the possible extremes.

The general causes of pain may be conceptualized on a continuum from pain that is totally psychogenic to pain that is totally physical. "Pure" psychogenic pain may be defined as a localized sensation of pain caused solely by mental events, with no physical findings to initiate or sustain the pain. Pure psychogenic pain is extremely rare. However, the term *psychogenic* is used loosely, and this leads to misunderstandings about its frequency.

For example, in the literature, tension headache is often referred to as psychogenic headache. Yet when a stressful situation is followed by a headache, it does not mean that the person's brain perceived the stressful environment and immediately converted it into a pain in the head. It is not pure psychogenic pain. Very soon after the stress is perceived, physical changes occur, usually in the form of contraction of the muscles in the neck and scalp, ischaemia, accumulation of toxins, and further muscle contraction. Thus what may be called psychogenic headache is actually caused by both mental and physical events, not one or the other. In this instance, the intensity of pain – pain perception – is influenced by both physical and mental events.

By contrast, pure physical pain is a localized sensation of pain caused solely by physical events not accompanied by mental events. Again, this is extremely rare. It is unusual to have a cut or burn that hurts and to have no thoughts or feelings about it. The person is going to think something about the pain. The accompanying mental events may render the pain more bearable if the patient thinks that the pain will be relieved and he/she will recover. However, if the mental events involve the fear that no help will be available and that death is imminent, pain may be very difficult to tolerate. In this instance, pain tolerance, as opposed to pain intensity, is influenced by both physical and mental events.

The most successful approach to pain control is to assess and treat both the physical and mental causes. Most localized sensations of pain are a combination of *both* physical and mental events (Fig. 2.1). No pain is

Fig. 2.1 Most pain results from a combination of both physical and mental events. Rarely is pain purely psychogenic (mental) or purely physical in origin. Pain results from a total body response.

imaginary, and calling pain imaginary certainly does not make it go away. The final word on imaginary versus real pain may well be a quote from a collection of letters to the *New England Journal of Medicine* (Moskow, 1987, p. 68): "Pain occurring in unicorns, griffins, and jabberwockies is always imaginary pain, since these are imaginary animals; patients on the other hand, are real, and so they always have real pain."

7. Pain behaviour: acute pain model vs. adaptation

Misconception: Visible signs, either physiological or behavioural, accompany pain and can be used to verify its existence and severity.

Correction: Even with severe pain, periods of physiological and behavioural adaptation occur, leading to periods of minimal pain or no signs of pain. Lack of pain expression does not necessarily mean lack of pain. How must the patient behave for us to believe pain is being felt?

In the acute pain model, certain signs of pain exist at the onset of sudden, severe pain. Physiologically the patient may have increased heart rate, perspiration, pallor, or increased blood pressure. Behaviourally, the patient may talk about the pain, cry, moan, tense the skeletal muscles, or rub the painful part. However, the acute pain model usually exists only briefly. Both physiological and behavioural adaptation occur, sometimes within seconds or minutes. In other words, the patient may continue to hurt just as badly, but behavioural and physiological signs of pain will cease to exist, at least for certain periods (Fig. 2.2).

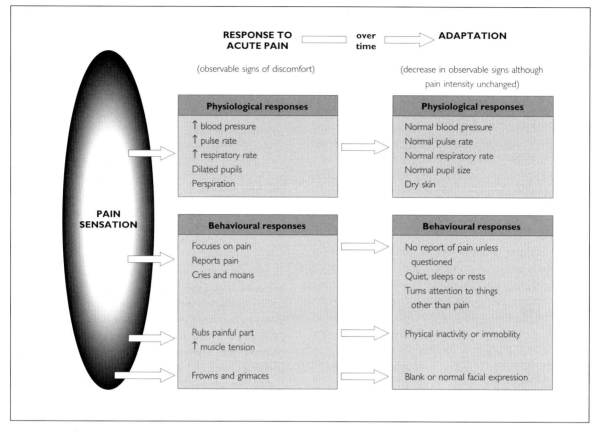

Fig. 2.2 Acute pain model vs. adaptation. Modified from Brunner, LS, and Suddarth, DS: *Textbook of Medical-Surgical Nursing*, 6th edn., Philadelphia, 1988, JB Lippincott.

Physiologically, the body seeks equilibrium. Certain physiological responses could not be sustained without there finally being physical harm to the person. Thus these parameters usually return to near normal for periods. Occasionally, a patient may go into shock from severe pain, but most patients show physiological adaptation.

Behaviourally there is also adaptation. The pain may continue to be just as severe as it was at its onset, but if the pain remains at that level of severity for days, the patient is not likely to continue to scream for the entire time. Patients minimize their controllable behavioural expressions of pain for a number of reasons, including the following:

- To be a "good patient." The patient may realize that the health-care team is more or less responsible for keeping him/her quiet and that they do not like to hear crying or persistent requests for pain relief.

- To avoid being a "sissy," i.e. to maintain a favourable self-concept. If the patient values a stoic response to pain or notes that those around do, it may be embarrassing to even talk about the pain except to selected individuals and only at certain times. A sudden increase in pain may lead to a gasp or grimace, but the patient may strive to bring this under control quickly.

- Exhaustion. Pain is fatiguing. After the patient has been in pain for hours, or certainly for days, he/she becomes too tired to talk and cry about the pain and so tired that sleep intervenes. Many health-care team members are taught to equate sleep with pain relief. While sleeping patients may not have a conscious awareness of pain, they may have a dream-state awareness, and more importantly, they will be in pain when they awaken—unless there has been a miracle cure. Double-blind analgesic studies have been done since the 1950s, and in these studies when patients in hospital are evaluated for pain relief at hourly intervals, they are awakened because it is well known that even patients with severe pain may sleep. Or patients with pain may close their eyes and remain very still, appearing to be asleep, but actually may only be trying to make the pain bearable by conserving energy or concentrating on something else. Many types of behaviour diminish as a result of sheer exhaustion.

- Distraction. The patient may laugh and joke with visitors, walk them to the elevator, and then walk to the nurse's station to request an analgesic. If distraction is not understood, this patient will be misunderstood. As discussed in Chapter 6, distraction is a potent method of making pain more bearable, but it does not make pain go away. While the patient made the effort to distract him/herself with the visitors, he/she probably became exhausted from this plus the on-going pain. Now that the distraction has ceased, the pain is back in the centre of the awareness, difficult to tolerate, leading to tiredness. The patient now needs another form of pain relief that allows rest, and hence an analgesic is requested.

For a variety of reasons, adaptation will occur, and the patient's behavioural and physiological response to pain will become minimal or cease to exist for periods, even if the pain is severe. Lack of response to pain does not necessarily mean a lack of pain. If we adhere to the acute pain model in assessing a patient with pain, at some point we are likely to think or say "The patient doesn't act like he/she's in pain." Whenever you think or say this or hear others say it, ask "How would this person have to act for us to believe he/she has pain?" This is not an easy question to answer honestly. One of the first things that most people acknowledge is that laughter is not appropriate. The patient who smiles when asking for a narcotic is not very likely to be believed. It usually seems more appropriate if the patient frowns or becomes tearful. Decreased activity is also preferred. In home care, patients who go to work usually finds this is held against them in the form of people saying "If they can go to work, it couldn't be that bad." In the hospital, the patient who walks the halls and visits other patients is not likely to be freely given a

strong analgesic. The likelihood of receiving a narcotic injection is increased, however, if the patient goes to bed, curls up in the fetal position, and frowns.

It is apparent that we do not really wish to reinforce, encourage, or require the behaviour patterns that are apt to convince us that the patient hurts. In fact, we actually want to encourage the behaviour that ordinarily makes us doubt the patient. Requiring patients to act as if they are in pain is embarrassing to them, but many learn that they must alter their behaviour to be believed and helped by the health-care team and their own families. If we require patients to look or act like they are in pain, we may even help reinforce a disability. By doubting patients' pain when they go to work but believing them when they stay in bed, we inadvertently reinforce inactivity and lower the quality of life.

For many years it has been known in pain research that behavioural and physiological signs are unreliable indices of pain severity, and the patient's self-report of pain has been accepted as the most successful way to quantify pain (Houde, 1982). Unfortunately, in daily clinical practice we seem reluctant to follow this simple guideline.

Occasionally, behavioural management techniques, such as operant conditioning, are used to minimize the patient's expression of pain. However, this is not to be confused with pain relief and is done only in carefully selected patients who understand and consent to such an approach. For example, it may be clear that a patient focuses on his/her pain and discusses it to such an extent that others take avoiding action or that the patient is unable to focus attention on other ways of handling problems. In some pain management programmes this is discussed with the patient, and the importance of focusing on other approaches to life's problems is explained. With the patient's understanding and cooperation, discussion of pain by the patient may be limited to a certain time of day or to one particular person, focusing the rest of the time on other solutions to problems.

8. Pain perception: predictability vs. variability

Pain perception may be defined as the least experience of pain that a person can recognize. Simply, it is the point at which a given stimulus is felt as painful and the amount of pain felt beyond that point.

Misconception: Comparable physical stimuli produce

comparable pain in different people. The severity and duration of pain can be predicted accurately for everyone on the basis of the stimuli for pain.

Correction: Comparable stimuli in different people do *not* produce the same intensities of pain. Comparable stimuli in different people produce different intensities and durations of pain. There is no direct and invariant relationship between any stimulus and the perception of pain.

It is tempting to believe that we can predict severity and duration of pain, probably because we like to know what to expect. However, such a belief will produce erroneous conclusions. Patients who experience more pain for longer periods may be erroneously judged as exaggerating. Any health-care team member with experience in caring for patients with certain painful procedures or diseases will be able to develop some fairly accurate conclusions about the range of intensity and duration of pain for most people exposed to a certain painful condition; however, this is merely a range of possibilities and there will always be exceptions.

Health-care team members tend to expect that postoperative pain following cholecystectomy, laminectomy, or thyroid lobectomy will be moderate to severe for 1–2 days and subside substantially or be resolved within 3 to 4 days. A study of 88 patients on a typical post-surgical unit revealed that in 31% of patients, pain persisted beyond the fourth day because of complications and that the patients received inadequate analgesia for this (Melzack et al, 1987).

The fact that pain intensity and duration vary, sometimes considerably, between individuals exposed to comparable painful conditions may be best appreciated by a review of current theories of the underlying mechanisms of pain. For example, the gate control theory (pp. 46–47) clearly indicates that a comparable stimulus in different people will be subject to a variety of different factors that influence whether that stimulus will reach awareness and be felt as painful. Pain may be decreased, or the gate partially closed to pain, so to speak, if there is stimulation over the large-diameter afferent fibres such as rubbing, inhibition from the brain stem due to sensory input from distraction, or inhibition from the cortex due to knowledge that the pain will end soon. In a person exposed to the same stimuli but without inhibition from these areas, the pain is much greater.

Similarly, the endorphins (see pp. 47–48) help explain why pain intensity and duration vary from one person to another. The endorphins are familiar to both lay persons and health-care team members and provide a fairly easily understood explanation of why people feel pain differently. For example, simply knowing that different people have different levels of natural narcotics in their bodies and that these levels may be influenced by a variety of factors, such as duration of pain and stress, helps us realize that individuals having the same disease or surgical procedure are likely to feel different intensities of pain and require different amounts of narcotic for relief. Those with high levels of endorphins probably will feel less pain and need less narcotic than those with a low level.

9. Pain tolerance: high vs. low

Pain tolerance may be defined as the duration or intensity of pain that a person is *willing* to endure. A high pain tolerance means that pain must be very intense or last a long time before the person finds it intolerable or wants pain relief. A low pain tolerance means that mild or brief pain is intolerable to the person and results in a desire for relief.

Misconception: People with pain should be taught to have a high tolerance for pain. The more prolonged the pain or the more experience a person has with pain, the better the tolerance for pain.

Correction: Pain tolerance is the individual's unique response, varying between patients and varying in the individual patient from one situation to another. People with prolonged or recurrent pain tend to have an increasingly low pain tolerance. The patient's tolerance for pain is not a matter to be judged as right or wrong by the health-care team. Respect for the patient's pain tolerance is crucial for adequate pain control.

Pain tolerance may be stable for the individual, but there seem to be great variations between individuals. However, pain tolerance may vary considerably within the individual. Under certain circumstances a person's pain tolerance may increase or decrease. For example, if an analgesic makes the patient drowsy, then pain may be tolerated during visiting hours so he/she can be alert to converse with family members, but there may be unwillingness to tolerate the same degree of pain at bedtime or during meals.

Pain tolerance may also be affected by the patient's

own goals or by what it is thought others value. For example, during childbirth the mother may tolerate what she rates as severe pain without any anaesthesia or analgesia either because she wants to be alert for the delivery and spare her unborn baby any possible ill-effects of medications or because she believes that her husband would be ashamed of her if she requested analgesia.

Pain tolerance is probably also influenced by the specific combination of pain intensity and duration for the particular situation. The patient may tolerate mild pain for a long time but tolerate severe pain for only a brief period.

Prolonged or recurrent experience with pain tends to lower pain tolerance because pain tends to be inadequately controlled. If the patient with prolonged pain had repeated experiences of having pain quickly and adequately controlled, the patient might be confident about pain management and be able to learn to use non-invasive or self-management pain-relief methods. However, the patient who goes into accident and emergency with recurrent migraine headaches or who is hospitalized for recurrent sickle cell crises or exacerbations of low back pain is likely to learn two things that decrease pain tolerance: (1) how severe the pain may be, and (2) how difficult it is to get pain relief. With many memories such as these, the patient with prolonged or recurrent pain faces each period of pain with increasing fear and depression and fewer resources with which to bear the pain.

Pain tolerance is an important aspect of adequate pain control. Patients are often asked to rate their pain on a scale such as 0–10, discussed in this chapter in the section on assessment tools (pp. 30-37). The patient is also asked to identify the rating that represents an acceptable level of pain. This is a significant index to the patient's pain tolerance, i.e. the severity of pain he/she is willing to endure. In titrating analgesics or identifying the effectiveness of other pain-relief measures, the patient's tolerance for pain is extremely important. Although we would like to reduce pain to zero at all times, this is not always possible. By identifying the level of pain relief that is satisfactory to the patient, it may be possible to identify a more realistic immediate goal.

The following are distinct entities in the individual patient but are often very difficult to assess separately:

- Pain intensity (perception).
- Pain tolerance.
- Pain expression.

Whenever possible, the nurse distinguishes between these, remembering that pain tolerance is probably more relevant to establishing pain control than either the intensity of pain or the manner in which the patient expresses pain. For example, two patients may rate their pain at 4 on a scale of 0–10. Both may be lying in bed watching television. These data cover pain intensity and pain expression but do not tell us if that level of pain is tolerable to either patient. Therefore we do not know if further pain relief is needed. Obviously one patient may find pain of a 4 rating easily tolerated, but the other patient may find it unbearable. Further, although we do not know if the rating of 4 in both patients means equal pain, this does not matter, since our intention is not to compare one patient with another, nor is it our purpose to judge whether the patient should tolerate the pain.

In many cultures a value judgment is placed on pain tolerance. Often a high pain tolerance is admired. Men are usually expected to tolerate more pain than women, and adults to tolerate more pain than children. Although each of us is entitled to our personal value regarding pain tolerance in ourselves and others, as health professionals we have no right to impose that value judgment on the patient. Inadvertently imposing our personal values or cultural beliefs may lead to erroneous conclusions, such as believing that men who report pain need relief more desperately than do women who report pain.

10. Placebos: faked or imagined pain vs. real pain

A placebo may be defined as any medical treatment (medication or procedure, including surgery) or nursing care that produces an effect in a patient because of its implicit or explicit intent and not because of its specific nature or therapeutic properties (physical or chemical properties). When a patient responds to a placebo in accordance with its intent, that patient is said to be a placebo reactor for that occasion. The response is called a positive placebo response.

Misconception: When the patient reports relief following a placebo, this means that the patient is a malingerer or the pain is "all in the head."

Correction: There is no evidence in the literature to justify using a placebo to determine the presence or absence of pain or to determine whether pain is physical or psychogenic in origin; in fact, to do so raises serious ethical and legal questions. The only accurate conclusion about a person who reacts positively to a placebo is that he/she very much wants pain relief and that he/she trusts something or someone to help him/her obtain it (Goodwin et al, 1979; McCaffery, 1979).

Using a placebo in this inappropriate way usually requires the nurse to lie to the patient about what medication is being received. This deception may destroy the patient's trust in the health-care team and, ultimately, the hospital. The question of damage to the nurse-patient relationship is important to consider, because although the physician may prescribe a placebo, it is the nurse who gives it and often must answer the patient's questions about it. Each nurse must personally decide how to react if asked to administer a placebo under these circumstances.

However, placebos are appropriate and important in research situations. In these instances, the patient is told about the placebo and gives informed consent to its use.

Suggestions for dealing with a prescription for a placebo may include the following strategies:

- Discuss with the doctor the reason for using a placebo.
- Use research to reinforce the point that using a placebo to diagnose pain is inappropriate.
  Fact: A minimum of a third of all people with obvious physical stimuli for pain (e.g. abdominal surgery, cancer pain) report adequate relief from use of a placebo (Lasagna et al, 1954; Goodwin et al, 1979).
  Fact: Although the mechanism underlying placebo analgesia is not well understood, it does have a physiological basis, possibly involving an increase in endorphins (Grevert et al, 1983; Levine et al, 1978).
- Suggest other strategies to better control the patient's pain. For example, implement a pain continuous assessment sheet (p. 38) or daily diary (see Appendix) to plan for changes or alternatives.
- If the physician continues to insist that a placebo be given, you have the right to refuse to give it. Let your senior nurse know about your action so that you will have administrative support.

Table 2.2 summarizes some of the myths about placebos. How many of these statements can you answer correctly? Take responsibility for correcting these myths among the health-care team members in your clinical setting.

MYTHS ABOUT PLACEBOS	
Are the following statements True or False ?	Answer
When a person reports pain relief from a placebo, it may be concluded that: a) the person is a malingerer b) there is no physical reason for the pain c) the person is easily duped or is neurotic.	False False False
Placebos are capable of relieving severe pain caused by obvious physical stimuli.	True
Patients who benefit from placebos may be intelligent, educated, and mentally healthy.	True

Table 2.2 Myths about placebos.

PATIENTS WITH PAIN WHO DENY PAIN OR REFUSE PAIN RELIEF

People who hurt may have a variety of reasons for denying pain or refusing analgesics. Strong indications that such patients might indeed have pain include patient behaviour such as frowning or rigid posture, pathology such as tumour encroachment on a nerve, or knowledge about the stimuli involved such as the discomfort usually reported from a procedure. This possibility should be explored with the patient. Usually the nurse or another health-care team member must initiate conversation with the patient about this, since the patient, for whatever reason, is avoiding discussion.

The definition of pain that we propose, "Pain is whatever the experiencing person says it is, existing whenever the experiencing person says it does," (McCaffery, 1968, p. 95) is appropriate for patients who indicate that they have pain. When a patient denies pain despite other indications, it is important not to take the patient's word for it without exploring the reasons for the denial.

Following are examples of frequent reasons why patients may deny or refuse analgesics. In each case, the nurse must introduce the subject and explore reasons along with possible solutions to the problems that are causing the patient to deny pain or refuse analgesics.

Communication/language problems

Some patients may not ordinarily use the word *pain*; therefore they may deny pain when asked about it. To avoid misinterpretation of terms, use other words such as *hurt, discomfort, aches, soreness,* or *pressure*.

Language barriers in patients who do not speak English, who are retarded, who have a physical disability which impairs speech and communication, or who are too young to verbalize may also result in denial of pain or need for analgesics. For example, one mentally retarded adult used the word "headache" for all pain. The nurse took this description literally and failed to realize that the patient had abdominal pain.

Fears Related to Analgesics

Some patients may be so afraid of analgesics, especially narcotics, that they refuse pain medications. Patients have the right to choose to feel pain or refuse analgesia; however, it is important that this decision is based on accurate information and not on unfounded fears and misconceptions.

Following are possible reasons why, and some suggested solutions for, patients who refuse pain medication (each of these is discussed in more detail in Chapter 4). The patient may not readily articulate these concerns, in which case the nurse may need to initiate a discussion about the issues presented below. A helpful question to begin the discussion with is "How do you feel about taking medications for relief of your pain/discomfort?"

- Fear of addiction. Stress to the patient that addiction does not happen when people take narcotics to relieve appropriate types of pain. Ask the patient "Would you want to take medication if you were not in pain?" If the patient answers no, then you may assure him/her that addiction is very unlikely. For the patient with prolonged pain, it is important to define addiction, distinguishing the psychological dependence from the physiological problems that might occur (see Chapter 4, pp. 76–79).
- Fear that taking pain medication now will result in it not working later on. This is a very common fear in patients who have prolonged pain, such as those with cancer. Explain that tolerance to analgesia can be handled. It is appropriate to take whatever the pa-

tient needs now to control pain. Later, if needed, the dose can be increased safely and effectively.
- Fear of sedation. If sedation does occur, it often stops after several days of the same dose of medication. If, however, it continues, dose adjustments and reassessment of the components of the pain may be tried.
- Fear of loss of control and/or "strange feelings." Try to identify and address specific fears. Explain that narcotics are not a "truth serum," which result in the patient doing or saying things against his/her will. If the patient experiences any feelings that are not liked, a different narcotic may be switched to. Stress that the patient's response to medication is continuously monitored and that he/she is never started on medication and then expected to just "put up with" whatever happens.
- Fear of injections. Injections scare many people, and some would rather put up with the pain than have an injection. Explore the possibility of using other routes of administration, e.g. PO, SL, IV infusion, or rectal suppositories. Many times the IM route is prescribed because it is what the doctor is most comfortable with, when in fact the patient could easily tolerate an alternative route. If there is no choice but to administer an injection, application of ice or local analgesic patch to the site before injecting the medication may reduce discomfort.

Inadvertent denial

Some patients may state that they feel fine in the presence of members of the health-care team, especially the doctor. They do not want to take up the doctor's time or divert him/her from other more important symptoms. The patient often feels better when the doctor is present. In fact visitors of any sort may improve the patient's mood. The latter does not mean to deny pain, but because a visit may be distracting and reassuring, when asked at that time the patient may claim to feel fine.

It may be helpful to describe the patient's behaviour before and after the appointment with the doctor. The doctor may then talk with the patient about inconsistencies between statements and behaviour and encourage him/her not to hesitate to share reports of pain.

Some patients are simply *not able to isolate pain as part of their total discomfort*. This is especially true in the person who is chronically debilitated with prolonged pain that has gradually increased. For example, an older person may experience joint pain and stiffness which have slowly increased over many years. The patient may have many additional physical and emotional miseries such as constipation, nausea, grief, and fear. It may be difficult to determine that physical pain constitutes part of these miseries. The nurse may be instrumental in assessing this by asking the patient about inconsistencies between behaviour and denial of discomfort. Ask the patient to agree to a trial dose of analgesics for 24 hours to see if any improvement is noticed in general comfort. Stress that these medications can always be stopped, but that they may make a tremendous difference if part of the patient's general discomfort is pain.

In some patients, the desire to recover or live longer is so strong that they may deny any negative symptom, such as pain. Some may deny to themselves that they have pain. They may try to convince themselves that they are really doing much better. The nurse may encourage a fighting spirit, but may also address the fact that comfort is an appropriate goal to work toward so that the patient will have the energy to continue to fight. Careful discussion and probing is important; other members of the health-care team, such as a chaplain or psychologist, may be consulted.

Deliberate cover-up

A patient may desire to please the doctor or nurse. Because they have tried to help, the patient wants to express gratitude by fulfilling a "good patient" role. Express your desire to know the truth. Discuss with the patient that you, the patient, and other health-care team members are working together as a team to control the pain, but you depend on him/her to give you accurate information about the effects of a treatment. Make assurances that you will not abandon the patient.

Some patients deliberately deny pain because they do not want to look like "a sissy." These may be people who are uncomfortable with saying "I hurt, please help me." Discuss what part of this acknowledgment bothers the patient. Reassure the latter that pain is appropriate for whatever condition is present or procedure that has been undergone. Emphasize that the use of analgesics and other measures will help to increase function

and/or speed recovery. Administer analgesics on a regular schedule or routinely offer them to the patient.

Some patients fear that the consequences of admitting pain may lead to diagnostic procedures, prolonged hospitalizations, and additional expenses. It is important to discuss the risks involved and options available.

A patient may say different things about the pain felt to different people: *do not assume manipulation*. In some instances, the patient may be trying to protect his/her family. He/she may only admit pain to certain members of the health-care team because they are trusted or are known better. In an attempt to avoid being a sissy, the patient may try not to talk with everyone about the pain.

In other cases, the family may report pain, while the patient denies it. The patient may be in awe of the health-care team and/or the family may feel helpless. Discussion with the family and patient may be helpful.

In summary, after exploration of the possible reasons for denial of pain, we may find that, in fact, the patient does not hurt. However, if the patient does have pain, he/she still has a right to choose to hurt. Hopefully, this decision will be based on accurate information and not on myths and misconceptions.

MAJOR TYPES OF PAIN: CLASSIFICATION AND TREATMENT APPROACHES

Pain specialists usually classify pain in two major categories—acute and chronic. Some type of classification system for various types of pain is helpful in the assessment of the patient with pain, since it provides a framework for understanding the major differences in patients' pain experiences and for identifying differences in approaches to pain relief recommended by pain specialists.

Classification of types of pain

Several classification systems for types of pain exist, and each tends to reflect a philosophy or concept of treatment approaches (e.g. Classification of Chronic Pain, 1986; Crue, 1985). The classification system that we use is a simplified adaptation of several others. There are two major categories of pain:

1. Acute pain

The critical, distinguishing characteristics of acute pain are that:

- It subsides as healing takes place, i.e. it has a predictable end.
- It is of brief duration, less than 3 months.

In most clinical areas the terminology *acute pain* means sudden, severe pain. In any discussion of pain as a speciality, it is important to remember that this customary definition does not apply. In fact, in the language of the pain specialist and throughout this text, acute pain not only has the above characteristics but also may be either sudden or slow in onset and may be of any intensity, ranging from mild to severe. Acute pain may include anything from a simple pin-prick to a traumatic amputation of a limb. Other examples include a fractured bone, streptococcal throat infection, and post- operative pain.

2. Chronic pain

Chronic pain is prolonged, usually for 3 months or longer (according to the International Association for the Study of Pain), but there is disagreement about how long pain should exist before being called chronic. It is clear that several distinctly different types of chronic pain exist, but there is controversy over exactly how they should be defined and classified. Following is one way to distinguish between different types of prolonged pain:

(a) Recurrent acute pain with potential for recurrence over a lifetime or a prolonged period, e.g. migraine headaches and sickle cell crises; these are self-contained episodes of pain that can be predicted to end. However, they tend to recur. In some people the recurrence may be frequent, e.g. a migraine once a week. In between episodes, the patient is virtually pain-free.

(b) Ongoing time-limited pain, or chronic acute: this pain has the potential for lasting months, perhaps years, but has a high probability of ending. It occurs almost daily over a long period. Examples may include cancer or burn pain. Such pain may last for many months before the condition is cured or controlled and pain subsides, or may end only with the death of the patient.

(c) Chronic non-malignant pain, sometimes referred to as chronic "benign" pain (discussed in Chapter 7): when the patient is severely disabled by the pain, the condition may be called chronic intractable benign pain syndrome. This type of pain usually occurs almost daily and has existed for 3 months or longer. Intensity may range from mild to very severe. Critical, distinguishing characteristics of this type of pain are that it:

- Is due to non-life-threatening causes.
- Is not responsive to currently available methods of pain relief.
- May continue for the remainder of the patient's life.

Examples include a wide variety of very different pain problems such as rheumatoid arthritis, peripheral neuropathy, phantom limb pain, diffuse myofascial pain, vascular diseases of the limbs such as Raynaud's disease, ankylosing spondylitis, and low back pain from various causes.

Treatment approaches recommended by pain specialists

Following is a brief review of treatment approaches recommended by those who specialize in pain control. Considerable controversy exists among pain specialists regarding certain forms of treatment and the type of treatment appropriate for specific painful conditions. Therefore this overview is a general guideline to the differences in pain control for the different categories of pain problems.

Perhaps the most important characteristic of pain that tends to determine recommended approaches to pain relief is whether an end to the pain can be predicted. If pain has a fairly predictable end, either by control of the cause or by death, a more aggressive approach to pain control is used than when the pain has no predictable end. Thus in the relief of post-operative pain, recurrent acute pain of sickle cell crises, chronic cancer pain, and the pain of any terminal illness, many pain specialists recommend an aggressive approach that includes liberal use of narcotics for opiate-responsive pain. When narcotics are used, an appropriate dose and interval is strongly encouraged. Thus the patient should receive as much narcotic as often as needed to relieve the pain.

When the pain has no predictable end and is not life threatening, a more conservative approach is advised. Traditionally narcotics have been avoided, although recently there have been reports of the successful use of narcotics in selected patients. Certainly surgical procedures for pain relief are avoided unless the procedure is clearly indicated. Until recently, far too many patients had the unfortunate experience of having multiple laminectomies for the purpose of relieving low back pain, only to find that the pain had become much worse after these procedures.

IMMEDIATE HELP FOR ASSESSMENT

Quick Assessment in Situations where Patients are Unable to Tolerate Lengthy Questions

Time involved: Reading time, 5 minutes; implementation time, about 10 minutes.

Sample situation: Mr M., 65 years old, with lung cancer and widespread metastases is admitted to your ward. He is not able to concentrate long enough to answer many questions. He grimaces frequently and cries out saying "It hurts, please give me something." His wife states that he is not swallowing anything by mouth.

Possible solution: Assess pain with minimal number of questions in order to give initial analgesic safely.

Expected outcome: Patient states he is comfortable. Further pain assessment is completed at a later time so that a detailed plan of care may be implemented.

Tell the patient that you are going to work to get him comfortable as quickly as possible but that you must get some information first:

1. Point (on his body) to where the pain is.
   Mr M. points to his lower back.
2. Is this the same location for the pain over the last several days?
   Mr M. says that this is the same area that has bothered him over the last week, but it has become much worse since yesterday evening.

3. On a 0–10 scale (0 = no pain, 10 = worst pain), what number would you give your pain right now?
   Mr M. becomes very agitated and yells "It is unbearable." This is a good enough answer under the circumstances.
4. What medication were you taking at home, and did it help the pain?
   Mrs M. tells you that her husband was taking oral morphine 90mg 4-hourly with ibuprofen 400mg 6-hourly. He has not been able to swallow anything since late last night, so he has had nothing for pain relief since then. Prior to this, the medication was keeping the pain well controlled.

Due to Mr M.'s condition, it was appropriate to ask only the most essential questions to initiate an analgesic regimen. The above four questions give you important baseline data and establish an initial narcotic d00ose.

Using a flow sheet, the immediate goal is to establish pain control quickly. Using Mr M.'s words ask "Is the pain more bearable now?" Once Mr M. is comfortable, additional questions from the initial pain assessment tool may be filled in, and a long-term plan of care may be reviewed with the patient and his wife.

One current concept of the treatment of pain distinguishes between a centralist and peripheralist view of chronic pain (Crue, 1985). The centralist view suggests that the mechanism for certain chronic pain conditions is in the central nervous system, not in the periphery as the peripheralist would believe. The centralist view maintains that there is no longer any stimulus for pain originating at the site of pain, and therefore treatment should not be aimed at the periphery. Nerve blocks, for example, would be inappropriate. This view does, however, recognize the peripheral input of chronic pain in certain conditions such as cancer, in which a nerve block might well be helpful. The merit of the centralist view is that some types of pain, such as phantom limb pain and other neuralgias, respond well to drugs that act centrally, such as the anticonvulsants.

ASSESSMENT TOOLS

In the assessment process, the nurse gathers information from the patient that allows an understanding of the experience and its effect on the patient's life. The information obtained guides the nurse in planning and evaluating strategies for care. Pain is rarely static; therefore its assessment is not a one-time process but is ongoing.

The assessment of pain is an initial step in understanding and working toward the patient's goals. Unfortunately, this crucial step may be neglected. In a study of 353 hospitalized medical and surgical patients who had experienced pain, less than half of the patients recalled a health-care team member asking them about their pain (Donovan et al, 1987).

Some patients are too ill to participate in in-depth pain assessment. "Immediate Help for Assessment" opposite gives an example of how this problem can be approached.

There are numerous methods of assessing pain. The McGill Pain Questionnaire is one well-known method; however, it is complex, time-consuming, and appropriate for research situations, not general clinical use (Melzack, 1975). More recently, a short form of the McGill questionnaire has been developed for use in research when time with patients is limited (Melzack, 1987). Several articles review other tools commonly used (Chapman et al, 1985; Karoly, 1985; McGuire, 1984; Syrjala and Chapman, 1984).

The purpose of this section is to present two tools that are *practical* in any clinical setting and *easily adapted* to an individual patient's needs: (1) initial pain-assessment tool and (2) continuous-assessment sheet for pain.

Initial pain-assessment tool

Ten sections comprise this tool (Figure 2.3, copyright McCaffery, 1982b; also appeared in Meinhart and McCaffery, 1983), which provides initial information from which a plan of care may be developed. The authors encourage the reader to adapt this tool according to the forms already used in your clinical setting. All information is obtained directly from the patient whenever possible; no one else really knows the location, intensity, and other characteristics of the pain. If anyone other than the patient provides information, it should be noted, e.g. wife states patient is restless when he sleeps. Each of the ten sections is discussed in detail below.

I. Location

Using the front-, back-, and side-view figures, ask the patient to place a mark where the pain is. If there is more than one site of pain, use letters, e.g. A, B, C, to distin-

KEY POINT: When asking a patient about the location of pain, do not rely solely on a verbal description of the location. Ask the patient to point to or trace with two fingers the area of pain. Verbal descriptions of pain location can be confusing and nonspecific.

guish the different sites. If the patient is unwilling or unable to mark the figures on the tool, ask him/her to trace or point to the areas on the body that hurt, and then you or a family member can mark the figure for the patient.

II. Intensity

Naturally the person experiencing the pain is the only one who knows its intensity. In this step of the assessment process, the goal is to translate the patient's description of intensity into numbers or words that provide as objective a description as possible for a subjective experience.

Various numerical scales may be used and include 0–5, 0–10, or 0–100, where 0 equals no pain, and the largest number equals the worst pain. The patient is asked "What number would you give your pain right now?" Additional questions include "What number on a 0–10 scale would you give your pain when it is the worst that it gets and when it is the best that it gets?" "At what number is the pain at an acceptable level for you?" This last question is particularly important because it acknowledges each person's individuality in tolerating pain. On a 0–10 scale, 3 may be an acceptable level of pain control for some people but unacceptable for others. The number that is acceptable to the patient then becomes the goal that you both work toward initially, perhaps hoping to do better eventually. The goal is to relieve as much pain as possible. A pain rating of 0 twenty-four hours a day is the ideal but is not always realistic.

Advantages of using a numerical scale to describe pain intensity include:

- Consistency in interpretation and communication of pain rating. Verbal or written statements of a patient's exact numerical pain rating, e.g. 8 on a 0–10 scale, are likely to be more consistently reported among health-care team members than a word description, e.g. "a lot of pain."
- Clearer understanding of the patient's experience. A patient who rates pain at 100 when asked to rate it on a 0–10 scale clearly communicates its severity through exaggeration and helps us understand far better than with a descriptive phrase such as "the pain is very bad."

INITIAL PAIN-ASSESSMENT TOOL   Date _____

Patient's Name _____   Age _____ Ward _____

Diagnosis _____ Doctor _____

                                     Nurse _____

I.   LOCATION: Patient or nurse mark drawing.

II.   INTENSITY: Patient rates the pain. Scale used: _____

Present: _____

Worse pain gets: _____

Best pain gets: _____

Acceptable level of pain: _____

III.   QUALITY: (use patient's own words, e.g. prick, ache, burn, throb, pull, sharp)
        _____
        _____

IV.   ONSET, DURATION VARIATIONS, RHYTHMS: _____
        _____

V.   MANNER OF EXPRESSING PAIN: _____
        _____
        _____

VI.   WHAT RELIEVES THE PAIN? _____
        _____
        _____

VII.   WHAT CAUSES OR INCREASES THE PAIN? _____
        _____
        _____

VIII.   EFFECTS OF PAIN: (Note decreased function, decreased quality of life.)

Accompanying symptoms (e.g. nausea) _____

Sleep _____

Appetite _____

Physical activity _____

Relationship with others (e.g. irritability) _____

Emotions (e.g. anger, suicidal, crying) _____

Concentration _____

Other _____

IX.   OTHER COMMENTS: _____
        _____

X.   PLAN: _____
        _____

■ May be duplicated for use in clinical practice. From McCaffery, M; Beebe, A; and Latham , J (ed.): *Pain: Clinical Manual for Nursing Practice*, London, 1994, Mosby, an imprint of Times Mirror International Publishers Ltd. '

Fig. 2.3 Initial pain-assessment tool.

• Method of evaluating the effectiveness of an intervention. Using a numerical rating scale clearly documents the effectiveness of interventions, e.g. pain reduced from 7 to 3 when a relaxation technique is used in addition to pain medication. On the other hand, if a patient's pain is the most severe at 9, and the least severe it gets is 7 two hours after oral pain medication, it is quickly evident that more effective interventions need to be explored with the patient.

When asked to use a numerical scale to rate their pain, some patients may ask "What is the right answer?" It is important to stress that there is no "right or wrong" answer, that the patient is the one experiencing pain, and therefore is the only one who knows what the rating should be.

Some patients are unable to use a numerical scale to rate their pain; the numbers do not make sense to them, or it is too hard for them to apply numbers to their experience. In this case, the following choice of descriptive words may be helpful for the patient to use:

• No pain.
• A little pain.
• A lot of pain.
• Too much pain.

These four phrases may then be converted to a 0–3 scale for documentation and communication among healthcare team members: 0 equals no pain, 1 equals a little pain, 2 equals a lot of pain, and 3 equals too much pain.

A visual analogue scale is considered to be a more sensitive and reliable method of measuring pain intensity (Chapman et al, 1985; Syrjala and Chapman, 1984; Wallenstein et al, 1980). However, it has been our experience that progression is not as easily understood horizontally as it is vertically. A vertical progression, i.e. from bottom to top, may be a more familiar concept to patients and therefore easier to apply to pain intensity. For example, the temperature on a thermometer increases from bottom to top, and a container fills with fluid from bottom to top. If a patient has trouble verbalizing a numerical scale, Fig. 2.4 may be shown to help in understanding the concept. If necessary the patient can mark the rating directly on the scale.

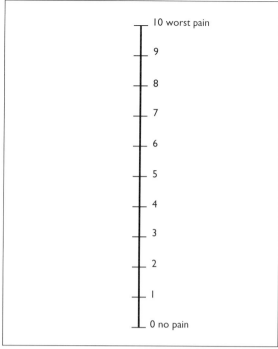

Fig. 2.4 Vertical visual analogue scale.
■ May be duplicated for use in clinical practice. From McCaffery, M; Beebe, A; and Latham , J (ed.): *Pain: Clinical Manual for Nursing Practice*, London, 1994, Mosby, an imprint of Times Mirror International Publishers Ltd.

KEY POINT: Which scale or phrase used to rate pain intensity is not as important as applying the following guidelines:
• Use what makes sense to the patient.
• Use the same scale every time with the same patient.
• Specify the parameters of whatever scale is used each time it is used so that the meaning of the pain rating is clear. For example, a rating of 5 is meaningless unless it is followed by a statement of the scale used, e.g. 5 on a scale of 0–10 (0 = no pain, 10 = worst pain) or 5 on a scale of 0–5 (0 = no pain, 5 = worst pain).

How do you get health-care team members to use a pain-rating scale? If you are just beginning to implement a pain-rating scale in your clinical setting, one of the best ways is to be a role model. Use the scale whenever you communicate verbally or on paper with doctors, other nurses, or other health-care team members. The specific, concise, and consistent data gained from a scale will be one of its selling points.

III. Quality

Ask the patient to describe the pain felt. This may be very difficult to do. Questions such as "What words would you use to describe your pain?" or "What would you do to me to have me feel the pain that you have?" may help the patient if he states that the pain is indescribable.

If the patient still has trouble describing the pain, the 15 descriptors used in the short-form McGill Pain Questionnaire may be helpful (Melzack, 1987):

- Throbbing.
- Shooting.
- Stabbing.
- Sharp.
- Cramping.
- Gnawing.
- Hot–burning.
- Aching.
- Heavy.
- Tender.
- Splitting.
- Tiring–exhausting.
- Sickening.
- Fearful.
- Punishing–cruel.

Descriptions of the pain may be helpful in determining its origin and implementing effective measures for its control. For instance, burning, shocklike pain may indicate injury to the nerve tissue. This type of pain often does not respond to narcotic analgesics (see Chapter 4).

IV. Onset, duration, variations, and rhythms

Assessment of this section might include such questions as "How long have you had this pain?" "Has its intensity or quality changed since you first noticed it?" "Is there any event or activity that changes the nature of the pain; for example, movement, being involved in a hobby, or visiting with family?" "Is the pain better or worse at certain times during the day or night?"

V. Manner of expressing pain

Learning the patient's expression of pain is particularly important if the patient cannot communicate, is very young, or is unable to hear. Family members who know the patient's expression of pain will be able to tell you what clues they look for, e.g. a facial expression or body posture. In patients who cannot verbally communicate, these indications may be all we have to assess pain and evaluate interventions. However, for the patient who can communicate, facial expressions or body posture should be used only as clues to the presence of pain, not as sole indicators. Ask the patient and trust what he/she tells you. However, remember some patients hesitate to admit pain.

VI. What relieves the pain?

If a patient is in hospital, there may be specific pain-relieving methods that were used successfully at home. The patient may assume that these are not possible to continue upon admission. Discussing these methods may result in their being easily incorporated into the plan of care. For instance, listening to music to enhance the effects of a bedtime analgesic can easily be included by using headphones on a portable cassette tape player.

VII. What causes or increases the pain?

Knowledge of the things that make pain worse allows planning care so that these increases in pain are avoided. For instance, if lying on the hard table used for radiation treatments increases the pain, a patient may plan to take an extra dose of analgesic beforehand so that it has taken effect by the time treatment begins.

VIII. Effects of pain

Asking the patient what effect the pain has on each of the areas listed on the chart indicates the extent that it is interfering with daily life. Answers to these questions also indicate any need to control other symptoms. It is helpful to be specific when asking questions about the effects of pain. For example, "Is physical activity limited because of pain?, if so, how?" "Does pain interfere with sleep?" "How does it interfere?" "Is getting to sleep at night a problem?" "How many consecutive hours do you sleep?" "Do you awaken throughout the night because of pain?"

INITIAL PAIN-ASSESSMENT TOOL   Date *10/4/94*

Patient's Name   *Mr T*   Age **45**   Ward *Surgical Unit*

Diagnosis *Splenectomy 12 hrs post op pin insert* Doctor

for fractured (L) femur Nurse

I.   LOCATION: Patient or nurse mark drawing.

II.   INTENSITY: Patient rates the pain. Scale used: *0-10 (0 = no pain, 10 = worst pain)*

Present: *Site A = 8; Site B = 6 2 hours after Pethidine 75mg IM*

Worse pain gets: *Site A=10 when cough; Site B = 10 when try to shift position*

Best pain gets: *Site A and B = 6 when lies totally still*

Acceptable level of pain: *2-3 could move more and sleep*

III. QUALITY: (use patient's own words, e.g. prick, ache, burn, throb, pull, sharp)

A - deep aching. B - sharp throbbing

IV.   ONSET, DURATION VARIATIONS, RHYTHMS: *Pain in site B felt right after accident*

Movement increases pain at both sites.

V.   MANNER OF EXPRESSING PAIN: *Clenching side rails, grimacing, PT, readily*

describes pain and states he is not comfortable.

VI.   WHAT RELIEVES THE PAIN?   *Has not felt relief since coming out of surgery*

Lying totally still decreases pain from 8 to 6

VII. WHAT CAUSES OR INCREASES THE PAIN?   *Movement coughing increases pain ↑to 9-10.*

VIII. EFFECTS OF PAIN: (Note decreased function, decreased quality of life.)

Accompanying symptoms (e.g. nausea) *Nausea when got OOB, pain ↑to 9*

Sleep *Difficulty falling asleep, wakes up approximately every hour due to pain.*

Appetite *Just started clear liquids.*

Physical activity *Been in chair once Pain ↑ to 9*

Relationship with others (e.g. irritability) *Can't talk to wife because of pain.*

Emotions (e.g. anger, suicidal, crying)

Concentration

Other

IX.   OTHER COMMENTS: *Knows importance of getting OOB, but states can't stand pain.*

X.   PLAN: *Evaluate response to Pethidine IM. Suggest change to higher*

dose or different route. Goal: pain rating of 2-3.

Fig. 2.5 Initial pain-assessment tool completed for Mr T.

INITIAL PAIN-ASSESSMENT TOOL Date **5/2/94**

Patient's Name **Mrs P** Age **62** Ward **Home care**

Diagnosis **Breast cancer with bone metastases** Doctor

to (R) rib and lumbar spine. Arthritis in both knees Nurse
and shoulders

I. LOCATION: Patient or nurse mark drawing. **A = Rib pain B = Back pain C = knee pain D = Shoulder Pain**

II. INTENSITY: Patient rates the pain. Scale used: **Unable to use numbers, prefers to use: no pain, a little Pain**

Present: **A little pain** **a lot of pain, too much pain**

Worse pain gets: **a lot of pain**

Best pain gets: **a little pain**

Acceptable level of pain: **a little pain**

III. QUALITY: (use patient's own words, e.g. prick, ache, burn, throb, pull, sharp)
A and B are constant aching pain. C and D are inconsistent throbbing pain.

IV. ONSET, DURATION VARIATIONS, RHYTHMS: **A and B started about a week ago. "X-ray shows**
I have more cancer in the bones there." C and D – had for about 15 years. Worst when first wakes up

V. MANNER OF EXPRESSING PAIN: **Reluctant to "bother" nurses.**

VI. WHAT RELIEVES THE PAIN? **A and B – medication. Movement of R arm makes rib pain worse –**
Lying still helps. Heated pad to shoulder pain helps a bit.

VII. WHAT CAUSES OR INCREASES THE PAIN? **Movement makes rib pain worse – sitting upright**
in chair ↑ back pain. Damp weather makes shoulders and knees ache more.

VIII. EFFECTS OF PAIN: (Note decreased function, decreased quality of life.)

Accompanying symptoms (e.g. nausea) **None**

Sleep **Falls asleep easily. Awakens every 1-2hr because can"t get comfortable**

Appetite **Not much interest in food since chemotherapy treatments 4 months ago.**

Physical activity **Tries to sit in recliner in living room as much as possible.**

Relationship with others (e.g. irritability) **Feels a "bother" to daughter who she lives with**

Emotions (e.g. anger, suicidal, crying) **Tries to "keep going".**

Concentration **Alert, pain interferes with interest in her grandchildren**

Other

IX. OTHER COMMENTS:

X. PLAN: **Evaluate pain medication. Possibly add non-steroidal anti inflammatory**
medication. Improve sleep by improving pain control.

Fig. 2.6 Initial pain-assessment tool completed for Mrs P.

IX. Other comments

It may be helpful to ask the patient "Is there anything else that you can tell me that may help us work with you to get the best possible control of your pain?"

X. Plan

This communicates the initial plan for pain control. Examples of using an initial pain assessment tool in the hospital and home situations are shown in Figs 2.5 and 2.6.

Continuous-assessment sheet for pain

The assessment sheet (copyright McCaffery, 1982b; also appeared in Meinhart and McCaffery, 1983) allows ongoing evaluation of pain (see pp. 38–40). Although it is most frequently used to evaluate the safety and effectiveness of analgesics, it is also appropriate for non-pharmacological methods of pain control. Columns may be added for the latter purpose, or such methods may be included in the "other" column.

The only safe and effective way to administer an analgesic is to monitor the patient's response to the medication and make changes based on these responses. The flow sheet is a tool that allows quick documentation of such responses along with easy retrieval of information for continuous evaluation.

Appropriate uses of the assessment sheet

Situations in which the use of an assessment sheet may be appropriate include the following:

- Initial doses of any new prescription of analgesic. Although initial doses are based on as much pharmacological knowledge and individual history as possible, initial doses are still "educated guesses" because each person reacts differently to medication. However, follow-up with an assessment sheet so that changes can be made immediately results in a guess being tailored or titrated into a safe and effective analgesic regimen. A new prescription of analgesic not only includes any change in choice of drug but also any change in dose, interval, or route of administration.
- Some part of the analgesic regimen is causing the health-care team to be unsure of or fearful of its administration. For example, a high dose of narcotic may cause nurses to hesitate giving what is prescribed. An assessment sheet that provides easy access to the patient's respiratory rate can be quickly reassuring. If you suggest to a doctor a new route of narcotic administration, reassuring the doctor that the patient will be closely monitored using a flow sheet may be a helpful strategy.
- A patient's pain changes, or a complicated pain situation results in ineffective pain control. Documentation of responses according to time and specific analgesic given may help the team gain a clearer picture of adjustments that need to be made.

Characteristics of the pain-assessment sheet

The assessment sheet provides a quick and easy evaluation tool. It is a tool that can be used in the home setting where the patient or family member may fill in information in the columns.

A suggested format for a continuous-assessment sheet is located at the end of this chapter. However, the form may be changed according to the individual patient's needs or the setting in which it is used. The columns that would probably remain regardless of the situation would be Time, Pain Rating, and Plan and Comments.

An explanation of the assessment sheet columns follows:

- *Time.* Initially most routes are assessed hourly, if possible, except for IV, which is monitored more frequently until safety and effectiveness are established.
- *Pain rating.* A footnote about this column appears at the bottom of the form. It is important to explain which scale is used at the top of the form so that everyone is consistent and clear about its meaning.
- *Analgesic.* This column should include the name of the drug, dose, and route. If this form is used to evaluate non-pharmacological pain control methods, simply use "Pain Control Method" instead.
- *Respiration, pulse, blood pressure, level of arousal.* Respiratory status is the most important physiological parameter to monitor in acute pain management to determine safety of a narcotic analgesic. A dramatic decrease in respiratory rate, e.g. from 12 to 6, 30 minutes after a narcotic is given IM requires immediate dose reduction with close patient evaluation. A less dramatic decrease in respirations, e.g. from 12 to 10 may occur when the patient sleeps and requires no dose adjustment. The flow sheet clearly documents these different responses.

CONTINUOUS-ASSESSMENT SHEET FOR PAIN

Patient _____   Date _____

*Pain rating scale used _____

Purpose: To evaluate the safety and effectiveness of the analgesic(s).
Analgesic(s) prescribed: _____

Time	Pain rating	Analgesic	R	P	BP	Level of arousal	Other†	Plan and comments

*   *Pain rating*: A number of different scales may be used. Indicate which scale is used and use the same one each time. For example, 0–10 (0 = no pain, 10 = worst pain).

†   *Possibilities for other columns:* bowel function, activities, nausea and vomiting, other pain-relief measures. Identify the side effects of greatest concern to patient, family, doctor, nurses.

■ May be duplicated for use in clinical practice. From McCaffery, M; Beebe, A; and Latham , J (ed.): *Pain: Clinical Manual for Nursing Practice*, London, 1994, Mosby, an imprint of Times Mirror International Publishers Ltd.

CONTINUOUS-ASSESSMENT SHEET FOR PAIN FOR MR T.

Patient *Mr T*   Date *10/4/94*

Pain rating scale used 0 to 10 (0 = no pain, 10 = worst pain)

Purpose: To evaluate the safety and effectiveness of the analgesic(s).

Analgesic(s) prescribed: *Pethidine 75mg IM 4 hrly prn Later changed to morphine*

Time	Pain rating	Analgesic	R	P	BP	Level of arousal	Other†	Plan and comments
10/4 9am	A = 8 B = 6	pethidine 75mg IM	22			Awake "Really hurts" clenching side rails		Site A = splenectomy
930am	A = 7 B = 6		18			Ask if he can have more pain med		Site B=femur change to different
9.45am	A = 8 B = 7	morphine 10mg IV bolus	22			Alert Asking about new med		analgesic to ↓ pain Evaluate
		paracetomol suppository 500mgs						morphine + paracetomol
10am	A = 5 B = 3		18			States pain is easing somewhat		
10.30 am	A = 5 B = 3	morphine 10 mg IV bolus	16			Eyes closed. Open immed. when		IV bolus repeated only last 45-50min
						name called		+ pain rating remains high
11am	A = 3 B = 1		14			Eyes closed opens imed when name called		
						feels much better		
11.15	A = 3	morphine infusion	18			Alert talking with wife		
1pm	A = 2 B = 1		16			Answers questions easily.		
2pm		morphine 10mg IV bolus	22			Alert. Anxiety with effort to get		Bolus given to get pt in chair
						into chair		
2.15pm	A = 4 B = 3	20mg/hr continues paracetamol	18			Sitting in chair states pain much		Continue current Plan
		supp. 500mg				better		

* *Pain rating*: A number of different scales may be used. Indicate which scale is used and use the same one each time. For example, 0–10 (0 = no pain, 10 = worst pain).

† *Possibilities for other columns*: bowel function, activities, nausea and vomiting, other pain-relief measures. Identify the side effects of greatest concern to patient, family, doctor, nurses.

CONTINUOUS-ASSESSMENT SHEET FOR PAIN FOR MRS P.

Patient **Mrs P**   Date **5/2/94**

*Pain rating scale used **No pain, a little pain, a lot of pain, too much pain. Unable to use a numerical scale.**

Purpose: To evaluate the safety and effectiveness of the analgesic(s).
Analgesic(s) prescribed: **morphine 5-10mg orally, 4-hourly ATC**

Time	Pain rating	Analgesic	R	P	BP	Level of arousal	Other†	Plan and comments
10am	A lot of pain	morphine 10mg orally	18			Sleepy answers questions appropriately		Improve pain relief without sedation
12n			14			Eyes closed		
1pm	A little pain		16			Talking with family falls back to sleep easily		
2pm	A little pain	morphine 10mg orally	16					
3pm	A little pain					Opens eyes when name called		
6pm	No pain	morphine 5mg orally	14			Eyes closed Easily awakened		↓morphine to try to ↓ sedation
10pm	No pain	morphine 5mg orally	14			More awake but sleeping comfortably when able		

*   *Pain rating:* A number of different scales may be used. Indicate which scale is used and use the same one each time. For example, 0–10 (0 = no pain, 10 = worst pain).

†   *Possibilities for other columns:* bowel function, activities, nausea and vomiting, other pain relief measures. Identify the side effects of greatest concern to patient, family, doctor, nurses.

Pulse and blood pressure are rarely monitored unless a patient's respiratory status becomes unstable. A certain amount of sedation may be noted initially; however, it usually subsides. Unless respiration changes, the presence of sedation does not automatically warrant a change in analgesic regimen.

- *Other.* Additional parameters may need to be assessed and evaluated. Examples of these are noted at the bottom of the form and depend on the individual patient situation.
- *Plan and comments.* This column may include strategies for improving or maintaining pain control.

Examples of using a pain continuous assessment sheet are shown on pp. 39 and 40, which show continuing asessment and evaluation of Mr T. and Mrs P.

Additional assessment tool

Instead of the tools discussed above, a daily record kept by the patient or family may be helpful in gathering data, especially if the patient is at home. In the Appendix is a suggested format for the daily diary (copyright McCaffery, 1980; also appeared in Meinhart and McCaffery, 1983). As with the tools mentioned previously, it may be altered to adjust to an individual situation. It may be accompanied by the patient/family teaching point.

The record may be particularly helpful for the patient to bring to the next surgery visit or to show to the community nurse. Every hour does not need to be recorded; however, it is important to note when medication is taken or when an activity alters a previous pain rating. A completed daily record for Mrs A. is shown at the end of this chapter.

SUMMARY

This chapter has addressed the important components of pain assessment. Misconceptions that hamper accurate assessment have been discussed, and three practical assessment tools, appropriate in any clinical setting, have been presented.

REFERENCES AND SELECTED READINGS

Cancer Pain Relief, World Health Organization, 1986.

Chapman, DD, Casey, KL, Dubner, R, et al: Pain measurement: an overview. *Pain,* **22**:1–31, 1985.

Classification of chronic pain. *Pain* (suppl.) **3**:S1–S226, 1986.

Cleeland, CS: Assessing pain in cancer: the patient's role. In: *Management of Cancer Pain*, pp. 17–21, HP Publishing Co, Inc., New York, 1984.

Crue, BL, Jr.: Multidisciplinary pain treatment programmes: current status. *Clin. J. Pain*, 1:31–38, 1985.

Daut, RL, Cleeland, CS: The prevalence and severity of pain in cancer. *Cancer,* 50:1913–1918, 1982.

Donovan, MI: Clinical assessment of cancer pain. In: McGuire, DB, Yarbro, CH, eds: *Cancer Pain Management*, pp. 105–131, Grune & Stratton, Orlando, 1987.

Donovan, M, Dillon, P, McGuire, L: Incidence and characteristics of pain in a sample of medical–surgical inpatients. *Pain,* 30:69–78, 1987.

Dworkin, RH, et al: Unraveling the effects of compensation, litigation, and employment in treatment response in chronic pain. *Pain,* **23**:49–59, 1985.

Goodwin, JS, Goodwin, JM, Vogel, AA: Knowledge and use of placebos by house officers and nurses. *Ann. Intern. Med.,* **91**:106–110, 1979.

Grevert, P, Albert, LH, Goldstein, A: Partial antagonism of placebo analgesia by naloxone. *Pain,* **16**:129–143, 1983.

Hendler, N: Depression caused by chronic pain. *J. Clin. Psychiatr.,* **45**:30–38, Mar 1984.

Houde, RW: Methods for measuring clinical pain in humans, *Acta Anaesth. Scand.* (suppl.) **74**:25–29, 1982.

Infante, MC, Mooney, NE: Interactive aspects of pain assessment. *Orthoped. Nurs.,* 6:31–34, 1987.

Karoly, P: The assessment of pain: concepts and procedures. In: Karoly, P, ed.: *Measurement Strategies in Health Psychology*, pp. 461–519, Wiley Interscience, New York, 1985.

Lasagna, L, Mosteller, F, von Felsinger, JM, Beecher, HK: A study of the placebo response. *Am. J. Med.,* 16:770–779, 1954.

Leavitt, F, Sweet, JJ: Characteristics and frequency of malingering among patients with low back pain. *Pain,* 25:357–364, 1986.

Levine, JD, Gordon, NC, Fields, H: The mechanism of placebo analgesia. *Lancet,* **2**:654–657, 1978.

McCaffery, M: *Nursing Practice Theories Related to Cognition, Bodily Pain, and Man-Environment Interactions*, University of California at Los Angeles Students' Store, Los Angeles, 1968.

McCaffery, M: Nursing Management of the Patient with Pain, ed. 2, JB Lippincott Co, Philadelphia, 1979.

McCaffery, M: Unpublished material, 1980.

McCaffery, M: Would you administer placebos for pain? *Nursing,* **12**:80–85, Feb 1982.

McCaffery, M: Unpublished material, 1982b.

McGuire, DB: The measurement of clinical pain. *Nurs. Res.,* **33**:152–156, 1984.

McGuire, DB: Comprehensive and multi-dimensional assessment of pain. *J. Pain and Symptom Management,* **7(5)**:312–319, July 1992.

Meinhart, NT, McCaffery, M: *Pain: a Nursing Approach to Assessment and Analysis*, Appleton-Century Crofts, Norwalk, Conn., 1983.

Melzack, R: The McGill pain questionnaire: major properties and scoring methods. *Pain*, 1:275–299, 1975.

Melzack, R: The short-form McGill pain questionnaire. *Pain*, 30:191–197, 1987.

Melzack, R, Abbott, FV, Zackon, W, Mulder, DS, Davis, MWL: Pain on a surgical ward: a survey of the duration and intensity of pain and the effectiveness of medication. *Pain*, 29:67–72, 1987.

Melzack, R, Katz, J, Jeans, ME: The role of compensation in chronic pain: analysis using a new method of scoring the McGill pain questionnaire. *Pain*, 23:101–112, 1985.

Miser, AW, McCalla, J, Dothage, JA, Wesley, M, Miser, JS: Pain as a presenting symptom in children and young adults with newly diagnosed malignancy. *Pain*, 29:85–90, 1987.

Moskow, SB: *Hunan hand and other Ailments*, Little, Brown & Co., Boston, 1987.

Perry, SW, Cella, DF, Falkenberg, J, et al: Pain perception vs pain response in burn patients. *Am. J. Nurs.* 87:698, 1987.

Reesor, KA, Craig, KD: Medically incongruent chronic back pain: physical limitations, suffering, and ineffective coping. *Pain*, 32:35–45, 1988.

Sanford, KD, Schlicher, CM: Pain management, are your biases showing? *Nurs. Life*, 6:47–51, 1986.

Shacham, S, Reinhardt, LC, Raubertas, RF, Cleeland, CS: Emotional states and pain: intraindividual and interindividual measures of association. *J. Behav. Med.*, 6: 405–419, 1983.

Syrjala, KL, Chapman, CR: Measurement of clinical pain: a review and integration of research findings. In: Benedetti, C, Chapman, CR, Moricca, G, eds.: *Advances in Pain Research and Therapy*, pp. 71–101, vol. 7, Raven Press, New York, 1984.

Wallenstein, SL: Measurement of pain and analgesia in cancer patients. *Cancer*, 53:2260–2264, 1984.

Wallenstein, SL, Heidrich, G, Kaiko, R, Houde, RW: Clinical evaluation of mild analgesics: the measurement of clinical pain. *Br. J. Clin. Pharmacol.*, 10:319S–327S, 1980.

DAILY DIARY

Name *Mrs A*   **Date** *10/3/94*

Time	Pain-rating scale 0-10 (0=no pain, 10=worst pain)	Medication type & amount taken	Other pain-relief measures tried or anything that influences your pain	Major activity being done: lying sitting standing/walking
12 MIDNIGHT				Sleep (10pm)
1 AM				
2				
3				
4				⇓
5				
6	6 very stiff	ibuprofen 4 x 400mgs paracetamol 500mg	Heating pad to low back.	Remains in bed
7.30	3		Aim shower head at low back x 5 min	Shower & Dress
8				Breakfast
9				Standing + walking for light housework
10	4	paracetamol 500mg		↓
11				Listen to radio -reclining on sofa
noon 12		ibuprofen 4 x 400mg		Sitting -Lunch
1	3			↓
2				Shopping-standing/walking
3				↓
4	5	ibuprofen 4 x 400mgs paracetamol 500mg	Does stretching exercises	Swimming in heated pool
5	3		Ice pack to lower back	Reclining on settee
6	2			Watch TV - reclining
7.30	2			Supper -sitting
8				Read + watch TV
9				↓
10		paracetamol 500mg		Bedtime
11				

Comments *Since I'm taking so much additional paracetamol, is it possible to increase ibuprofen*

* Daily diary for Mrs A.: Mrs A. has rheumatoid arthritis. Stiffness in her lower back is especially bad upon awakening early in the morning. Heat to the area helps first thing in the morning, while cold packs help later in the day after exercise. Recording activities and medication helped the nurse and Mrs A. determine that an increase in ibuprofen might help. No side effects from lower dose were noted, so ibuprofen was increased to 6-hourly.

43

3

The Process of Nursing People with Pain

NURSING PROCESS:
A PROBLEM-SOLVING APPROACH

The process of nursing involves a systematic, scientific approach to care for patients and families. In order to deliver effective and safe care to patients with pain, the nurse collects appropriate information; identifies the problem; plans, implements, and evaluates nursing interventions; and makes appropriate modifications based on evaluation. Problem-solving in this manner is referred to as the nursing process.

The nursing process allows the nurse to be responsive to individual human needs. The components of this process are not mutually exclusive; they overlap, and each provides information for the other, sometimes resulting in a readjustment or revision of a previous step in the nursing process (Fig. 3.1). Following are the five components of this process (Campbell, 1984; Carpenito, 1983).

1. Assessment

Subjective information, i.e. symptoms, and objective information, e.g. signs, are gathered that include not only physical information but also psychological and social aspects of the individual patient which may influence his/her perception of and response to pain. Assessment is an ongoing process that is carried out by history taking, observation, interviewing, and physical examination.

2. Problem Identification

Gathering information helps the nurse decide on the nature of the problem. Once the existence and extent of a problem are identified, a nursing diagnosis is made (see "Nursing Diagnosis Related to Pain" in this chapter).

3. Planning

The approach, or planning step identifies the goals and sets the priorities that both the patient and the nurse decide to work toward.

4. Intervention

Implementing an intervention involves performing a nursing measure that will diminish, resolve, or prevent the defined problem. A nursing measure for a patient with pain may include:

a. Nursing treatments, e.g. facilitating hygiene, initiating a relaxation technique, and coordinating community care.
b. Nursing observations, e.g. baseline respirations before administering a narcotic.
c. Health education, e.g. correcting a patient's or family's misconceptions about pain and its treatment, and teaching the concept of patient-controlled analgesia.
d. Medical treatments performed by the nurse, e.g. administering a prescribed narcotic.

5. Evaluation

This step determines the effectiveness of nursing care in diminishing, resolving, or preventing the defined problem and predicts the need for future nursing actions. For example, evaluation of the safety and effectiveness of a narcotic analgesic includes monitoring a patient's response using an assessment. Evaluation includes ongoing assessment and may involve revisions of the plan of care.

In this book the major components of the nursing process are discussed primarily as follows: assessment in Chapter 2, nursing diagnosis in Chapter 3, and nursing interventions in Chapters 4–7. Chapters 8 and 9 identify

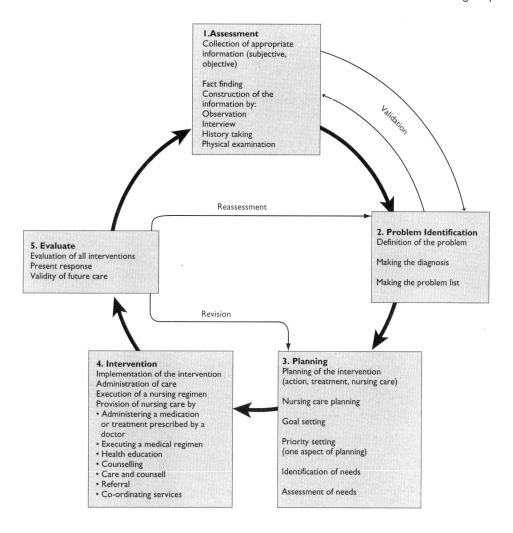

Fig. 3.1 Conceptualization of nursing practice using the nursing process.
Modified from Reeder, SJ, and Martin, LL: *Maternity Nursing*, ed. 16, JB Lippincott, Philadelphia, 1987.

special considerations in these areas for children and the elderly, respectively.

The nursing care plans in this book are set up to incorporate the five components of the nursing process. Column I is assessment, column II is potential nursing diagnoses, column III is planning/intervention, and column IV is evaluation/expected outcomes.

NURSING DIAGNOSES RELATED TO PAIN

Whilst the actual process of "Nursing Diagnosis" is not practised as such in Great Britain, the principles behind the concept are very pertinent to the care of patients with pain, and can be applied to practices such as the nursing process carried out in Great Britain.

When a problem is identified and possible aetiology established, a nursing diagnosis is stated. Nursing diagnoses allow nurses to identify changes in the health of individuals in a systematic manner. Nursing diagnosis is defined as:

...a statement that describes a health state or an actual or potential alteration in a person's life processes (physiological, psychological, sociocultural, developmental, and spiritual). The nurse uses the nursing process to identify and synthesize clinical data and to order nursing interventions to reduce, eliminate, or prevent health alterations which are in the legal and educational domain of nursing

(Carpenito, 1983, p. 4).

45

As of 1988 (Proceedings of the Eighth National Conference of the North American Nursing Diagnosis Association), 98 diagnoses have been approved by the North American Nursing Diagnosis Association for use in nursing practice. The following two are directly associated with the care of patients with pain:

• Chronic pain.
• Pain.

Because pain, especially if it is prolonged, may affect all aspects of a person's life, the following 18 diagnoses may be especially appropriate for patients with pain:

• Anxiety.
• Constipation.
• Ineffective individual coping.
• Diversional activity deficit.
• Fatigue.
• Fear.
• Knowledge deficit (specify).
• Impaired physical mobility.
• Powerlessness.
• Feeding self-care deficit.
• Bathing/hygiene self-care deficit.
• Dressing/grooming self-care deficit.
• Toileting self-care deficit.
• Sexual dysfunction.
• Sleep pattern disturbance.
• Social isolation.
• Spiritual distress (distress of the human spirit).
• Altered thought processes.

This is by no means an exhaustive list, but as the nurse collects information and evaluates the plan, this list should alert him/her to the potential for pain to disrupt many aspects of a person's life.

PAIN THEORIES

Although the exact mechanism for the transmission and perception of pain is not known, neurophysiological, psychological, and sociological research has contributed to the formation of pain theories. By definition, a theory does not represent actual fact; instead it stimulates thought and provides a basis for research. For the nurse who cares for patients with pain, pain theories offer a conceptual framework for research and for specific pain-relieving methods.

Although several theories exist, three will be briefly reviewed below. Those wishing further discussion and study are referred to the selected readings at the end of the chapter.

I. Gate control theory as a conceptual framework

The gate control theory, originally proposed in 1965 (Melzack and Wall, 1965), is not presented from a neurophysiological standpoint; instead parts of the theory that are especially useful in clinical practice are discussed below as a *conceptual framework*.

The gate control theory is particularly relevant to nursing practice in that it presents:

• An integrated conceptual model for appreciating the many factors that contribute to individual differences in the experience of pain.
• A conceptualization of categories of activity that may form a theoretical base for developing various pain-relief measures.

Table 3.1 summarizes aspects of the theory that are useful in clinical practice. The middle column of the table shows three general categories of activity that may contribute to pain relief, i.e. three ways to close or partially close the gate so that impulses felt as painful are less likely to reach the level of awareness. These three aspects of the theory are discussed below in relation to pain control measures.

1. Cutaneous stimulation may relieve pain.

The gate control theory proposes that activation of large-diameter nerve fibres may alleviate pain. Since the skin is heavily endowed with such fibres, many types of tactile stimulation have the potential for pain relief. Specific types of cutaneous stimulation, such as massage or vibration, are obvious examples of the direct application of this theory. However, an element of touch and cutaneous stimulation also may be involved in other pain-relief measures. Distraction may include rhythmic rubbing of a body part experiencing pain, or relaxation may be enhanced by a back-rub.

2. "Normal" or excessive sensory input may relieve pain.

It appears that the reticular system in the brainstem can inhibit incoming stimuli, including pain, if the person is receiving sufficient or excessive sensory input. The brainstem may then project inhibitory impulses that help close the gate to the transmission of impulses felt as painful. To accomplish this, elaborate distraction strategies may be devised. Sensory restriction, especially monotony, is avoided. This may enable the patient to "tune

Table 3.1 Nursing Practice Aspects of the Gate Control Theory of Pain

Major Contributions

1. An integrated conceptual model for appreciating the many factors that contribute to individual differences in the experience of pain.
2. Conceptualization of categories of activity that may form a theoretical base for developing various pain-relief measures.

Nature of the Gate

The transmission of potentially painful impulses to the level of conscious awareness may be effected by a gating mechanism, possibly located at the spinal cord level of the CNS in the dorsal horn.

Structures Involved	No Pain or Decreased Intensity of Pain	Pain
Spinal cord ? nerve fibres	Results from CLOSING THE GATE by: 1. Activity in the *large diameter nerve fibres*, e.g. caused by skin stimulation.	Results from OPENING THE GATE by: 1. Activity in the *small diameter nerve fibres*, e.g. caused by tissue damage.
Brainstem	2. Inhibitory impulses from the *brainstem*, e.g. caused by sufficient or maximal sensory input arriving through distraction or guided imagery, or	2. Facilitatory impulses from the *brainstem*, e.g. caused by insufficient input from a monotonous environment, or
Cerebral cortex and thalamus	3. Inhibitory impulses from the *cerebral cortex* and *thalamus*, e.g. caused by anxiety reduction based on learning when the pain will end and how to relieve it.	3. Facilitatory impulses from the cerebral cortex and *thalamus*, e.g. caused by fear that the intensity of pain will escalate and will be associated with severe illness, disability, and/or death.

out" pain. Most pain-relief methods involve some degree of sensory input. Some are excellent sources of sensory stimuli. Guided imagery, for example, involves intense concentration on imaginary sensory experiences. It is even possible that the enigma of causing brief pain to relieve chronic pain can be explained on the basis of brainstem activities. Intense stimulation of trigger points, by needling, for example, could increase input to the brainstem, which would close the gates to pain from other body areas (Melzack, Stillwell and Fox, 1977).

3. Accurate information about the cause and relief of pain, a sense of control, or a decrease in anxiety or depression, may relieve pain.

The gate control theory suggests that pain can be alleviated by inhibitory signals from the cerebral cortex and thalamus. Thoughts, emotions, and past experiences stored in these structures may result in impulses that affect the transmission of pain impulses. Therefore pain may be relieved by reducing unnecessary sources of anxiety about pain and by increasing the patient's feeling of confidence and control with respect to pain

relief. Often this is accomplished through the nature of the nurse's relationship with the patient with pain or through certain patient teaching. Of course, most other methods of pain relief also contribute, directly or indirectly, to anxiety reduction and increased understanding of the pain experience.

2. Endorphins and non-opioid pathways

In the mid 1970s, the body's own internally secreted narcotic-like substances called endorphins were identified (Snyder, 1977). The term *endorphin* is a combination of the words "endogenous" and "morphine," meaning morphine within. It is believed that an impulse from the brain triggers the release of endorphins. They lock into the narcotic receptors at nerve endings in the brain and spinal cord to block the transmission of a pain signal, preventing the impulse from reaching consciousness.

Endorphin research has helped us understand that pain perception and the need for analgesia vary from one individual to another. Differences in the amount of endorphin present in different individuals and the probability that other factors increase or decrease endorphin levels help explain the differences in pain perception (Janal et al, 1984; Tamsen et al, 1982).

Preliminary research suggests that the following factors tend to increase or decrease endorphin levels (Clark et al, 1986; Emrich, 1981; Janal et al, 1984; Tamsen et al, 1982; Terenius, 1984; Whipple and Komisaruk, 1985):

↓ Endorphins	↑ Endorphins
Prolonged pain	Brief pain
Recurrent stress	Brief stress
Prolonged use of	Physical exercise
morphine or alcohol	Massive trauma
	Acupuncture, some types
	Transcutaneous electrical
	nerve stimulation, some types
	Placebos, possibly
	Sexual activity

It may be tempting to assume that because endorphins are "natural" substances, they therefore have more benefits and fewer side effects than the narcotics that we administer. In fact we have not isolated anything that might be of more benefit than the narcotics presently administered. This certainly raises the question of the benefit of spending considerable time, energy, and expense to increase the patient's own endorphin levels.

Although there was considerable excitement initially over the endorphins, there are few clinically useful conclusions arising from this research (McGrath and Unruh, 1987). There remains hope for the discovery of new analgesic drugs based on these narcotic-like substances (Terenius, 1984).

Endorphin-mediated analgesia appears not to be the only system that may produce pain-relieving effects. There is evidence that non-opioid pathways may produce relief in patients with clinical pain (Janal et al, 1984; Walker and Katz, 1981; Young and Chambi, 1987).

3. Multiple opioid receptor theory: practical aspects

How can a drug relieve pain in the same manner as a narcotic but also wipe out or antagonize another narcotic? The theory of multiple opioid receptor sites helps explain such events, and is one of the most recent theories related to pain relief. Like all theories, it is not fact; it is an idea generated by the need to explain something and is meant to stimulate thought and research. However, the reality is that narcotics relieve pain in a variety of ways – ways that may complement, compete, or be specific in ways we do not fully understand.

For definitions of terms used in this section see box below.

Definitions: Opioid Receptor Site Theory

Opioid: Narcotic- or opiate-like drug; includes natural, synthetic, and endogenous drugs.

Receptor site: That portion of a nerve cell to which a drug can bind. There are several different opioid receptor sites, e.g. mu, kappa, and sigma.

Agonist: In large enough doses this type of drug binds to a specific receptor site and initiates activity at that receptor site. Types of agonists:

a. *Pure agonist:* Binds tightly to the receptor site and produces the near maximal activity possible at that receptor site.

b. *Partial agonist:* Binds to the receptor site less tightly than a pure agonist, producing less effect than the latter.

Antagonist: In large enough doses this type of drug binds to a specific receptor and blocks activity at that receptor; or it displaces the agonist at the receptor site, thereby stopping the receptor's activity. Types of antagonists:

a. *Pure antagonist:* Binds tightly to the receptor site and stops or blocks activity at that site.

b. *Partial antagonist:* Binds to the receptor site less tightly than a pure antagonist, stopping or blocking less of the activity at that site.

Spinal analgesia: Pain relief with awareness; results from binding of opioids to receptor sites at the spinal level. The kappa opioid receptor provides spinal analgesia.

Supraspinal analgesia: Pain relief that affects awareness and other cortical and brainstem functions such as respiration; results from binding of opioids to receptor sites at the supraspinal level. The mu opioid receptor provides supraspinal analgesia.

Overview of Multiple Opioid Receptor Theory

In the central nervous system (CNS) at the spinal and supraspinal levels, theory suggests that narcotics may bind to, or occupy, multiple opioid receptor sites at the ends of nerves (Buprenorphine, 1976; Houde, 1979; Jaffee and Martin, 1985; Martin et al, 1976; Millan, 1986; Offermeier and Van Rooyen, 1984; Physicians' Desk Reference, 1987; Rogmagnoli and Keats, 1980; Wood, 1982; Yaksh et al, 1987). Three receptor sites have practical implications for effective use of narcotics. Table 3.2 lists three opioid receptor sites and their activities as follows:

1. *Mu* (μ) receptor site. Activity consists of supraspinal and probably spinal analgesia, respiratory depression, physical dependence, tolerance, constipation, and euphoria.
2. *Kappa* (κ) receptor site. Activity consists of spinal level analgesia and sedation, but no respiratory depression and no physical dependence.
3. *Sigma* (σ) receptor site. Activity consists of vasomotor stimulation and probable psychotomimetic effects (mimics psychosis, e.g. hallucinations).

Drugs bind to opioid receptor sites with varying degrees of affinity, or strength, i.e. some bind very tightly, referred to as "pure," and others bind less tightly, referred to as "partial." When a drug binds to a receptor site, the action may be pure or partial agonist or antagonist (Table 3.2):

> **KEY POINT:** Effective use of all groups of narcotics, e.g. agonists and agonist-antagonists (or partial agonists), depend on a basic understanding that there are three opioid receptor sites – mu, kappa and sigma.

1. When an *agonist drug* binds to the receptor site, activity occurs, i.e. an agonist *turns on the activity*, or
2. When an *antagonist drug* binds to the receptor site, activity is antagonized or blocked, i.e. an antagonist *turns off or blocks the activity*.

Table 3.2 lists analgesia as an activity at the mu and kappa receptor sites. Therefore when an agonist drug binds to either of these sites, pain relief will occur. Table 3.2 shows morphine, pethidine, and several other narcotics binding as agonists at the mu receptor site and not binding as agonist or antagonist to the other two receptor sites. Thus these drugs relieve pain mainly by action at the mu receptor.

When an antagonist drug attaches to the mu or kappa sites, analgesia at these sites will be blocked; or an antagonist drug can displace an agonist drug that is attached to the mu or kappa site, reversing analgesia along with other effects such as respiratory depression.

The purest narcotic antagonist is naloxone (Narcan). This antagonizes, or blocks, activity at all three opioid receptor sites, but its strongest antagonist effect is at the mu and kappa sites. Naloxone is com-

Table 3.2 Practical Summary of Actions at Opioid Receptor Sites

Opioid Receptor Site	Activity	Drug Action	
		Agonist (On)	**Antagonist (Off)**
Mu (μ)	Analgesia, respiratory depression, physical dependence, tolerance, constipation, euphoria	Pure: e.g. morphine, methadone, codeine, fentanyl, diamorphine, meperidine Partial: buprenorphine	Pure: naloxone Partial: nalbuphine, pentazocine
Kappa (κ)	Analgesia, sedation, no physical dependence, no respiratory depression	buprenorphine, nalbuphine, pentazocine	Pure: naloxone
Sigma (σ)	Vasomotor stimulation, psycholomimetic effects (e.g., hallucinations, paranoia)	pentazocine	Antagonists not very effective at this site

monly used as an antidote for narcotic overdose, particularly to reverse respiratory depression and sedation, but it also reverses analgesia and other activities at the mu and kappa sites.

Table 3.2 shows that two drugs, nalbuphine and pentazocine, result in analgesia by binding as agonists at the kappa site. Thus they relieve pain mainly by action at the kappa, not the mu, site. Nalbuphine and pentazocine are also shown as partial antagonists at the mu site, meaning they can antagonize some of the analgesia and other effects of morphine and other pure agonists at the mu site. Buprenorphine is shown as an agonist at both the mu and kappa sites, so it relieves pain at two receptor sites.

Clinical application of opioid receptor theory

Two Groups of Narcotics. Pain relief from narcotics can result from drug occupation of receptors of more than one type. Currently, two types of narcotics are marketed in the UK:

1. Pure narcotic agonists, such as morphine and codeine, occupy the mu site and do not antagonize activity at other receptor sites.
2. Narcotic agonist-antagonists occupy the kappa site for pain relief and antagonize the effects of pure agonists at the mu site. Only two are available in the UK:
   • nalbuphine
   • pentazocine (this drug is now not widely used or recommended in current clinical practice).

Buprenorphine is also a narcotic agonist-antagonist but is unlike the others in this group. It does not antagonize at the mu site except at very high doses in very physically dependent persons. Also, although respiratory depression is rare with this drug, this is the only narcotic-induced respiratory depression that cannot be completely reversed by naloxone.

Potential problems with narcotic agonist-antagonists

If the narcotic antagonist property of nalbuphine and pentazocine is not understood, these drugs may cause the following difficulties:

• *They may precipitate withdrawal in a person who has been on pure narcotic agonists for a week or more.* After a course of narcotic agonists, the person may become physically dependent, i.e. if the narcotic is abruptly discontinued, the person experiences withdrawal. Narcotics with an antagonist property may precipitate withdrawal by abruptly blocking the action of the pure agonist. Therefore the two narcotic agonist-antagonists mentioned must be used with caution after a person has been on pure narcotics for a week or longer. A physically dependent person may be carefully switched from a narcotic agonist to an agonist-antagonist, but it may take up to 10 days or longer of small, daily decreases in the agonist accompanied by small, daily additions of the agonist-antagonist.

• *Given along with pure narcotics, they may eventually antagonize analgesia from the pure narcotics.* Initially, giving the two narcotic groups together may be additive, and it is difficult to predict when the agonist-antagonist will begin to reverse analgesia of the agonist. Early in narcotic therapy, a decision should be made about which group of narcotics will be used. A person can be switched from a narcotic agonist-antagonist to a narcotic agonist without much difficulty, except for some possible initial decrease in analgesia until the agonist-antagonist is excreted.

Benefits of the narcotic agonist-antagonists

Because all of the narcotic agonist-antagonists (buprenorphine, nalbuphine, and pentazocine) act mainly at the kappa site where there is no respiratory depression, they usually cause only limited respiratory depression, on which there is a ceiling. Beyond a certain dose, additional respiratory depression does not occur; therefore an increase in dose usually results in more pain relief without more respiratory depression. For further explanation and clinical examples, see Chapter 4.

Future applications of multiple opioid receptor theory

Greater understanding of the actions, location, and other characteristics of the various opioid receptor sites may play an important role in developing a more perfect analgesic and in refining methods of using analgesics. Perhaps it will be possible to identify an opioid receptor site with excellent analgesia and no side effects and then develop a drug that would attach to that site only.

Understanding of the opioid receptor sites may enable us to determine the most appropriate drug for a certain route of administration. For example, an analgesic with affinity for spinal opioid receptor sites only might be the most logical choice for epidural or intrathecal administration.

Tolerance to analgesia may be more easily controlled by identifying which drugs act at the various opioid receptor sites. Alternating drugs that act at different opioid receptor sites may delay tolerance. Of course, further research may yield unexpected findings. Already the search for the understanding of endorphins and opioid receptor sites has revealed that there are non-opioid analgesic systems. Humans apparently also have natural nonnarcotic substances that provide pain relief. The current status of research into human analgesic systems has been called the "tip of the iceberg".

GUIDELINES FOR PAIN CONTROL

Following is a general introduction to the pain-control methods discussed in Chapters 4–9. Certain attitudes and approaches that are important to communicate to a patient with pain and his/her family are summarized in the box at the top of the page. Occasionally the nurse must accept the fact that the desired relationship between nurse and patient is unlikely to develop. The nurse does not desert the patient but makes every effort to promote a relationship between the patient and someone else.

Deciding which pain-control measures to use with which patient can be difficult. Because pain experience is highly individual, its treatment must be likewise. In-depth discussions of the goals and guidelines for individualizing pain-control measures are discussed in each of the chapters that follow. The box on the right summarizes these guidelines.

> **Important Attitudes Communicated by the Nurse to the Patient and Family**
> 1. I care.
> 2. I believe you about your pain.
> 3. I respect the way you are reacting to the pain.
> 4. I want to explore with you what you think will help relieve your pain.
> 5. I want to discuss with you what your pain means to you.
> 6. I am willing to stay with you even if I fail to help control your pain.
> 7. If you cannot relate to me, I will try to find someone else for you.

> **Summary of Guidelines for Using and Individualizing Pain-Control Measures**
> 1. Be open-minded about what may control pain.
> 2. Include what the patient believes will be effective.
> 3. Consider the patient's ability or willingness to be active or passive in the application of pain-control measures.
> 4. Use pain-control measures before pain becomes severe.
> 5. Use a variety of pain-control measures.
> 6. Institute and modify pain-control measures on the basis of the patient's response.
> 7. If the pain-control measure is ineffective the first time it is used, consider encouraging the patient to try it at least one or two more times before abandoning it.
> 8. Keep trying.
> 9. Do no harm.

REFERENCES AND SELECTED READINGS

Buprenorphine: *Med. Lett. Drugs Ther.* 28–56, May 23, 1986.

Campbell, C: *Nursing Diagnosis and Intervention in Nursing Practice*, 2nd edn., John Wiley & Sons, New York, 1984.

Carpenito, LJ: *Nursing Diagnosis: Application to Clinical Practice*, JB Lippincott, Philadelphia, 1983,

Clark, WC, Yang, JC, and Janal, MN: Altered pain and visual sensitivity in humans: the effect of acute and chronic stress. In: Kelly, DD, (ed.): Stress-induced analgesia, *Ann. N.Y. Acad. Sci.* **467**:116–129, 1986.

Emrich, HM, ed.: The role of endorphins in neuropsychiatry. In: Ban, TA, et al, (eds.): *Modern Problems of Pharmacopsychiatry*, pp. 1–292, vol. 17, Basle, New York, 1981.

Hoffert, M.: The gate control theory re-revisited, *J. Pain Sympt. Manag.* 1:39–41, Winter 1986.

Houde, RW: Analgesic effectiveness of the narcotic agonist-antagonists, *Br J Clin Pharmacol* **7**:297S-308S, 1979

Jaffee, JH and Martin, WR: Opioid analgesics and antagonists. In: Gilman, AG, et al (eds.): Goodman and Gilman's *The Pharmacological Basis of Therapeutics*, ed. 7, pp. 491–553, Macmillan Publishing Co., New York, 1985.

Janal, MN, Colt, EWD, Clark, WC, and Glusman, M: Pain sensitivity, mood and plasma endocrine levels in man following long-distance running: effects of naloxone. *Pain,* **19**:13–25, 1984.

Kim, MJ, McFarland, GK, and McLane, AM: *Pocket Guide to Nursing Diagnoses,* 3rd edn., The CV Mosby Co., St Louis, 1989.

Kosten, TR, and Kleber, HD: Control of nociception by endogenous opioids. In: Aronoff, GM (ed.) *Mediguide to Pain,* **8**:1–5, DellaCorte Publications, New York, 1987.

Martin, WR, Eades, CG, Thompson, JA, et al: The effects of morphine and nalorphine-like drugs in the nondependent and morphine-dependent chronic spinal dog. *J. Pharmacol. Exp. Ther.,* **197**:517–532, 1976.

Melzack, R, Stillwell, DB, and Fox, EJ: Trigger points and acupuncture points for pain: correlations and implications. *Pain,* **3**:3–23, 1977.

Melzack, R, and Wall, PD: Pain mechanisms: a new theory. *Science,* **150**:971–979, 1965.

McGrath, PJ, and Unruh, AM: *Pain in Children and Adolescents,* Elsevier, Amsterdam, 1987.

Millan, MJ: Multiple opioid systems and pain. *Pain,* **27**:303–347, 1986.

Offermeier, J, and Van Rooyen, JM: Opioid drugs and their receptors: a summary of the present state of knowledge. *S. Afr. Med. J.,* **66**:299–305, Aug 1984.

Pasternak, GW: Multiple morphine and enkephalin receptors and the relief of pain. *JAMA,* **259**:1362–1367, Mar 1988.

Physicians' Desk Reference, 41st edn., Medical Economics Co Inc., Oradell, NJ, 1987.

Proceedings of the Eighth National Conference of the North American Nursing Diagnosis Association, St Louis, Mar 13–16, 1988.

Rance, MJ: Multiple opiate receptors—their occurrence and significance. *Clin. Anaesthesiol.,* **1**:183–199, Apr 1983.

Riordan, MP: Validation of the defining characteristics of the nursing diagnosis, alteration in comfort: pain. In: McLane, AM (ed.): *Classification of Nursing Diagnoses: proceedings of the seventh conference,* pp 221-228, The CV Mosby Co., St Louis, 1987.

Rogmagnoli, A, and Keats, AJS: Ceiling effect for respiratory depression by nalbuphine. *Clin. Pharmacol. Ther.,* **27**:478–485, Apr 1980.

Snyder, SH: Opiate receptors and internal opiates. *Sci. Am.,* **236**:44–56, 1977.

Tamsen, A, Sakurada, T, Wahlstrom, A, et al: Postoperative demand for analgesics in relation to individual levels of endorphins and substance P in cerebrospinal fluid. *Pain,* **13**: 171–183, 1982.

Terenius, L: The endogenous opioids and other central peptides. In: Wall, PD, and Melzack, R (eds.) *Textbook of Pain,* pp. 133–141, Churchill Livingstone, Edinburgh, 1984.

Walker, JB, and Katz, RL: Non-opioid pathways suppress pain in humans. *Pain,* **11**:347–354, 1981.

Whipple, B: Methods of pain control: review of research and literature. *Image: J. Nurs. Scholar,* **19**:142–146, Fall 1987.

Whipple, B, and Komisaruk, BR: Elevation of pain threshold by vaginal stimulation in women. *Pain,* **21**:357–367, 1985.

Wood, PL: Multiple opiate receptors: support for unique mu, delta and kappa sites. *Neuropharmacology,* **21**:487–497, 1982.

Yaksh, TL, Durant, PAC, Gaumann, DM, Stevens, CW, and Mjanger, E: The use of receptor-selective agents as analgesics in the spinal cord: trends and possibilities. *J. Pain Sympt. Manag.* **2**:129–138, Summer 1987.

Young, RF, and Chambi, VI: Pain relief by electrical stimulation of the periaqueductal and periventricular gray matter. Evidence for a non-opioid mechanism. *J. Neurosurg.,* **66**:364–371, 1987.

Pharmacological Control of Pain

A Multidisciplinary Approach

Relevant Patient/Family Teaching Points (see Appendix):
- Antidepressant medications to help with pain control.
- Common side effects of narcotics.
- Instructions for using non-narcotic analgesics at home.
- Preventive approach with pain medication.

What is your role and responsibility in this situation?

Mrs M. has end-stage breast cancer. She is admitted to your unit for pain control. The admitting doctor has requested pethidine 50mg IM 4-hourly PRN for pain.
You have already assessed Mrs M.'s pain. You know the dose of pethidine is inadequate and the route and drug choice are inappropriate.

It is unacceptable for health-care professionals to allow this kind of under-treatment of pain and inappropriate prescribing to continue. As professionals with a knowledge base in assessment, treatment and evaluation, nurses must articulate their suggestions for optimal pain control to all members of the health-care team. It is our responsibility to obtain the best pain control possible for patients, and it is part of our role to work toward this in whatever clinical setting we practice.

The responsibility for pharmacological control of pain rests with the *entire* health-care team. Each member possesses a unique body of information, but some knowledge is shared by all. The key people involved are most often the physician, the nurse, and the patient. Usually all three possess some information about the pharmacology of analgesics, yet each makes a unique contribution to pharmacological control. For example, the doctor's prescription of analgesic is influenced by the patient's physical pathology; the nurse's recommendations about changes in analgesics are based on an assessment of the patient's responses; and the patient, who is the only one who can feel the pain, contributes by communicating information about the pain felt.

For these reasons, this chapter addresses pharmacological control of pain as a multidisciplinary process. Since the information and recommendations in this chapter are pertinent to all members of the health-care team, they are not labelled as nursing care guidelines (as they are in other chapters).

The nurse's immediate role and responsibility in the above situation is to communicate effectively the assessment reached and suggestions to the doctor so that Mrs M. can begin a medication regime that satisfies her and that effectively controls the pain.

To assist the nurse in making a significant contribution to the multidisciplinary approach, this chapter presents specific information that enables the nurse to:
- Be knowledgeable of the pharmacological control of pain.
- Be able to effectively communicate this knowledge with the doctor and other health-care team members.

■ Generic drug names are used throughout the text.

- Cite research and articles that are particularly helpful in documenting a point or backing up a suggestion.

THE ROLE AND RESPONSIBILITY OF THE NURSE

The nurse plays a key role in assuring good pain control for people with unrelieved pain. The nurse is with the patient more than any other health-care team member and is in a position to constantly assess and evaluate the effectiveness of the pain treatments.

Nursing behaviour that results in an *active role* in the use of medications for pain control includes:
- Choosing the appropriate analgesic.
- Determining whether to give it.
- Evaluating its effectiveness.
- Obtaining a change in analgesic prescriptions if needed.

This behaviour involves the application of assessment skills and knowledge about analgesics to each individual patient situation. Table 4.1 elaborates on the nurse's role in relation to medications for pain relief.

Table 4.1 Nurse's responsibility in relation to medication for pain relief

Nurse is expected to:	Comments
1. Determine whether the analgesic is to be given and, if so, when.	1. Many analgesics are given on a PRN basis (PRN means use clinical judgement). Assess and apply knowledge. Based on this assessment, a PRN analgesic order may be given on a regular basis, e.g. every 3 hours.
2. Choose the appropriate analgesic(s) when more than one is prescribed.	2. More than one analgesic is often available. Which one does the nurse give? Two at the same time? Avoid one? This decision is based on pharmacological knowledge along with skills in assessment and evaluation
3. Be alert to the possibility of certain side effects as a result of the analgesic.	3. The nurse plays a key role in identifying life-threatening side effects, e.g. respiratory, depression and identifies "unwanted" side effects, e.g. constipation, which can seriously influence the patient's comfort as much as the pain itself.
4. Evaluate effectiveness of the analgesic at regular frequent intervals following each administration, but especially the initial dose.	4. This is a vital step in ensuring effective pain control. Assessment and evaluation are continuous processes. A flow sheet is recommended.
5. Report promptly and accurately to the doctor when a change is needed.	5. Every new prescription of analgesic for the individual patient is merely a "calculated" guess that must be evaluated. Too small a dosage should be changed as quickly as too large a dosage.
6. Make suggestions for specific changes, e.g. drug, route, dosage, and interval	6. The nurse has a unique blend of knowledge: pharmacological information and direct observation of patient. The result is that the nurse is in an ideal position to make an educated guess about what may work better for the individual patient.
7. Advise the patient about the use of analgesics, both prescription and non-prescription.	7. The nurse has a key educational role about dosage, side effects, addressing misconceptions, preventive regimes and how to talk with a doctor or nurse about questions or problems concerning medication.

Nurses also often suggest changes in analgesics. To accomplish this effectively, the following areas must be addressed:

1. *Communicate a concise pain assessment.* Continuing with the example on p. 53, the nurse might report "Mrs M. rates her pain at 9 on a 0–10 scale (0 = no pain, 10 = worst pain). Upon movement her pain increases to 10. The least the pain gets is 6 when she lies totally still. Pain does not get below 6 even after she takes pethidine 50mg IM 4-hourly. She has been without sleep for the last 2 days because of the pain.

2. *Use an equianalgesic chart when suggesting dose changes.* This is discussed in detail starting on p. 70 and pp. 82–87. Tables 4.4 and 4.10 list equianalgesic doses for mild to moderate and moderate to severe pain. Share a copy of these tables with doctors and other health-care team members. Have them available so that they are easily accessible, e.g. display one in a central place such as the treatment room or drug cupboard in your clinical setting.

3. *Supply reference and research articles to back up suggestions.* For example, in Mrs M.'s case, and for any patient receiving pethidine, the following articles might be made available to the doctor and other health-care team members:
   Pyle, BJ, et al: Toxicity of Norpethidine in sickle cell crisis. *BMJ*, **304**:1478–1479, 1992.
   Geller, RJ: Meperidine (pethidine) in patient-controlled analgesia – a near fatal mishap. *Anaesth. Analg.*, **76**:655–657, 1993.
   Kaiko, R, et al: Central nervous system excitatory effects of meperidine (pethidine) in cancer patients. *Ann. Neurol.* **13**:180–185, Feb 1983. This article discusses the potential toxic effects and mood changes associated with pethidine.
   McCaffery, M: Problems with meperidine (pethidine), *Am. J. Nurs.* **84**:525, Apr 1984. Reviews Kaiko's article and discusses clinical implications of inappropriate use of meperidine (pethidine).
   McCaffery, M: Giving meperidine (pethidine) for pain – should it be so mechanical? *Nursing* **17**:61–64, Apr 1987.

4. *Address misconceptions held by the health-care provider, patient, and family.* In Mrs M.'s case, or any patient receiving opioids, these might include the following (both of these misconceptions are discussed in greater detail later in this chapter):
   Misconception: Injections are the most effective route of medication for severe pain.
   Correction: Oral route is the first choice and can control severe pain *if:*
   • Patient can swallow.

• Nausea and vomiting is controlled.
• Preventive approach is used.
• High enough dose is used.

Misconception: Pain medication taken regularly will result in Mrs M. becoming addicted.

Correction: Addiction does not occur when people are taking pain medication to relieve pain. The majority of people stop taking pain medication when the pain stops.

5. *Never give up approaching doctors.* Although the ultimate power to change analgesic regimes lies legally with the doctor, nurses must continue to suggest changes based on assessment, consistent evaluation of the patient's response, and knowledge of pharmacology, supported by current references from the literature. It is our responsibility as professionals to assure that the control of pain is a priority in health care. Re-education is difficult and frustrating. However, persistence is the key, with the ultimate goal being effective pain control through the appropriate use of analgesics and adjuvant medications.

KEY CONCEPTS IN ANALGESIC THERAPY

How an analgesic is used is probably more important than which one is used. The following three key concepts for effective analgesic therapy apply to both acute and chronic pain.

1. Use a Preventive Approach

Stay on top of the pain. This approach has been the mainstay for treatment of prolonged pain from cancer (Foley and Inturrisi, 1987; Levy, 1985). It is also recommended for acute pain, such as the control of post-operative pain (Rutter et al, 1980). A preventive approach means that the analgesic is given before pain occurs or before it increases, i.e.:

• Regularly. If pain occurs consistently and predictably throughout a 24-hour period, then regular administration is appropriate. This may mean waking the patient at night to take the analgesic if pain usually awakens him/her at night or if he/she awakens in the morning with pain out of control.

• PRN (as needed, requires nursing assessment and evaluation). PRN dosing should be used to prevent pain from occurring or increasing. Some pain cannot be predicted, so occasional dosing rather than regular dosing may be appropriate, but it too should be used preventively *as soon as* pain begins and *before* it gets out of control.

IMMEDIATE HELP FOR PHARMACOLOGICAL CONTROL OF PAIN

Making the Best of Inadequate Analgesics

Time involved: reading time, 10 minutes; decision time, 10–15 minutes; implementation time, variable.

Sample situation: For Mr R., 25 years old, this is the fifth day following surgical repair of a gunshot wound to the abdomen. The surgical site is infected, drains were inserted at 8:00 am, and the patient's pain has not been well controlled during the 8 hours since then.

Analgesics ordered: pethidine 50mg IM 3-hourly PRN for severe pain; paracetamol 500mg 4-hourly PRN for pain or fever; dihydrocodeine 30mg; one tablet 4-hourly PRN for mild to moderate pain.

It is 4:00 pm and you have just seen the patient for the first time. He is alert, breathing well (respiration 16 per minute), and tells you his pain is awful now and that today the injections help even less than before. The medication record shows that he received both pethidine at 7:30 am and 12 noon. The chart includes a note, made about 1 hour following each injection, that the pain was not relieved. The doctor was notified both times, but the orders have not been changed. No side effects were noted. Paracetamol and dihydrocodeine have also been given separately on previous days with poor pain relief but no side effects noted.

Possible solution: While you continue to try to contact the doctor, make better use of the available prescriptions.

Expected outcome: Better pain relief, although it probably will not be satisfactory.

DON'Ts

1. Do not tell the patient that the analgesics given should have relieved his pain.
2. Do not tell the patient he simply must endure the pain.
3. Do not tell the patient that post-operative pain should not be severe after 3 days.
4. Do not tell the patient nothing else can be done to help him.
5. Do not tell the patient that narcotics must be tapered to avoid addiction.

DOs

1. Assure the patient you know he hurts as much as he says he does.
2. Tell the patient you will continue to try to contact the doctor to get the prescriptions changed.
3. Tell the patient that in the meantime you will try to use the present analgesics in a way that provides somewhat better pain relief.
4. Answers to the following questions are basic to getting better results from inadequate prescriptions. Here they are answered in relation to Mr R. Use your patient's responses and charted information to document your assessment and the rationale for your actions.
   • Is the patient experiencing any undesirable side effects from the present analgesics? No side effects were noted from pethidine, paracetamol or dihydrocodeine.
   • After the administration of each analgesic, is the patient still in pain? Yes. Document in the chart that following administration of each analgesic no side effects are noted but pain is not relieved, e.g. following pethidine IM, pain is still mild to moderate. State that dihydrocodeine and/or paracetamol need to be added to relieve the remaining mild to moderate pain. Therefore it appears both safe and necessary to give two or more analgesics at the same time.
   • How often can the analgesics be given, and can pain be predicted to continue? The prescription allows pethidine every 3 hours and dihydrocodeine and paracetamol every 4 hours. Yes, pain can be expected to be ongoing, i.e. it will return. Document that the PRN prescriptions are needed to relieve and prevent the return of severe pain, and they need to be implemented regularly, given as often as the prescription allows.
   • Are any of the analgesics incompatible? That is, are there any analgesics ordered that would be dangerous to combine?
   Giving two or more pure narcotic agonists, such as pethidine and dihydrocodeine, at the same time results in additive analgesia and depressant effects. Document that additive analgesia is needed and that additive depressant effects, e.g. decreased respirations are not expected since no depressant effects have been noted from the single administration of a narcotic, but that both analgesic and depressant effects will be monitored hourly.
   Combining non-narcotics with narcotics is a safe and pharmacologically sound method of pain relief.
   • What can the patient have right now? All of them.
   • Which analgesics are the most effective? Probably, in descending order, pethidine, dihydrocodeine, and paracetamol.
5. Plan to give as many available analgesics as often as is allowed, as long as it appears to be safe to do so. Keep a continuous assessment sheet (p. 38) to document safety and degree of pain relief. Following is the plan for Mr R.
   4:00 pm—Pethidine 50mg IM; dihydrocodeine one tablet; paracetamol 500mg orally.

Continued.

Making the Best of Inadequate Analgesics – cont'd.

6:00 pm—Enough time has elapsed to evaluate the effect of the analgesics administered at 4:00 pm.

7:00 pm—Pethidine 50mg IM (continued 3-hourly at 10 pm, 1:00 am, etc.).

8:00 pm—paracetamol 500mg orally (continued every 4 hours at 12 midnight, 4:00 am, etc.).

6. Adjust the number and frequency of analgesics given on the basis of the patient's response regarding pain relief and side effects. If he has no side effects and if pain relief is better but still inadequate, continue the above plan of administering as many analgesics as often as possible and continue to try to contact the doctor.

7. Show the results of the flow sheet to the doctor and to other nurses.
   - Encourage the nurses to continue to use your plan.
   - Encourage the doctor to use the information to provide better analgesic prescriptions. Suggest a longer acting narcotic at a more effective dose, e.g. morphine 10mg IM 4-hourly. Suggest regular administration of all analgesics at frequent enough intervals to keep pain from increasing.

Summary of Guidelines: When Available Analgesics Result in Inadequate Pain Relief, How Can the Nurse Temporarily Make Them Work as Well as Possible?

Caution: Never use these guidelines as a substitute for contacting the patient's doctor, persistently presenting to the doctor an organized assessment of the patient's response to present analgesic prescriptions, and providing appropriate references that support changes that seem appropriate for the patient.

Purpose of these simple guidelines: To provide *temporary* assistance when available analgesics are not providing adequate pain relief. In reality there are times when a patient is in pain and access to appropriate analgesics is not possible. Multiple reasons for this exist, in both hospital and home care. The doctor may not agree to change the prescriptions, he may be temporarily unavailable for consultation, or he may prescribe analgesics that are not available in that area or at that time (nights and weekends are especially difficult). The patient may have lost his medication or run out because he failed to obtain a further supply.

Simple guides to improving pain relief when existing analgesics are inadequate revolve around two questions:

1. *What are the logical choices?*
   - *Look at all medications the patient is currently taking.*
   - *Identify all narcotic and non-narcotic analgesics.* If they have been prescribed they can usually be given simultaneously or alternately, but review exceptions below.

   - *Identify any narcotics that are incompatible.* This is rarely a problem. All pure narcotic agonists may be given simultaneously. Such practice is safe and fairly common, but it is not necessarily rational. Simply be aware that over time narcotic agonist-antagonists (e.g. buprenorphine) given along with pure narcotics may reduce the analgesia of pure narcotics, so discontinue one or the other. Most of the time, after a few days of administration, it is best to choose the pure narcotic, but not always.
   - *Identify any non-narcotics that are incompatible.* Although most of the current concern is that one non-narcotic, especially aspirin, will decrease the effectiveness of another, the most serious danger is that chronic simultaneous use of more than one non-narcotic will increase side effects. Certainly, for a few days there seems to be little danger in simultaneous administration of non-narcotics, especially paracetamol with any other non-narcotic.
   - *Identify any drug given as a "potentiator" of narcotic analgesia, and consider eliminating it.* Most popular "potentiators" are most accurately viewed as sedatives, tranquillizers, or anti-emetics. Some popular potentiators merely sedate, and some, such as the phenothiazines e.g. chlorpromazine actually increase pain and potentiate narcotic-related side effects. When additional analgesia is needed, most of the time the most effective and safest approach is simply to increase the narcotic dose, rather than add a so-called potentiator. Never confuse sedation with pain relief.
   - *Give narcotics with non-narcotics.* This is logical and safe, particularly if the patient has taken both without incident.

If a given non-narcotic is safe for the individual and if a given narcotic is safe for the individual, there is absolutely no known reason to suspect that simultaneous administration of both narcotic and non-narcotic will pose any danger. There is every reason to suspect that the combination will be beneficial and safe.

2. *Once you identify the rational choices, what do you do?*
   - Give narcotics and non-narcotics on a regular basis, maintaining the best analgesic blood level you can.
   - Evaluate safety and effectiveness with the flow sheet, and adjust dose, interval, and drug choice accordingly.

If on-going pain can be predicted, the analgesic that is prescribed PRN should be implemented regularly and should be re-written for regular administration.

Patient Example

Postoperative prescription for Mrs A. includes pain medication every 3–4 hours PRN. By assessing Mrs A.'s pain, the nurse establishes that it regularly returns about every 3 hours. Based on this information, the nurse gives the pain medication on a regular 3-hourly regime. To ensure the safety and effectiveness of this regime, assessment and evaluation of Mrs A.'s pain and response continue.

> **KEY POINT**: Teach patient to request pain medication as soon as pain occurs or *before* it increases.

Patient Example

Mr S. is scheduled for total hip replacement. The nurse teaches Mr S. the 0–10 scale (0 = no pain, 10 = worst pain) pre-operatively so that he is familiar with the scale and can use it post-operatively to rate his pain. It is apparent that at a rating of 4, Mr S.'s pain begins to escalate quickly. He asks for pain medication at this rating and finds he is able to stay comfortable. The nurse regularly evaluates this plan with Mr S., thereby assuring continuous and effective pain control.

> **Benefits of a Preventive Approach with Analgesics**
> 1. Patient spends less time in pain.
>   *Result:* Can direct energy to restoring health, e.g. physiotherapy, immediate post-operative activities of turning, coughing, and deep breathing.
> 2. Doses of analgesic can be lower than if pain is allowed to increase or become severe.
> 3. Fewer side effects due to lower dose.
> 4. Decreased anxiety about return of pain, erases memory of pain and stops fearful anticipation of its return.
> 5. Decreased concern about obtaining relief when needed.
>   *Result:* Decrease in craving the drug for pain relief, prevents "clockwatching behaviour"
> 6. Overall increase in activities.

The box above summarizes the benefits of a preventive approach in the prescribing of analgesic medication.

2. Titrate to effect

Adjust and individualize the analgesic for each patient. The effect desired is pain relief with the fewest side effects. This involves tailoring analgesics by adjusting the following.

Dose

Patient Example

After a dose of medication, Mrs A. rates her pain at 8 on the 0–10 scale, and her respiration has remained stable between 18 and 20. The next time it is administered the narcotic dose is increased to obtain better pain control.

Route of administration

Patient Example

Mr B. is admitted to hospital because his pain suddenly increases at home and oral morphine did not relieve the pain below 9. For the past 2 days he has been unable to sleep because of the pain. The goal now is to get Mr B. comfortable quickly with an SC continuous infusion of narcotic while diagnostic studies are being done. Allow him to get some sleep without pain, then titrate back onto an appropriate equivalent oral narcotic and non-narcotic in preparation to discharge home.

Choice of drug

Patient Example

Mr F. states that pethidine 75mg IM helps his post-operative pain, but that the effect wears off in 2 hours. He also notices that he feels "jumpy" and that this same feeling resulted from the analgesic he received during his last surgery. Because of the short duration of analgesia felt by Mr F. and the possible cumulative effects of an active metabolite of pethidine in his system (see pp. 89–91), the pethidine was stopped. Using an equianalgesic chart, the doctor prescribed a dose of morphine more effective than pethidine, i.e. 15mg morphine IM, and a non-narcotic analgesic, paracetamol 1g, was added.

KEY POINT: The only safe and effective way to administer analgesics is to watch the individual's response to the drug. Use a pain-medication continuous assessment sheet to monitor these responses (see p. 39 for an example).

3. Patient-controlled analgesia (PCA)

The person who feels the pain is the person who must have, wherever possible, control of all measures to relieve it. It is essential to remember that pain can only be felt by the person who has it.

In its broadest sense, the key concept of PCA may be defined as the patient's self-administration of all forms of pain control by methods that consider safety, as well as the patient's ability and willingness to exercise control. The person with pain is not always able to understand or do much regarding pain control, but with guidance and safety precautions, the following aspects of pain control are determined by the patient as a result of his/her direct action, directions to others, or carefully monitored indications of need:

- Start or stop a form of pain relief.
- Increase or decrease the amount of pain relief.

Clinical implementation and patient teaching

Although the key concepts of a preventive approach, individualizing the medication and enabling patients to control their care, are used in virtually all health–illness situations, their application to pain control often sounds like a totally new idea. Unlike many other health-care problems, pain is subjective—it cannot be objectively measured, touched, or seen. Further, people have exaggerated fears about one of the major methods of controlling pain—narcotics. For these reasons it is often difficult to implement concepts for pain control that are commonly used elsewhere.

An analogy is sometimes helpful in explaining to the health-care team the wisdom of prevention of pain and individualizing pain relief, especially with narcotics. Controlling diabetes may be compared with controlling pain. Health professionals and most laymen are aware that diabetes may need to be controlled by daily doses of insulin. These doses are given preventively to avoid a return of the symptoms of the disease. The dosage of insulin is carefully titrated in accordance with the individual's response. Hence, it would be insulting to

approach health professionals about the care of the diabetic by reminding them that insulin should be given before the patient develops diabetic coma and that the same dose of insulin should not be given to every diabetic. Equally absurd is the reminder that we do not tell diabetics that no matter how high their blood sugar level is, they cannot receive any more insulin and they must handle this some other way.

What is done in the care of the person with diabetes is not very different from what is advocated in the care of the person with pain. We want to provide pain relief before pain returns and individualize the dosage. A reminder of the analogy of the diabetic is sometimes helpful when a preventive approach or titration of a drug fails to be implemented clinically. For example, when health professionals are tempted to put an arbitrary limit on the dosage or frequency of narcotic, the analogy with insulin can be used. Telling a patient who is in severe pain but alert and breathing well that he/she cannot have any more narcotic is just as senseless as placing a limit on the insulin dosage regardless of the blood sugar level.

Another example of applying the diabetic analogy is in relation to using a preventive approach with narcotics. If the patient is on doses of narcotic regularly, the nurse giving the change of shift report may tell you that the last dose of narcotic due 2 hours previously was not given because the patient was not in pain. This nurse might be reminded of the diabetic analogy. You may add that just as we do not wait for the diabetic to feel poorly before giving insulin, we try not to wait until the patient is in pain before giving the narcotic. If the reason for not giving the narcotic is that the patient was sleeping, you may add that if the prescription had been for insulin (or antibiotics or digoxin), 2 hours would not have elapsed before giving the dose. The patient would have been woken up because we have a better appreciation of preventing the return of symptoms and maintaining a blood level with other drugs than we do with narcotics.

Some of the most common misunderstandings about the key concepts of prevention and titration are related to the high doses of narcotic that may occur and the reasons for regular versus PRN dosing. These areas concern both the health-care team and the patient and family. They are explained more fully here, along with patient/family teaching tools (see Appendix).

Dosage of narcotic—is there a limit?

Question: The authors are frequently asked "What is the highest dose of narcotic that I can give?"

Answer: There is no answer to that question in terms of milligrams, because there is no set optimal or maximal dosage of narcotic (Levy, 1985). The dosage that should be used is the one that controls the pain to the satisfaction of the patient with minimal side effects. For some patients this may be 10mg morphine orally 4-hourly, for others it may be 480mg/hr IV morphine (Portenoy et al, 1986).

The fear behind this question on dose really concerns safety, i.e. "What is the highest dose of narcotic that I can *safely* give?" Again, because each patient reacts to medication differently, there is no maximal number of milligrams that will apply to every individual. The following points can, however, facilitate the safe administration of narcotics.

Use a pain continuous assessment sheet (p. 38) to monitor the patient's responses, specifically pain rating and side effects, e.g. respiratory rate. Nurses readily titrate down when a narcotic dosage is too high for the individual patient. All we are suggesting is that titration be in the upward direction when analgesia is inadequate, and it is safe for the individual. For example, if you give morphine 10mg IM and the patient has complete pain relief, becomes sedated, and the respiration rate drops from 12 to 6, you would no doubt *lower* the next dose of morphine. Conversely, if you give that same dose of morphine 10mg IM and the patient has minimal relief, is fully alert, and maintains the previous respiratory rate of 14, you should *increase* the next dose.

Specific aspects of "titrate to effect" are explained in the box on the right and a tool for patient/family teaching is provided in the appendix.

Regular dosing vs. PRN (as required)

Pain that continuously recurs requires analgesics on a regular basis (see p. 55). The purpose is to stay on top of the pain, keeping the patient as comfortable as possible all of the time and preventing the pain from escalating out of control. A successful preventive approach breaks the cycle of pain and anxiety and eases the fearful anticipation of pain. Figs. 4.1 and 4.2 illustrate the concept of a continuous level of analgesia vs. the peaks and troughs that can occur with PRN dosing.

Titrate to effect: dose and interval

What is it? Titrating the analgesic dose and interval means finding the lowest dose and longest interval of a drug that relieves pain to the patient's satisfaction with minimal side effects.

How do you do it? Use a flow sheet and look at the following patient responses, in the following order:

- First, respiratory function, e.g. rate.
- Second, pain rating.
- Third, based on the above, determine what should be done with the number of milligrams of analgesic the patient is receiving. *The last thing you look at are the milligrams being given; look at effect first.*

Example of titrating up: If the patient is breathing well, e.g. 12/minute, with a pain rating of 8 on a 0–10 scale, the milligrams of analgesic should be increased probably by 50% to 100% (see p. 98 for discussion of percentages).

Example of titrating down due to problems with respiratory function: If the patient's respiratory rate has dropped from 12 to 6/minute following narcotic administration, the milligrams of analgesic should be decreased, probably by 50%, and possibly even discontinued until the respiratory rate improves.

Example of titrating down due to excessive pain relief or side effects: If the patient's respiratory rate is 14/minute, he/she complains of sedation, i.e. he/she cannot continue a conversation without falling asleep, and he/she rates his pain at 0–1 on 0–10 scale, reduce the milligrams of analgesic, e.g. by 20%.

KEY POINT: (1) Patients are usually not aware that they must ask for pain medication. If PRN dosing is used, initiate teaching about this early in the course of treatment, e.g. pre-operatively. (2) When narcotics are withheld from people who need them for pain relief, the result is clock-watching behaviour (see p. 77 for further discussion).

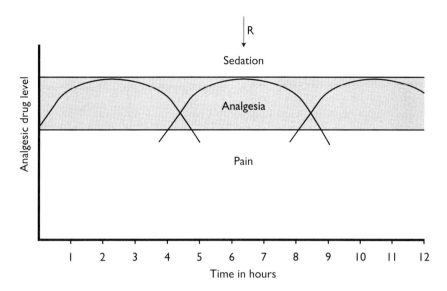

Fig. 4.1 Illustration of the relatively smooth analgesic level that can be obtained by individualizing the dose and using regular administration of analgesic IM or SC. Analgesics are administered before the pain returns; ideally no noticeable peaks and troughs occur. That is, the drug level does not rise above what is required for analgesia, which would cause side effects such as sedation and respiratory depression; and the drug level does not fall below what is required for analgesia, which would cause increasing pain.

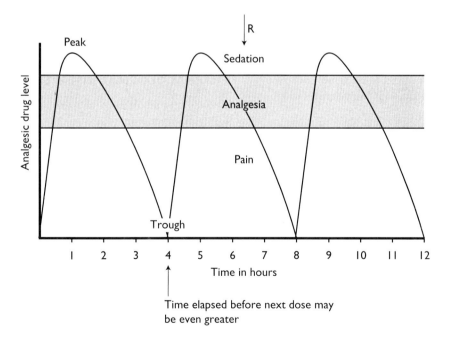

Fig. 4.2 Illustration of the peaks and troughs that often occur when analgesia by the oral, IM, or SC route is given in the traditional PRN manner that requires the patient to wait for the return of pain before requesting or obtaining the next dose of analgesic.

Taking medication on an "as needed" or PRN regime may be appropriate in instances when the pain is incidental, intermittent, or unpredictable. However, even in this instance, education of patient and family is vital to effective analgesia. The individual must know to take or ask for the medication as soon as the pain begins and before the pain becomes severe. PRN medication may be used to supplement regular analgesic doses when a particular activity is known to cause pain. The following two examples illustrate this concept.

Patient Examples

1. During her hospitalization, Mrs J. begins radiotherapy treatments. Although her pain is well controlled on oral morphine 30mg 4-hourly, movement associated with the treatment increases her pain to 8 on a 0–10 scale (0 = no pain, 10 = worst pain). Morphine 15mg IV PRN before radiation therapy treatment helped prevent pain on movement from increasing above 4. The IV route was chosen for PRN medication because treatment time changed each day and something was needed that started to work immediately.
2. Mobilization increases Mr T.'s pain to 6 on the 0–10 scale. The district nurse encouraged his wife to give him an extra dose of co-dydramol about 1 hour before his daily walk. With further assessment, the additional co-dydramol dose was stopped because of dizziness during walking. Mr T. had fewer side effects and the pain was well controlled by taking only plain paracetamol 500mg before his walk.

Patient Example

Analgesics continue to be prescribed "PRN for pain" on a surgical unit despite the nurses' attempt to educate doctors to change to regular dosing for the first 48 hours post-operatively. Doctors' prescriptions for an analgesic every 3 hours/PRN were *implemented* in the nursing-care plan as regular doses after assessment of each individual's response to the first dose.

To assure effective analgesia, the nurses used a pain medication flow sheet, consistent assessment, and concise documentation to support their administering PRN medication on a regular basis. For example, if pain relief was adequate but lasted no longer than 3 hours, the following was written in the nursing care plan:

Give analgesic regularly 3-hourly to prevent severe pain for the next 24 hours: 9 am–12 n-3 pm-6 pm-12 mn-3am-6am. Re-evaluate patient's pain rating at 9 am.

Patient teaching regarding PCA

Not all patients are candidates for PCA, especially via IV, SC, or spinal routes. Some patients are not able to understand instructions, and others do not feel confident handling their own analgesia or the technical aspects of the pump. However, our belief is that patients should be given as much information as they can understand about the analgesic delivery system, even when it is not in their direct control.

Certainly, when patients are given direct control, e.g. to initiate boluses, they should be told how often they can administer the bolus, whether they will receive a dose each time they make an attempt, what the drug is, and the dose. (Some pumps deliver a dose in proportion to the amount of time that has elapsed if the full lockout interval has not elapsed.) Bell tones or other noises that occur when a bolus is initiated should never be used to fool patients into thinking they have received a dose when they have not.

In addition, explain the concept of prevention to patients and instruct them to keep their pain under control by administering additional medication as soon as pain begins to return or increase or prior to a painful event, e.g. pain on mobilization. Leave instructions for whom to notify if the medication seems excessive or if pain relief is not satisfactory.

PHARMACOLOGICAL INTERVENTIONS

This chapter discusses three main types of pharmacological interventions for pain relief: (1) non-narcotic analgesics or non-steroidal anti-inflammatory drugs (NSAIDs), (2) narcotic analgesics or opioids, and (3) adjuvant analgesics. A summary of these three analgesic groups can be found in the box above. Certainly not all of these are appropriate for all patients with pain, and for each drug there are specific contra-indications. However, general suggestions for situations or patients with painful problems most likely to benefit from various pharmacological approaches along with possible problems and limitations are listed at the beginning of the discussion of each of the three groups. These suggestions are based on the definitions and classifications of pain appearing in Chapter 2 on assessment.

Non-narcotic analgesics (NSAIDs)

Indications for non-narcotics

Examples of situations in which non-narcotics, especially NSAIDs, may help relieve pain are:

- Highly inflammatory conditions such as rheumatoid arthritis.
- Mild to moderate acute or chronic pain of peripheral origin, e.g. low back pain caused by muscle strain; headache.
- As co-analgesic providing a baseline of non-narcotic analgesia in severe acute or chronic pain requiring narcotics.
- Conditions associated with excessive prostaglandin at the site of injury or pain, e.g. dysmenorrhea, certain malignant tumours, certain cancer therapies, bone metastasis, and postoperative pain.
- Desire by the patient to avoid drugs that affect thinking or emotions ("mind-altering" drugs) or the desire to be fully alert.

Disadvantages of non-narcotics

Examples of possible disadvantages or limitations of some non-narcotic analgesics are:

- Undesirable side effects in certain patients (e.g. allergic response, increased bleeding time, fluid retention, tinnitus, GI upset) may occur, necessitating changing administration, dosage, or drug.
- Analgesic ceiling: beyond a certain dosage, increased analgesia will not occur.
- Impossibility of predicting which non-narcotic (especially those with a strong anti-inflammatory effect) the individual patient will respond best to or tolerate. Matching patient to drug is done by trial and error.
- In most instances, if non-narcotics are used alone, they relieve only mild to moderate pain, not severe pain.
- Daily use for months or longer of high doses or combinations of non-narcotics could lead to organ damage.
- Although recommended regimes are available, some patients will require careful titration to arrive at a safe and effective dosage.
- Some analgesia will usually occur within a few hours, but the full benefit may not be realized until days or weeks of regular administration.

- Effectiveness is under-rated. Health-care team members tend not to be educated about uses of non-narcotics, especially NSAIDs, for conditions other than arthritis.

Mechanisms underlying effects of NSAIDs

NSAIDs* are non-narcotics that usually have three effects:

1. Anti-inflammatory.
2. Analgesic.
3. Anti-pyretic.

However, the NSAIDs differ in the degree to which they produce these effects. For example, paracetamol is effective as an analgesic for mild to moderate pain and as an anti-pyretic but has little anti-inflammatory effect. On the other hand, diflunisal has anti-inflammatory and analgesic effects but minimal anti-pyretic effects.

Reasons for the important differences between these drugs are not clear but may be due in part to variation in the sensitivity of enzymes in the different tissues and the fact that different drugs have different modes of inhibiting the inflammatory process. Most likely the NSAIDs reduce inflammation and pain by inhibiting the synthesis of prostaglandins. The significance of this is obvious when one considers the following discoveries about prostaglandins:

- They have been detected in almost every body tissue and fluid.
- They are formed as a result of the action of enzymes on substances released from damaged cells.
- There are numerous prostaglandins, and they have diverse effects.
- Some are important contributors to the signs and symptoms of inflammation, e.g. swelling and redness.
- Some sensitize the afferent nerve endings to bradykinin (a pain substance) and other effects of chemical or mechanical stimuli, i.e. they amplify the system for producing pain.
- Even low concentrations can cause hyperalgesia, a state in which pain is caused by stimulation (e.g. touch) that is normally painless.

*Except where noted otherwise, the information on NSAIDs is obtained from Chapters 28 and 29 of Goodman and Gilman's *The Pharmacological Basis of Therapeutics*, ed 7, Macmillan Publishing Co. New York, 1985,

Most NSAIDs probably prevent the synthesis of prostaglandins from arachidonic acid by inhibiting the cyclo-oxygenase enzyme that is necessary for the formation of the cyclic endoperoxides (Fig. 4.3). When cyclo-oxygenase is inhibited, so is the synthesis of all products beyond this step in the pathway of inflammation. This accounts for some of the side effects of NSAIDs. The synthesis of thromboxane, an important factor in platelet aggregation, is blocked by many NSAIDs, and this leads to increased bleeding time.

Not all NSAIDs inhibit platelet aggregation, however. The non-acetylated salicylates apparently have little effect on platelet aggregation. For this reason and others, it is thought that they inhibit the synthesis of prostaglandin somewhere after the production of the endoperoxides but prior to the formation of the prostaglandins involved in pain. Blockage of prostaglandin formation and other possible modes of action of NSAIDs in inhibiting inflammation, relieving pain, and producing side effects are shown in Fig. 4.3.

The exact mode of action for paracetamol, which has weak anti-inflammatory action, is not clear. Except for paracetamol, NSAIDs probably should not be combined due to increased risk of side effects, especially gastric and renal damage.

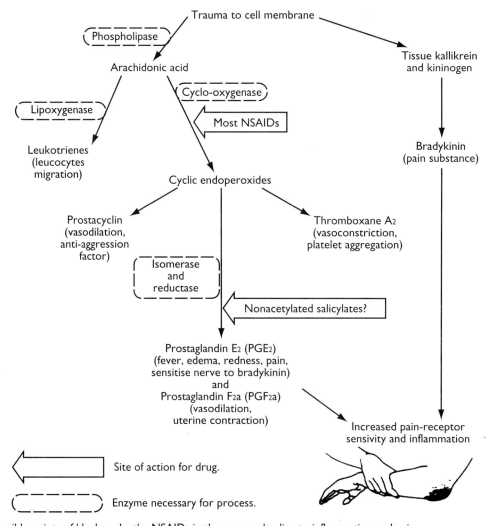

Fig. 4.3 Possible points of blockage by the NSAIDs in the process leading to inflammation and pain.

Selection of an NSAID for analgesia

Selecting an NSAID for use as an analgesic is certainly a simpler matter than selecting one for the long-term treatment of a highly inflammatory condition such as rheumatoid arthritis. Yet, using NSAIDs simply as analgesics, not necessarily for their anti-inflammatory effects, is a relatively new idea. Aspirin and paracetamol have been used as simple analgesics for many years but only recently have the other NSAIDs been studied as analgesics. Thus existing guidelines for selecting NSAIDs for the individual patient are primarily based on the need for an anti-inflammatory effect and the need for a drug that would be tolerated over a long period. Such guidelines are not always relevant to the selection of a NSAID for analgesia alone.

Further, although the mechanism for analgesia may be separate from the anti-inflammatory mechanism, these two effects may very well overlap when a drug is given to the individual patient. The analgesic effect usually occurs within 2 hours of the initial recommended dose, but the maximal anti-inflammatory effect may not occur for a week or longer. When the anti-inflammatory effect does occur, however, it may very well provide increased analgesia.

Thus the question of how much the anti-inflammatory effect of the drug contributes to the analgesic effect complicates the issue. Add to this the fact that the effectiveness of NSAIDs in relieving pain depends on the type of pain, and the matter becomes fairly complex.

It has been said that no NSAIDs are superior to aspirin, and this may well be true if the patient can tolerate high enough doses of aspirin. One distinct advantage that some other NSAIDs have over aspirin is simply that they are better tolerated in that they produce fewer or less intense side effects; some NSAIDs are easier for the patient to take.

An overview of NSAIDs used as analgesics is presented in Table 4.2. Currently, numerous publications of research and clinical experience with the use of NSAIDs have resulted in vast and varied claims about the drugs as analgesics as well as anti-inflammatory agents. In an attempt to provide as accurate and as simple a guide as possible, one basic reference was used—the well-respected Goodman and Gilman's *The Pharmacological Basis of Therapeutics,* ed 8,

Macmillan Publishing Co. New York, 1990. Although it is tempting to add some recent findings, we decided to limit the table to information that seems to have an acceptable level of proof rather than risk premature inclusion of new information. Thus although the table may lack information that will eventually prove to be useful, the information that is currently in the table is likely to stand the test of time. Refer to the annotated references for additional, current information on the use of NSAIDs.

Doses are omitted from Table 4.2 because recommendations for doses change fairly often. Usually new recommendations are for higher doses, but a current reference should be used to determine a dose. Another point to bear in mind is that the recommended dose for analgesia is often lower than that recommended for an anti-inflammatory effect.

Certain NSAIDs are omitted from Table 4.2 because current data indicate that they *would not be good initial choices* of analgesics, although they may be good choices for their anti-inflammatory effect or as analgesics if other drugs are ineffective or intolerable. Those omitted, along with the reasons, are listed below:

- The pyrazolone derivatives, phenylbutazone and oxyphenbutazone are only available for the treatment of severe ankylosing spondylitis under hospital supervision, because of their severe toxic effects, e.g. aplastic anaemia.
- The pyrole acetic acid derivative, tolmetin, has been reported to cause severe anaphylactoid reactions in patients who are not sensitive to aspirin and other similar drugs.
- The fenamates, or anthranilic acid derivatives, e.g. mefenamic acid, are analgesic but cause side effects frequently, particularly severe diarrhoea, and are felt to have no advantages over other NSAIDs.

Based on the above reasoning, one may question the inclusion of indomethacin in Table 4.2. However, indomethacin is often used as a standard of comparison, in addition to aspirin. In addition, studies of its use rectally in the immediate postoperative period are very promising. Other NSAIDs given rectally may very well be as effective, but with the exception of diclofenac, there is not really sufficient data available to support their use.

TABLE 4-2 SELECTED NSAIDS USED FOR ANALGESIA*

Class/Medication Acetylated Salicylates	Formulations and Frequency†	Comments
Aspirin	Tablets, enteric-coated tablets, soluble/dispersible, rectal suppository; every 4–6hr initially	Non prescription. Tends to be the standard for comparison and evaluation of other NSAIDs. Platelets are especially susceptible to its acetylating action and so a single dose as low as 40mg per day of aspirin will inhibit platelet cyclo-oxygenase for the life of the platelet (8–11 days); a single dose of 600mg aspirin approximately doubles the mean bleeding time of normal persons for 4–7 days.
Benorylate (aspirin–paracetemol ester: 2g benorylate equivalent to approx. 1.15g aspirin and 970mg paracetamol)	Tablets, granules, sugar-free suspension:every 12hr	Concurrent use of other paracetomol or aspirin containing analgesics should be avoided. Broken down only after absorption from gastro-intestinal tract, gastric tolerance slightly better than with aspirin.
Nonacetylated Salicylates Diflunisal (As a group they are much better tolerated than aspirin and have little, if any, effect on platelet aggregation and bleeding time.)	Tablets; every 8–12hr	Prescription. Minimal antipyretic effect.
Para-Aminophenol Derivatives (e.g. paracetamol).	Capsules, tablets, liquids, rectal suppository; every 4 hr	Non prescription. Effective analgesic and antipyretic but weak anti-inflammatory. Well tolerated; lacks many of the side effects of aspirin, such as no gastric irritation and no effect on bleeding time. May be given with other NSAIDs. Total daily dose should not exceed 4000mg.
Propionic Acid Derivatives (As a group they are usually better tolerated than aspirin or indomethacin; they have similar, although less intense, unwanted side effects.)		
fenoprofen	Capsules, tablets; every 4-8hr.	Prescription.
ibuprofen	Tablets; every 4-8hr.	Nonprescription in doses of 200mg/tablet; prescription in doses over 200mg/tablet. More effective than aspirin for relief of dysmenorrhea.

TABLE 4-2 SELECTED NSAIDS USED FOR ANALGESIA* CONT'D

Class/Medication	Formulations and Frequency†	Comments
ketoprofen	Capsules; every 6–8hr; modified release 12-hourly. Injection. (Deep IM) 4-hourly for maximum of 3 days.	Prescription.
naproxen	Tablets, liquid; every 6–12hr.; Suppositories.	Prescription. More effective than aspirin for relief of dysmenorrhea. Better tolerated than ibuprofen, fenoprofen, and indomethacin. Similar to diclofenac.
naproxen sodium	Tablets; every 6–8hr.	Prescription. Similar to naproxen, but more rapid onset of analgesia.
Indole Acetic Acid Derivatives		
indomethacin	Capsules, sustained release, rectal suppositories; every 8–12hr. (Available IV for treatment of patent ductus arteriosus in neonates.)	Prescription. Use as analgesic probably should be restricted to a few days, if possible, e.g. postoperative pain (use cautiously if the patient is at risk for postoperative bleeding). High risk of side effects is associated with chronic administration, i.e. weeks. For unknown reasons, doses given at night are better tolerated. A useful way to employ the drug and avoid side effects is to give a large dose at night and use a better tolerated analgesic during the day. Always give with, or after, food.
sulindac	Tablets; every 12hr.	Prescription. Lower incidence of GI toxicity than indomethacin. Relative lack of effect on kidneys. Little or no placental transfer.
Oxicams		
piroxicam	Capsules; every 24hr, but may be given twice a day.	Prescription. Long acting, e.g. 24hr. Better tolerated than aspirin or indomethacin. Maximal Anti-inflammatory effect takes 2 weeks or longer.
diclofenac	Tablets, dispersible tablets, sustained release tablets, every 6–8hrs., maximum dosage 150mg/day. Suppositories, injection (IM use only).	Prescription. Injection is useful in renal colic (now considered drug of choice over pethidine) but must be given by deep intragluteal injection and for a maximum of 2 days. Also useful postoperatively with or without opioids.

Drug actions: All of the above are not only analgesic but also anti-inflammatory and antipyretic, unless noted otherwise.
†If this is duplicated, add to this column the correct recommended doses and date the entry.

General guide: The individual's response to these drugs is unpredictable. If a drug is ineffective or has intolerable side effects, it is often logical to try another. The drugs are grouped according to chemical categories to emphasize the point that they may share similar therapeutic actions and side effects but may be chemically unrelated. Significant differences exist even within a chemical category. Thus one should expect a large variation in response of individuals to the same drug and different drugs regarding pain relief and side effects.

Most of the data in this table are obtained from:
Flower, RJ, Moncada, S, and Vane, JR: Drug therapy of Inflammation, pp 674–715. In Gilman, AG, et al, eds: Goodman and Gilman's *The Pharmacological Basis of Therapeutics*, ed 7, Macmillan Publishing Co. New York, 1985.
Moncada, S, Flower, RJ, and Vane, JR: Prostaglandins, prostacyclin, thromboxane A_2 and leukotrienes, pp.660–673. In Gilman, AG, et al, eds: Goodman and Gilman's *The Pharmacological Basis of Therapeutics*, ed 7, Macmillan Publishing Co. New York, 1985.

Reasbeck, PG, Rice, ML, and Reasbeck, JC: Double-blind controlled trial of indomethacin as an adjunct to narcotic analgesia after major abdominal surgery, *Lancet* **2**:115–118, July 1982.

Adverse side effects

Comments on the side effects of NSAIDs are included in Table 4.2 and are discussed in the patient/family teaching point for home use of non-narcotic analgesics (Appendix 1).

Because the side effects of NSAIDs include fluid retention, gastric ulceration, bleeding, nephritis, and decreased growth of new bone (Amadio and Cummings, 1986; Ritter and Gioe, 1982), these drugs should be used with extreme caution in patients with ulcers, bleeding problems, low platelet count, oedema, high blood pressure, congestive heart failure, poor renal function, or joint replacements requiring generation of new bone. The presence of aspirin sensitivity or asthma in a patient also dictates caution, as the sensitivity may also apply to NSAIDs.

Promising uses of NSAIDs

Many times in clinical practice, NSAIDs are overlooked and underestimated as an effective analgesic choice. The following is an overview of selected painful conditions shown to be responsive to NSAIDs. With this information and specific references, nurses can be instrumental in suggesting these analgesics for the appropriate situation.

1. *Postoperative pain*. Research has shown that NSAIDs such as aspirin and ibuprofen are effective in the relief of pain following episiotomy, herniorrhaphy, orthopaedic surgery, and tooth extraction (Dionne and Cooper, 1978; Slavic-Svircev et al, 1984).

KEY POINT: A simple overall guideline to using NSAIDs as analgesics:

Paracetamol is the easiest to take; it has fewer side effects than any analgesic, but may be a less effective analgesic for more than mild pain.

Aspirin is a good analgesic for mild to moderate pain but is one of the most difficult to take; it has many side effects that may be intense enough to limit its use in some individuals.

Some of the other NSAIDs are likely to be better analgesics than paracetamol and at least equal to aspirin in analgesic ability, but they are usually easier to take than aspirin, i.e. have fewer or less intense side effects.

In post-orthopaedic surgical patients, ibuprofen 400mg was more effective, longer acting, and caused greater mood improvement than codeine 30mg plus paracetamol (Heidrich et al, 1985).

In post-thoracic surgery patients, indomethacin rectal suppository 100mg every 8 hours provided analgesia allowing patients to move and effectively perform deep breathing and coughing exercises. Many patients required no additional pain medication (Tejada, 1986). Another study of patients after major abdominal surgery who received indomethacin rectal suppository 100mg every 8 hours had less pain on each of the first 4 postoperative days than those who received intramuscular (IM) morphine (Reasbeck et al, 1982).

Diclofenac has been shown to be effective in relief of post-operative pain both alone and in combination with opioids.

2. *Cancer pain*. Kantor (1984) estimates that of all patients with cancer, probably about 50% have pain that could be controlled with NSAIDs alone, i.e. without the addition of a narcotic. NSAIDs can be particularly effective for pain from bone tumours and bone metastases. In addition to inhibition of prostaglandins in bone tumours, NSAIDs may actually inhibit the progress of bone tumours (Ventafridda et al, 1980). Many people with metastatic cancer may have hypercalcaemia, which increases pain. The NSAIDs can reduce serum calcium levels and thereby decrease pain (Kantor, 1984).

If cancer pain progresses, combining a narcotic with an NSAID can produce significant analgesia (Beaver, 1984b).

Patient Example (Hill, 1986)

Forty-seven-year-old man with metastatic adenocarcinoma with extreme pain from subcutaneous lesions and oedematous right leg. The following analgesics were tried with little success until a narcotic plus non-narcotic combination was used:

- Oral pethidine 50mg every 4 hours. Result: no relief.
- Oral pethidine 100–150mg every 4 hours. Result: minimal relief.
- Morphine 30mg orally every 4 hours plus diazepam 10mg orally every 6 hours. Result: side effects unacceptable to patient, i.e. a "wiped-out" feeling with confusion and nightmares.
- Oral pethidine 150mg every 4 hours. Result: no relief.

- Morphine 90mg orally every 4 hours. Result: controlled leg pain, not effective for subcutaneous lesions.
- Diflunisal 500mg b.d. plus morphine 90mg orally every 4 hours. Result: good pain control.

3. *Other conditions.* Many back disorders have no clearly or easily determined aetiology but are thought to be associated with greater or lesser degrees of inflammation (Kantor, 1982). Clinicians working with patients who have low back pain have noted that NSAIDs are sometimes effective in relieving the pain (Brena, 1983).

Various research has shown that NSAIDs may be effective in relieving the pain of, or as prophylaxis for, migraine, but not all patients respond well (Bernstein, 1982). This may reflect differences in types of migraine headaches, as well as differences in patients. Varied responses of migraines to NSAIDs may be due to insufficient doses prescribed because of fear of side effects. For example, a migraine patient may require up to 150mg of indomethacin daily.

Indomethacin in particular has been studied. It is thought to be 50–60 times more potent than aspirin in the inhibition of prostacyclin, a prostaglandin that causes cerebral vasodilation and plays a major role in inducing the pain of migraines. People with migraines seem to synthesize excessive amounts of prostacyclin. NSAIDs may also block the prostaglandin-mediated platelet aggregation and serotonin release associated with migraine. In addition to indomethacin, other NSAIDs such as mefenamic acid and naproxen have been effective (Bernstein, 1982). NSAIDs also seem particularly effective in treating menstrual-related migraines.

Painful menstrual cramps afflict many women, resulting in some being unable to function for a day or more once a month. For many women, NSAIDs provide very effective relief and replace the need for narcotics for pain control (Amadio and Cummings, 1986; Dingfelder, 1981; Wenzloff and Shrimp, 1984). Excessive concentrations of prostaglandins in the endometrium, menstrual fluid, and peripheral circulation is probably what leads to painful cramps, and prostaglandins can be decreased by NSAIDs (Anderson et al, 1978; Marx, 1979). Pre-treatment before the onset of menstrual flow is not necessary (Dawood, 1981).

Which NSAID to use

Unfortunately there is no absolute answer to this frequently asked question. It is impossible to predict which patient with a specific pain problem will respond favourably to NSAIDs and which patient will respond best to which NSAID. Factors considered in the selection of an NSAID are listed in Table 4.3.

Factor	Consideration
1. Individual patient problem a. History of ulcer disease	1. a. Consider propionic acid derivatives, non-acetylated salicylates or paracetamol. Avoid indomethacin, aspirin.
b. Poor renal function	b. Consider renal diflunisal NSAID, e.g. Dolobid, Clinoril.
c. Bleeding problems	c. Avoid pyrazolone derivatives. Consider non-acetylated salicylates or paracetamol.
2. Prior experience	2. Prior use of NSAID and resulting problems or success can help with present selection.
3. Ease of dosing and route	3. Liquid form for patients with trouble swallowing; e.g. Trilisate suppository form, e.g. indomethacin, diclofenac, naproxen, paracetamol; IV e.g. Indomethacin. Consider those which can be taken one or two times daily e.g. piroxicam, diflunisal, naproxen.
4. Cost	4. There is considerable variation in price between pharmacies and drugs. When this is an important factor, it may lead to the selection of one drug over another.

Table 4.3 Common Consideration in Selection of NSAIDs as Analgesics.

Guidelines for effective use of non-narcotics (NSAIDs)

To obtain the maximal benefit from non-narcotics, two general guidelines are:

1. If pain stays in the mild to moderate range of intensity, try a non-narcotic first rather than a narcotic. Occasional mild to moderate pain is usually treated with single doses of OTC products such as two aspirin or 1g paracetamol. If mild to moderate pain is continuous, e.g. 24 hours a day, day after day, it makes sense to give non-narcotics on a regular basis.
2. Even when pain relief requires narcotics because it is too severe to be relieved by non-narcotics, continue non-narcotics if possible. It is this guideline that is most commonly overlooked (implementation of this is discussed below).

Non-narcotics used alone

One of the main reasons for emphasizing these guidelines is that non-narcotics are more effective analgesics than most laymen and health-care professionals realize. For example, how effective do you think a dose of 600mg of aspirin or 1g paracetamol is compared with oral narcotics? A list of oral doses of narcotics that relieve no more pain than 650mg of aspirin or paracetamol are in the equianalgesic list in Table 4.4. Although there are individual differences in responses to medications, this table shows that in most people the following doses relieve only as much pain as 600mg aspirin or 1g paracetamol—or, conversely, 600mg aspirin or 1g paracetamol relieve as much pain as the following:

• codeine 32mg, orally.
• pethidine 50mg, orally.

Based on these findings it is evident that we underestimate the effectiveness of ordinary aspirin and paracetamol and overestimate that of low doses of oral narcotics. Obviously, we can relieve more pain with plain aspirin and paracetamol than most people realize.

Further, from a practical standpoint, non-narcotics are generally easier to obtain than narcotics. Doctors more readily prescribe non-narcotics than narcotics, providing the specific non-narcotic is not contra-indicated, and some non-narcotics require no prescription.

Analgesic	Oral Dosage (mg)
Non-narcotic Analgesics	
paracetamol	500–1000mg
aspirin	300–600mg
Narcotic Analgesics	
codeine	30mg
pethidine	50mg
pentazocine	30mg (available in 25mg tablets)
dextro-propoxyphene napsylate	100mg

*The equianalgesic doses in this chart are based primarily on recommendations of the Analgesic Study: Section, Sloan-Kettering Institute for Cancer Research, New York, based on double-blind analgesic research (Houde, 1979).

Table references:

Houde, RW: Systemic analgesics and related drugs: narcotic analgesics. In Bonica, JJ, and Vetafridda, V, eds: *Advances in Pain Research and Therapy*, vol 2, pp. 236–273, New York, 1979 Raven Press (see pp 84–85 for above list plus IM-Oral list.)

Moertel, CG: Relief of pain with oral medications, *Aust NZ J Med* (suppl 1) 6:1–8, 1976 (This double-blind study of ambulatory cancer patients suggests that the above list may be a conservative estimate of the potency of nonnarcotics, e.g. Moertel found it may take more than 65mg of codeine oral to equal 600mg aspirin. He also found that 10mg morphine oral was not as effective as 650mg aspirin.)

Rogers, AG, Pharmacology of analgesics, *J Neurosurg Nurs* 10:180–184, Dec 1978.

■ May be duplicated for use in clinical practice. From McCaffery, M; Beebe, A; and Latham , J (ed.): *Pain: Clinical Manual for Nursing Practice*, London, 1994, Mosby, an imprint of Times Mirror International Publishers Ltd.

Table 4.4 Equianalgesic Chart: Approximate Equivalent Doses of Oral Analgesics for Mild to Moderate Pain*

In the home-care setting, the nurse may teach the patient and family how to effectively and safely use OTC non-narcotics to enhance pain relief. Most combination products rely on aspirin or paracetamol or a combination of the two for pain relief. Since combination products are often more expensive than "straight" products, e.g. plain aspirin, the nurse may be able to help the patient who takes combination OTC analgesics analyse the ingredients and spend less money but obtain the same relief by using the less expensive "straight" products. For example, a substitute for the ingredients of two Anadin is simply two reasonable, plain aspirin containing 300mg each (any generic brand) plus a cup of tea or coffee (if the caffeine is actually desirable).

> **KEY POINT:** Pain-relieving effects of non-narcotic analgesics are under-estimated and under-used.

Regarding all NSAIDs, the degree of pain relief is variable, with some individuals with seemingly similar pathology being more responsive than others. NSAIDs in the same chemical class (Table 4.2) may affect individual patients differently. Several explanations have been suggested (Kantor, 1982):

1. There are probably differences in the way individuals absorb and metabolise these drugs.
2. There may be genetic differences in inflammatory responses of individuals.
3. Certain inflammatory pathways may be used preferentially over others at various stages of a disease process.

Although there is no research to verify this, some pain specialists suggest that when there is little analgesic response to one NSAID, it may be more helpful to *switch to another in a different chemical class* (Table 4.2) as opposed to selecting another from the same chemical class (Amadio and Cummings, 1986; Portenoy, 1987b). Suggested guidelines for effective use of non-narcotics are shown in Table 4.5.

Guideline	Comments
1. Weigh risk vs. benefits in selection.	1. e.g. aspirin; risk of GI upset but it is least expensive in this group. Paracetamol less anti-inflammatory effect but generally fewer side effects.
2. Start with a low dose to determine patient's reaction, e.g. side effects. Increase gradually to a dose that relieves pain, not exceeding maximal daily dose.	2. May need to increase to 1–2 times the starting dose. Ineffective analgesia may be due to inadequate doses.
3. If maximal anti-inflammatory effect is desired in addition to analgesia, allow adequate trial before discontinuing or switching.	3. An effective dose should provide pain relief within 2 hours. Maximal anti-inflammatory effect occurs later as drug accumulates. With regular doses for 1 week or longer, pain relief may increase.
4. If one drug becomes ineffective, but the pain is about the same, try a drug from a different chemical class (See Table 4.2 on NSAIDs).	4. The inflammatory process may have changed. A different drug may attack this process in another way.
5. If they do not relieve pain when used alone, combine with oral, SC, IM or IV narcotics for added analgesic effect.	5. Rationale: non-narcotic analgesics stop pain at the peripheral nervous system (PNS) level, and narcotics stop pain at CNS level. Combination of PNS plus CNS attack will provide added analgesic effect.

Table 4.5 Guidelines for Effective Use of Non-narcotic Analgesics

Non-narcotics in combination with narcotics

When pain cannot be relieved by NSAIDs alone, combine them with oral, IM, or IV narcotics. The rationale is:

- Non-narcotics are more effective than most people realize.
- Non-narcotic plus narcotic equals peripheral nervous system plus CNS effects.
- This combination produces an additive effect and reduces the narcotic dose needed, thereby decreasing narcotic side effects (Beaver, 1981).

Approaches to combining narcotics plus non-narcotics are:

1. PO narcotics plus non-narcotics.
   a. If the pain is continuous, consider regular doses of non-narcotic along with the narcotic, e.g. morphine 35mg orally 4-hourly regularly and Ibuprofen 400mg 4-hourly regularly.
   b. Some oral narcotics are already formulated with non-narcotics, but the non-narcotic dose is inadequate. Use the optimal therapeutic dose for effective analgesia. Refer to Table 4.6 to identify the amount and type of non-narcotic compounded with the narcotic in some commonly prescribed oral analgesics. For example:
      - Aspav tablets (papaveretum 10mg and aspirin 500mg), 1–2 tablets dissolved in water 4–6 hourly.
      - If several doses of this combination are given, be careful not to exceed the recommended total daily dose of aspirin.
2. IM, SC, IV narcotics plus rectal/IM non-narcotic.
   If the patient is receiving IM/IV or SC narcotics, it may be appropriate to add a non-narcotic (e.g. NSAID) to improve analgesia. Although several injectable NSAIDs are available, they have a relatively narrow range of indications, mainly based around acute exacerbations of inflammatory conditions. It may be worthwhile considering the use of a NSAID suppository, e.g. diclofenac 100mg or indomethacin 100mg, which only need to be given once a day.

If you are suggesting a non-narcotic plus narcotic combination to the doctor and other health-care team members, the following points and references will be helpful:

1. Many prescription analgesics already combine narcotic plus non-narcotic, e.g. co-codamol. Table 4.6 lists these common combinations.
2. Combining an *optimal* therapeutic dose of aspirin or paracetamol with a narcotic produces an additive analgesic effect (Beaver, 1981).
3. Research on cancer patients clearly indicates the benefit of combining narcotic and non-narcotic analgesics.
   - A clinical research study using double-blind technique with people with cancer pain found that giving 600mg of aspirin along with morphine 10mg IM provided significantly greater pain relief than morphine alone (Houde et al, 1960).
   - 400mg ibuprofen four times per day in addition to the cancer patient's prescribed oral narcotic resulted in greater analgesia than the narcotic plus placebo combination and no increase in side effects (Weingart et al, 1985).

Patient Example

On the evening following surgical removal of rectal polyps, Ms P., 74 years old, says her pain is poorly relieved with injections and she feels very drowsy. Her analgesic is nalbuphine 15mg IM. One hour after the injection, her pain is reduced from 7 to 4 on a scale of 0–10, and she is arousable and slightly confused, with respirations at 14 per minute.

Since increasing the nalbuphine would probably increase the sedation, a non-narcotic is added. Because of a history of ulcerative disease, paracetamol is chosen. PRN prescriptions are implemented regularly to prevent the return of pain. Attacking her pain centrally with the narcotic, nalbuphine 15mg IM every 6 hours, and peripherally with the non-narcotic paracetamol 500mg 4-hourly, her pain is reduced to 2 with no increase in sedation. She appears well oriented and says she feels more alert, probably because of better pain relief (Jain et al, 1986).

> **KEY POINT:** Combining two classes of analgesics, narcotic and non-narcotic, is a simple yet frequently overlooked strategy. This combination provides a safe and logical method of pain relief. They are two *different* analgesics:
> - They relieve pain in two different ways.
> - They have different side effects.
> - Giving them at the same time poses no more danger than alternating them, e.g. every 2 hours.

Brand Name	Generic Name	Ingredients
	co-dydramol	Paracetamol 500mg Dihydrocodeine tartrate 10mg
Remedeine		Paracetamol 500mg Dihydrocodeine tartrate 20mg
Remedeine Forte		Paracetamol 500mg Dihydrocodeine tartrate 30mg
Solpadol or Tylex		Paracetamol 500mg Codeine phosphate 30mg
Solpadol Effervescent		As Solpadol but also contains 16.8 mmol Na^+/tablet
Distalgesic, Cosalgesic	co-proxamol	Paracetamol 325mg Dextropropoxyphene hydrochloride 32.5mg
Fortagesic CD NHS		Paracetamol 500mg Pentazocine 15mg
Lobak NHS		Paracetamol 450mg Chlormezanone 100mg
Aspav Dispersible (Revised Formulation)		Aspirin 500mg Morphine 5mg Papaverine 600mcg Codeine 520mcg
Doloxene Compound NHS		Aspirin 375mg Dextropropoxyphene napsylate 100mg Caffeine 30mg
Equagesic CD NHS		Aspirin 250mg Meprobamate 150mg Ethoheptazine citrate 75mg
Robaxisal Forte NHS		Aspirin 325mg methocarbamol 400mg

CD   Controlled Drug

NHS Not prescribable under the NHS

Table 4.6 Common Combination Narcotic and Non-narcotic Oral Analgesics.

Patient/family teaching point

The patient/family teaching point (*Instructions for using non-narcotic analgesics at home* in the Appendix) may be duplicated, completed, and given to the patient who will be taking NSAIDs (other than paracetamol) as analgesics on an out-patient basis. When NSAIDs are used as analgesics in the hospital, some of the same points may need to be discussed with the patient, but unless the patient goes home with a prescription for them, use of the written form is probably unnecessary. The drugs are given by the nurses, and the patient can be directly observed for side effects.

In the "Additional Comments" section of the patient/family teaching form for home use of non-narcotic analgesics, the following should be included if the patient is on the particular drug:

Aspirin. Do not take if it has a strong vinegar smell. This means it has decomposed. Discard it and get a fresh supply.

Enteric-coated aspirin. Do not take with antacids or large amounts of milk because the coating may be destroyed.

Diflunisal. Has very little ability to reduce a fever.

Indomethacin. Urine or bowel movement may be green, but this is no cause for alarm. Always give with food or milk to minimise gastric upset. (If side effects are intolerable, consider the suppository form or a single oral dose at bedtime. Night-time doses or the rectal route are better tolerated for unknown reasons. During the day, another better tolerated analgesic, such as paracetamol, may be used.)

Naproxen. It is particularly important to avoid alcohol because naproxen may cause drowsiness and alcohol will increase the drowsiness.

Narcotic (opioid) analgesics

Examples of situations in which narcotics may be appropriate for pain relief:

- Moderate to severe acute pain, e.g. visceral trauma, orthopaedic fractures, post-operative pain.
- Recurrent, acute pain, e.g. sickle cell crisis.
- Prolonged, time-limited pain, e.g. terminal illness, cancer pain, burns.
- Desire for immediate relief of sudden, severe pain, e.g. renal colic, trauma. IV route provides relief in minutes.
- Selected patients with chronic non-malignant pain who do not benefit from other pain relief methods but are able to function well on a stabilized dose of narcotic for an opiate-sensitive pain.

Disadvantages of narcotics

A common misconception is that addiction will be a disadvantage in using narcotics; however, narcotic addiction as a result of treating pain with narcotics is very unlikely.

Examples of possible limitations or disadvantages of relieving pain with narcotics:

- Initial doses, changes in dosing, or a change in the patient's physical condition or pain require careful observation of the individual patient to arrive at a safe and effective dose.
- Failure to watch the individual's response to narcotic may lead to under-treating or over-treating pain. Needless suffering may occur that could be corrected by increasing the narcotic. Unnecessary side effects, such as respiratory depression or excessive sedation, may occur that need to be reversed with naloxone or eliminated by decreasing the dose.
- Even after careful titration, some patients will continue to experience undesirable side effects such as sedation, nausea, and vomiting, necessitating a change in narcotic or medication regime or additional medication, e.g. an anti-emetic.
- Re-education of health professionals, families, and patients is usually necessary if narcotics are to be used effectively. Under-use results from many misconceptions and exaggerated fears about narcotics.
- In certain chronic non-malignant pain conditions that would be more successfully treated with other modalities such as active physiotherapy behaviour modification, over-use of narcotics may result in increased sedation and depression along with decreased function.
- Inadequate relief may occur with neuropathic pain (e.g. lancinating nerve pain) or pain related to a highly inflammatory condition (e.g. rheumatoid arthritis).

- Prolonged use of narcotics may require an increase due to tolerance to analgesia and almost always requires measures to prevent constipation. This can be done safely and effectively, but it does require monitoring.
- Must be used with caution by persons engaged in potentially dangerous activities, such as driving a car, until degree of alteration of mood and level of consciousness are determined.
- Recovered substance abusers usually want to avoid narcotics since they do not want to be exposed to mind-altering drugs.

Mode of action of narcotics

Currently there are two broad types of narcotics available:

1. Narcotic agonists, pure agonists, e.g. codeine, oxycodone, morphine, diamorphine, Methadone, levorphanol and pethidine.
2. Narcotic agonist-antagonists, or partial agonists e.g. buprenorphine, nalbuphine, and pentazocine.

Narcotics, regardless of type, probably relieve pain at the level of the CNS by attaching to opioid receptor sites at the brain and spinal levels (Houde, 1979; Lim, 1967). In addition, the agonist-antagonists are also capable of blocking the analgesic effect of pure narcotics similar to the narcotic antagonist effect of naloxone. (The theory underlying these various actions is discussed on pp. 49–51.)

Forms of under-treatment with narcotics

Even when narcotics are clearly indicated, under-treatment of pain continues to be a pattern in health care today. The problem of under-treatment of pain is even greater in children. The result is needless suffering.

It is generally estimated that 85–90% of patients with acute pain or prolonged pain from end-stage disease could be comfortable if narcotics alone were used properly. However, it is apparent that people continue in moderate to severe distress from pain even when narcotics are used (Goman, 1991).

Nurses can make a difference in changing this unacceptable practice in health care. Being aware of the following specific forms of under-treatment of pain is a beginning.

1. *Doctors under-prescribe narcotics* (Angell, 1982; Charap, 1978; Grossman and Sheidler, 1985; Marks and Sachar, 1973; Sriwatanakul et al, 1983). This takes two forms:

a. Using less than the effective dosage of narcotic.

b. Allowing longer intervals between doses than the drug's duration of action.

Examples of under-prescribing are prescriptions for 50 and 75mg of pethidine 4-hourly PRN for pain. In fact for many people, especially younger patients, larger doses may be required for pain relief (Jaffee and Martin, 1985, p. 514). Although pethidine is cited as having a 2–4 hour duration of action (Jaffee and Martin, 1985, p. 505), in our experience, its duration is often only 2–3 hours.

2. *Nurses administer less* than what the patient could receive according to the doctor's prescription (Cohen, 1980; Fox, 1982; Marks and Sachar, 1973). This takes two forms:

a. Administering narcotics at longer intervals than allowed.

b. Administering less than the prescribed dose of narcotic. Legally this is a questionable practice.

In another now classic study in the pain literature, a person with chronic cholecystitis suffered unrelieved pain but received only 150mg of the 450mg of pethidine available to him over a 24-hour period (Marks and Sachar, 1973).

3. *People experiencing pain do not request or take narcotics* (Cleeland, 1987; Frank, 1980; Sriwatanakul et al, 1983). This takes three forms:

a. Taking the medicine at longer intervals than the duration of action.

b. Taking less than the prescribed dose.

c. Not taking the drug at all.

Why do these forms of under-treatment of pain exist? The four factors that often contribute to the under-treatment of pain are summarized in Table 4.7 and are discussed in the following section.

Misconceptions	Corrections
Health professionals, patients, and families fear causing: 1. Addiction (psychological dependence), e.g. relieving pain with narcotics, may lead to compulsive use in a large percentage of persons. 2. Physical dependence (withdrawal syndrome), e.g. hard to get the patient "off" narcotics, could be life-threatening.	1. No *evidence* supports fear of addiction as a reason for withholding narcotics when they are indicated for pain relief. All studies show that regardless of doses or length of time on narcotics, the incidence of addiction is *less than* 1%. 2. Withdrawal syndrome from narcotics is *rarely life-threatening* (except in infants born to physically dependent mothers). Most patients can be easily treated by gradually reducing the dose over 7–10 days. *Clinically it is rarely noticed* since pain usually subsides gradually with concomitant decrease in narcotic.
3. Tolerance to analgesia, e.g. if narcotics are started too soon or escalated too fast, pain relief will be impossible because doses will be fatal or a ceiling on analgesia will be reached.	3. Tolerance does not develop uniformly to all narcotic effects. Usually tolerance to analgesia is accompanied by even greater tolerance to respiratory depression and sedation. Hence, the *lethal dose is markedly elevated.* Further, there is no *ceiling on analgesia* of the strong narcotics, e.g. morphine.
4. Respiratory depression, e.g. large or frequent doses will be fatal, low doses are safe, or going beyond a certain dose in any patient is unsafe.	4. No *dose is automatically safe or fatal.* A low dose may be fatal for one patient, but 10 times that dose may be safe for another. The only safe way to administer a narcotic is to watch the first doses of each new amount given to the individual. A safe dose usually continues to be safe unless the drug accumulates or the patient's condition changes. *No patient need die of narcotic-induced respiratory depression.* It can be completely reversed with naloxone. (An exception is respiratory depression from buprenorphine.)

Table references:
Hodding,GC, Jann, M, and Ackerman, IP:Drug withdrawal syndromes-a literature review, *West J Med* **133**:383–391, Nov 1980.
Jaffe,JH:Drug addiction and drug abuse. In Gilman, AG, et al, eds: Goodman and Gilman's *The Pharmacological Basis of Therapeutics,* ed 7, pp. 532–581, New York, 1985, Macmillan Publishing Co.
Opiate abuse-Part I, *The Havard Medical School Mental Health Letter* **3**:1–4, Jan 1987.
Perry, s, and Heidrch, G: Management of pain during debridement: a survey of US burn units, *Pain* **13**:267–280, Jul 1982.
Porter, J, and Jick, H: Addiction rare in patients treated with narcotics, *N Engl J Med* **302**:123, 1980.
RAG: Clinical experience with in advanced malignant disease, *Int J Clin Pharmacol* **9**:184–198, 1974.

Table 4.7 Common Reasons for Under-Treatment of Pain with Narcotics

> **KEY POINT:** All groups, nurses, doctors, patients and families, tend to under-use narcotics and need to be re-educated.

Reasons for under-treatment with narcotics

Doctors, nurses, and patients and their family members have similar fears that result in the under-treatment of pain. Following are four common fears.

1. Fear of addiction

This appears to be the major reason for under-treatment among both health professionals and the public (Aguwa and Olusanya, 1978; Angell, 1982; Charap, 1978; Cohen, 1980; Frank, 1980; Trotter et al, 1981). The fear that *appropriate* use of narcotics causes addiction is irrational and undocumented. Increasing recognition of this fact is evidenced by an article in a substance abuse journal on "opiophobia" defined as "the irrational and undocumented fear that appropriate use of narcotics causes addiction" (Morgan, 1985–1986, p. 163).

A factual and unemotional approach to addiction requires that the term be defined and distinguished from other conditions related to narcotic use. In recent years the term *addiction* has been redefined. Not too long ago it was thought that addiction was both psychological and physiological dependence. Now physiological changes from repeated use of narcotics are recognized and treated as separate entities. Definitions and important differences between addiction and physiological conditions appear in Table 4.8.

Important aspects of the definitions in Table 4.8 are (Jaffe, 1985):

- Narcotic addiction, physical dependence, and tolerance are separate conditions. Each may occur alone, any two may occur together, or all three may be present at the same time.
- Physiological changes from repeated doses of narcotic are not the same as psychological dependence, and physiological changes do not automatically lead to psychological dependence. A patient may develop tolerance and require a higher dose, but this is not addiction. He/she may experience withdrawal syndrome if the narcotic is suddenly stopped, but again, this is not addiction.
- If a person is taking narcotics for the purpose of relieving pain, it is inappropriate to refer to him/her as an addict, no matter how much narcotic is being taken, how long, or how often. Pain relief is a legal, medical reason for prescribing and using narcotics.

Term	Definition	Differences
Addiction	*Behaviour* of overwhelming involvement with obtaining and using a drug for its psychic effects, not for approved medical reasons. High tendency to relapse back to continuing the drug once the pain is gone.	*Behaviour* that involves active, compulsive drug seeking and a tendency to relapse even after physical withdrawal subsides. Use of narcotics for pain relief is not addiction since pain relief is an approved medical use.
Tolerance	After repeated administration of a narcotic, a given dose begins to lose its effectiveness, resulting in the need for larger and larger doses. The first indication of tolerance is decreased duration, then decreased analgesia.	Involuntary behaviour based on *physiological changes*. The presence of drug tolerance does not mean the patient is addicted.
Physical dependence	After repeated administration of a narcotic, withdrawal symptoms occur if the narcotic is abruptly stopped.	Involuntary behaviour based on *physiological changes*. The presence of physical dependence does not mean the patient is addicted.

*Adapted from, Jaffe, JH:Drug addiction and abuse. In Gilman, AG, et al, eds:Goodman and Gilman's *The Pharmacological Basis of Therapeutics*, ed 7, p. 533, New York, 1985, Macmillan Publishing Co.

Table 4.8 Definitions of Addiction, Tolerance, and Physical Dependence.*

- Misuse of narcotics for pain relief is not the same as abuse or addiction. Some patients with pain may have narcotics mis-prescribed for them. For example, other forms of pain relief, such as physiotherapy or non-narcotics, may be more appropriate than narcotics. The patient with a mental illness such as endogenous depression may need psychotropic medication, not narcotics, to increase the ability to cope with pain. However, if a patient misuses narcotics because the physician inadvertently mis-prescribes, labelling the patient an addict is entirely inappropriate.

- The term *addiction* should be used with extreme care, since, in our society, to be addicted is often viewed as being a "bad person." When use of a drug is labelled addiction, considerable social stigma is attached.

Incidence of Addiction. The incidence of addiction as a result of taking narcotics for pain relief is extremely over-estimated. Addiction rarely occurs when a person takes narcotics for pain relief. Of major importance in dealing with exaggerated fears of addiction is to identify the following *research* about narcotic addiction:

1. Far less than 1% of hospitalized patients receiving pethidine 100mg 4-hourly regularly ever became addicted (Marks and Sachar, 1973).

2. Of almost 12,000 hospitalized medical in-patients who received at least one narcotic, only 4 patients could be reasonably well-documented as addicts (Porter and Jick, 1980).

3. The length of time a person is on narcotics does not increase the incidence of addiction (Foley and Rogers, 1981; Twycross, 1974).

Some people will disagree with these statements, but it is unlikely they can supply studies with different findings. Corrections to frequently expressed misconceptions about indicators of addiction are addressed in Table 4.9.

It is important to use appropriate guidelines and references when discussing fears of addiction with both other health-care professionals and patients and their families.

KEY POINT: The overwhelming majority of people stop taking narcotics when pain stops.

2. Fear of physical dependence (withdrawal syndrome)

This fear is related in part to the misconception that if withdrawal signs are present they are the result of addiction or will automatically lead to addiction. It is

Misconceptions about Indicators of Addiction	Comments/Corrections
1. Prolonged use of narcotics	1. Some pain is prolonged or lasts longer than expected. Length of time on narcotics does not increase likelihood of addiction.
2. Clock-watching	2. This usually results from inadequate pain relief. Some narcotics are short acting; some patients metabolise narcotics rapidly. The pain returns before the designated interval elapses.
3. Prefers "needle" to the tablet	3. This can be the result of not applying equianalgesic dosages when the route of narcotic is switched from injections to oral. The result is often under-medication. The effectiveness of a dose given IM may be 2–6 times greater than the same dose given orally.
4. "Enjoys his morphine" (or other narcotic)	4. Why not? If a person has been in pain, he will probably be happy to get relief.
5. Knows the name and dose of narcotic	5. This knowledge should be encouraged. It can be helpful information in assessing effective analgesics at a future time.
6. Requests narcotic in anticipation of pain	6. This can be an indication that the interval between doses is not timed correctly for individual pain. Reassess the pain and evaluate the interval; or the patient may have been instructed appropriately in the use of a preventive approach.
7. Requires higher and higher doses given more frequently	7. The underlying reason for the pain could be advancing, e.g. cancer metastasis. The other possibility is the development of tolerance.

Table 4.9 Misconceptions about Indicators of Addiction.

important to distinguish between physical dependence and addiction (Table 4.8). Other common misconceptions are that withdrawal from narcotics will be life-threatening, that the symptoms will be difficult to control, and that the occurrence of withdrawal symptoms will prevent decreases in doses as the pain subsides. However, as discussed below, physical dependence is rarely life-threatening, is easy to manage in most patients, and does not prevent decreases in narcotic doses as the pain decreases.

Incidence of Physical Dependence. The incidence of physical dependence is greater than most health-care professionals realise (Charap, 1978; Marks and Sachar, 1973). However, development of physical dependence is somewhat unpredictable. It probably begins to develop with the first dose of narcotic; after therapeutic doses of narcotic several times a day for 1 or 2 weeks, mild withdrawal symptoms may occur when the narcotic is stopped (Jaffe, 1985). These symptoms are so mild they are not usually recognized as withdrawal and certainly require no treatment. Clinical observations have shown that some patients on narcotics for long periods of time may demonstrate no recognizable withdrawal symptoms when the narcotic is stopped.

Symptoms of Narcotic Withdrawal. The symptoms of narcotic withdrawal are variable, ranging from mild to severe, and are less of a problem to manage than health-care professionals believe (Charap, 1978; Fox 1982). Symptoms of withdrawal and their severity depend on many factors, such as the particular narcotic used and the dose. In a survey of 72 hospital-based nurses, 83% erroneously feared that the hazard of withdrawal from morphine was as great or greater than withdrawal from barbiturates (Fox, 1982). However, even when symptoms of narcotic withdrawal are severe, they are rarely life-threatening (except in the newborn).

The following is a list of general characteristics of symptoms that may occur after abrupt discontinuation of a narcotic in a person who is physically dependent (Jaffe, 1985):

- *Approximately 8–12 hours* after last dose: yawning, lacrimation, rhinorrhea, and sweating.
- *Approximately 12–14 hours* after last dose: restlessness, irritability, tremors, dilated pupils, and anorexia.
- *Approximately 48–72 hours* after last dose: increasing irritability, violent yawning, severe sneezing, nausea and vomiting, diarrhoea, chills alternating with excessive sweating, muscle spasms, and low back pain.

- *Within 7 to 10 days,* these symptoms subside.
- *Abrupt withdrawal of methadone* may result in symptoms that develop more slowly and are more prolonged due to the long half-life of methadone.
- *Abrupt withdrawal of pethidine* can result in symptoms appearing within 3 hours of the last dose and subsiding after 4 to 5 days.

Treatment of Withdrawal Symptoms. The purpose of treatment is to suppress these symptoms and keep the person comfortable (exceptions are newborns of addicted mothers where the purpose is to maintain life). Treatment of withdrawal usually is not necessary because pain usually subsides gradually and narcotics are automatically gradually decreased.

If management of withdrawal symptoms is necessary, a formula to suppress withdrawal symptoms in a patient who does not need the narcotic for pain relief is (Foley and Inturrisi, 1987):

- Administer one-quarter of the previous narcotic daily dose in four divided doses for 2 days.
- Then decrease by one-half and continue to administer in four divided doses with 50% reductions every 2 days until a total daily dose of 10–15mg of morphine is reached.
- After 2 days at this dose, the narcotic can be discontinued.

Another common formula used for preventing significant withdrawal symptoms while narcotics are being reduced is to reduce the total daily dose by 10% a day over a 10-day period or by 5% a day over a 20-day period. α-blockers, e.g. clonidine have been used to supress the symptoms of withdrawal. However, in the UK, clonidine is not licensed for treatment of withdrawal. Lofexidine is the only α-blocker which has a licence (Guthrie, 1990; Washton et al, 1983).

Oddly, clinical experience suggests that sometimes the initial decreases are easier to tolerate than the final decreases. In other words, the patient may not feel any significant withdrawal symptoms during the first part of the detoxification process, but when low doses are reached, decreases may cause symptoms. The solution often is simply to maintain the patient on low doses for a little longer before further decreases are made.

The reassuring facts about physical dependence are:

- It is rarely life-threatening.
- It does not prevent decreases in doses.

- Symptoms can usually be easily treated by gradually reducing the narcotic dose.
- It is not the same as addiction and does not result in addiction.

> **KEY POINT:** The most frequent problem caused by withdrawal symptoms is misunderstanding their meaning. *Their presence is not to be interpreted as addiction.*

3. Fear of tolerance to narcotic analgesia

This tends to be of special concern in patients with prolonged pain, e.g. cancer, burns, and life-threatening illness. The doctor, nurse, patient, and family may be afraid to:

- Start narcotics "too soon" and/or
- Escalate the narcotic dose "too fast."

They fear, especially with patients in the end stages of a disease but with weeks or months to live, that if pain increases, pain relief will be impossible or lethal.

Reassurances for patients, families, and the health-care team

These include the following:

1. If tolerance does occur, it can usually be treated safely and effectively by increasing the narcotic dosage, or changing the route of administration.
2. The analgesic dose in a patient who has become tolerant to a narcotic is *not lethal* because the person also develops tolerance to the life-threatening side effect of respiratory depression as well as to sedation (Catalano, 1987; Foley, 1986; Jaffe, 1985; Twycross, 1974).
3. There is no such thing as the body becoming "immune" to analgesics. An adequate increase in dose or change in route of administration almost always results in increased pain relief.
4. There is *no ceiling* on the analgesic effects of strong narcotics such as morphine, diamorphine and methadone, (Levy, 1985; McCaffery, 1981; Miser et al, 1980).

Treatment of tolerance

Guidelines are:

1. Maintain the oral route as long as possible since tolerance develops slower than with the IM, SC or IV route (Foley and Rogers, 1981).
2. Increase the dose and/or decrease the interval between doses.

Patient Example

Mr R., 26 years old, has a history of sickle cell disease and painful crisis about once a year. In each of four admissions over 4 years, IV narcotics relieved pain and were titrated down after about 3 days using oral narcotics, and he was narcotic-free after 7 days. However, a crisis 6 months ago led to continuous pain due to multiple complications and more painful crises.

Initially, the painful crisis was relieved with a regime similar to previous ones, consisting of a total of 20mg morphine IV bolused over 30 minutes followed by continuous hourly infusion at 10mg/hr, titrated to oral morphine 80mg every 4 hours, regularly for ongoing, less severe pain. The dose and frequency of narcotics increased over the 6 months in a manner typical of tolerance to narcotic analgesia. Morphine was increased to 200mg every 4 hours. Sudden increases in pain required IV morphine boluses totalling 50–70mg over 30 minutes and 40mg infused hourly. During his fourteenth hospitalization lasting 3 weeks, Mr R's complications finally resolved and he was pain-free. As his pain subsided his narcotic dose decreased to zero, and he was discharged with no evidence of narcotic addiction.

This example is typical of the aggressive treatment that is needed for pain relief in complicated sickle cell crisis. The following articles may be helpful in getting the health care team to be willing to treat crises adequately:

Brozovic, M, Davies, SC, Yardumian, A, et al: Pain relief in sickle cell crises. *Lancet*, 2:624–625, Sept 13, 1986.

Cole, TB, Sprinkle, RH, Smith, SJ, and Buchanan, GR: Intravenous narcotic therapy for children with severe sickle cell crisis pain. *Am. J. Dis. Child.*, **140**:1255–1259, 1986.

Ives, T, and Guerra, M: Constant morphine infusion for severe sickle cell crisis pain. *Drug Intell. Clin. Pharm.*, **21**:625–626, July-Aug, 1987.

Payne, R: Pain management in sickle cell disease — rationale and techniques. *Ann. N.Y. Acad. Sci.*, **565**: 189–206, 1984.

Shapiro, B: The management of pain in sickle cell disease. *Paediatr. Clin. North Am.*, **36**:1029–1045, 1989.

> **KEY POINT:** Drug tolerance and physical dependence (withdrawal syndrome) are involuntary behaviours involving physiological responses. The person has no control over these conditions developing. The presence of tolerance or withdrawal symptoms does not mean the person is addicted.

4. Fear of respiratory depression

All narcotics are capable of producing respiratory depression and in fact to some extent affect all phases of respiratory activity. This is not life-threatening or even clinically significant in most patients. This capability in no way should prevent narcotics from being used to the fullest extent to relieve pain in all age groups. Studies show that equianalgesic doses of narcotic agonists produce about the same degree of respiratory depression (Jaffe and Martin, 1985). There is a ceiling to respiratory depression with narcotic agonist-antagonists. If narcotic-induced respiratory depression does occur, and if the patient is conscious, he/she can breathe if instructed to do so (Jaffe and Martin, 1985). An exception to this occurs with the use of fentanyl, which causes muscular rigidity along with respiratory depression.

Occurrence of Respiratory Depression. It is impossible to know what dose will produce clinically significant respiratory depression in a given patient. *Low doses cannot be assumed safe for all patients.* In a study of 3,263 hospitalized medical patients receiving pethidine IM in doses ranging from 25 to 100 mg, 3 patients had clinically significant respiratory depression. The doses were 50mg in two patients and 25mg in one patient (Miller and Jick, 1978).

Reassurances for Patients, Families, and the Health-Care Team. When people with severe pain and those who have developed tolerance need high doses of narcotic, respiratory depression usually is not a problem. High doses will usually be safe because:

- Severe pain appears to be nature's antidote since it counteracts the respiratory depressant effects of the narcotic.
- Tolerance to narcotic analgesia usually assures tolerance to respiratory depressant effects (Jaffe and Martin, 1985).

The pain flow sheet (opposite) is a tool that allows quick and easy monitoring of respiratory status.

> **KEY POINT:** The only safe and effective way to administer a narcotic is to *watch the individual's response*, especially to the first dose.

Patient Example

You are asked to administer Mrs D.'s pain medication, 150 mg oral morphine regularly. You question the dosage because your main concern is that the high dosage will cause her to stop breathing. You gather some facts to help you make your decision about the safety of giving this dose. The pain flow sheet for Mrs D. is shown above. By quickly scanning the respiratory column, the nurse sees that Mrs D.'s respiratory rate has remained stable despite this dose. In reviewing her prescriptions, you also note that she has been on this present dose for the past 2 weeks. With this information, you can confidently give the medication while continuing to monitor Mrs D.'s comfort level.

Treatment of Respiratory Depression. This is safe and effective (except in situations of overdose involving unknown quantities and substances). Many instances of narcotic-induced respiratory depression that occur in the clinical setting do not need any particular treatment other than decreasing the dose or frequency of narcotic. Following are guidelines for more aggressive treatment of respiratory depression, if required.

1. Naloxone is titrated slowly at 0.1–0.4mg IV over 2–3 minutes or 0.4mg in 10ml of saline as a slow bolus until respiration is normal.

   The purpose in most cases is to reverse the side effects, not the analgesic effect, of the narcotic. The most effective way to do this is to titrate the naloxone slowly. If the patient is conscious he/she can be instructed every 5–10 seconds to breathe.

   In the hospitalized patient, it is rarely necessary or appropriate to give rapidly IV 0.4mg (1ml) or 0.8mg (2ml) of naloxone. This practice is likely to eliminate all narcotic so that the patient has an abrupt return to severe pain. The ideal is both adequate ventilation and pain relief. Antagonize enough narcotic so that the patient breathes well again, but leave enough of the narcotic in the system to control pain.

2. Continue to observe the patient. Naloxone may wear off before the respiratory depressant effects of the narcotic decrease. The duration of action from IV naloxone may be as short as 30 minutes, and continuous infusions of naloxone may be required.

CONTINUOUS-ASSESSMENT SHEET FOR PAIN FOR MRs D

Patient *Mr s D*   Date

*Pain rating scale used   *0 to 10 (0 = no pain, 10 = worst pain)*

Purpose: To evaluate the safety and effectiveness of the analgesic(s).
Analgesic(s) prescribed: *Morphine 150mg orally 4 hours*

Time	Pain rating	Analgesic	R	P	BP	Level of sedation	Other†	Plan and comments
9am	3	Morphine 150mg	18			awake and alert		
10 am	1		16			States she is comfortable		
11am	1		12			Sleeping easily awakened		↓Resp due to PT sleeping
12n	2		16					
1pm	2	Morphine 150mg	18			Awake & alert		
5pm	2	Morphine 150mg	16			Talking with family members		
9pm	1	Morphine 150mg	12			Sleeping. Quickly awakens when name called		

This flow sheet is an example of the information that is useful to a nurse who is unfamiliar with the patient. No matter how large ar small the dose of narcotic prescribed, the patient's previous response is extremely helpful in determining the probable safety and effectiveness of the next dose. In this situation if the nurse is fearful of administering the prescription for oral morphine, 150mg 4-hourly regularly, information on this continuous assessment sheet reassures her that it has been given safely and effectively. She is therefore more likely to administer it.

Pain relief for narcotic addicts

Substance abuse disorder related to narcotics is the preferred terminology, but the term addiction is more commonly used. The term *narcotic addict* may refer to either recovered addicts or active users. In either case advice should be sought from a Drug Dependency Unit about clinical management. All management should be decided jointly by the primary clinicians, Drug Dependency Unit and the patient. It is important at all times that the patient feels in control of the situation.

Approaches to the recovered narcotic substance abuser with pain

With some patients who admit to former narcotic or other substance abuse, it may not always be clear to what extent they have recovered or are committed to remaining free of psychological dependence on narcotics or other drugs. However, when the patient receives health care for problems other than substance abuse, the patient's commitment to recovery from substance abuse is not questioned; it is respected and accepted.

Important considerations in providing pain relief with narcotics for a person recovering from narcotic or other substance abuse are:

- Explain to the patient the intent to use narcotics and why, e.g. that the pain is usually most effectively and efficiently relieved with narcotics.
- Ask the patient if there are any concerns about using narcotics for this episode of pain.

  Discuss more specific choices of narcotics including dose, frequency and duration if the patient is willing to proceed further.
- If the patient is not satisfied with the above approaches, consider non-narcotic alternatives, such as regional nerve blocks, TENS, NSAIDs, cold packs, acupuncture, or infiltration of the wound with a local anaesthetic.
- If the person is on methadone maintenance, i.e. a daily dose of methadone, for narcotic substance abuse, this dose must be continued. If oral methadone is not possible, approximately half the oral dose may be given IM in divided doses. For pain relief, *additional* narcotic is needed.
- Anticipate the need for larger than usual narcotic doses in the recovered addict or one who is on methadone maintenance. Either person may have tolerance to narcotic analgesia. Even the person who has not taken narcotics for months or years may quickly develop tolerance again if he/she was tolerant to analgesia previously, requiring larger than usual doses for pain relief. This should not be interpreted as addiction—it is a physiological change.

Approaches to the active narcotic substance abuser with pain

When an active narcotic addict, or other substance abuser, develops a painful condition, helping this person with pain control can be difficult. Why? Because health-care professionals may fear:

- Promoting the person's addiction by administering narcotics.
- Being manipulated by the addict to obtain additional narcotics.
- Lack of experience in dealing effectively with addicts.

The goal is to deliver humane care to a person with pain who happens to be a narcotic addict by:

1. Relieving the pain.
2. Keeping the person out of withdrawal.

Remember that long-term use of narcotics may have caused marked tolerance to narcotic analgesia. Therefore the person may require very large doses of narcotic for pain relief.

Considerations such as those discussed for recovered users should be taken into account. A clear plan of action including the drugs to be used and their dosages and time scale, followed by how the patient will be weaned off, and with what treatments, should be decided by the clinical teams and the patient. It is important at all times that there is one key medical prescriber to avoid the risk of multiple prescribing.

> **KEY POINT:** The narcotics addict has the same right to pain control as any other person. Narcotics should not be withheld as a punitive or rehabilitative measure. Treatment of the pain in this case requires different rules and expectations.

Equianalgesic doses of narcotics

Unfortunately, one of the best-kept secrets in all of pharmacology seems to be the equianalgesic dosage of narcotics by various routes for relief of moderate to severe pain, particularly the dose of narcotic required orally to equal the analgesic effect obtained by an IM dose. Lack of specific knowledge about this contributes to under-treatment as well as inappropriate conclusions about possible abuse and addiction.

> **KEY POINT:** The most common cause of under-medication in people with pain is the lack of knowledge of equianalgesic doses of drug (Foley, 1985b).

Patient Example

The analgesics prescribed are pethidine 50mg IM or oral PRN for pain. The patient refuses the pethidine tablets, saying that only the injection brings the pain from 9 to 5 on a 0–10 scale (0 = no pain, 10 = worst pain). The outcome of this situation is that the patient is unjustifiably labelled as a drug abuser because he "prefers the needle to the tablet."

Misconception: Patients who "prefer the needle to the pill" are abusers or potential addicts.

Correction: Narcotics given IM are two to six times more effective than the same dose given orally. The patient logically asks for the medication that effectively relieves the pain.

Using the same dose regardless of route in the above example is inappropriate and ignores the concept of equianalgesic dosing. Equianalgesic means approximately equal analgesia, i.e. doses of medication that provide about the same pain relief when:

- Switching from one route of administration to another, such as from IM to oral or IV to oral.
- Switching from one drug to another, such as pethidine to morphine.

Application of information about the equianalgesic doses in Table 4.10 is one of the important steps in tailoring an analgesic regime for each individual patient.

The following three annotated references may be helpful if you are caring for an active narcotic addict with pain:

1. Fultz, J, Senay, E, Pray, B, and Thornton, W: When a narcotic addict is hospitalized. *AJN,* **80**:478–481, March 1980. This article presents facts about medical complications, signs and symptoms of withdrawal, and doses for methadone maintenance. Extensive bibliography and factual presentation may be helpful to intellectually understand the process of controlling an addict's physical needs while hospitalized.
2. Leporati, NC, and Chychula, LH: How you can really help the drug-abusing patient. *Nursing,* **12**:46–49, June 1982. Five specific guidelines are suggested for interacting with a substance abuser who is in your care. Two scripts of nurse–patient dialogues to get the patient talking about his/her problem are included. A chart lists commonly abused drugs and their effects. This helpful article presents realistic and unrealistic goals for patient care.
3. Stimmel, B: *Pain, Analgesia and Addiction: the Pharmacologic Treatment of Pain,* New York, 1983, Raven Press. Excellent guidelines for the care of narcotic-dependent populations are presented on pp. 294-297. The management of pain in heroin addicts and in people on methadone maintenance programmes is discussed.

To become familiar with the equianalgesic chart in Table 4.10, note that there are four columns. Each column is discussed here, beginning with the left one.

1. *Analgesic* column lists the analgesics with morphine first, since it is the usual standard of comparison. The remainder of the analgesics are listed in alphabetical order by generic name. Only those analgesics and formulations available for human use are listed.
2. *IM Route (mg)* column lists the doses of analgesics by the IM or SC route that are approximately equal to each other in ability to relieve pain. Any dose in this column would be a reasonable initial dose to use to substitute for any other dose of analgesic in the same column or in the oral column.

For example, if the patient has a prescription for pethidine 75mg IM, and if you wish to switch the patient to a dose of morphine IM or SC that will relieve the same amount of pain, you would follow these steps:

- Locate pethidine, in the left column.
- Find the dose listed for pethidine for the IM column. In this case it is the dose you wish to change, 75mg.
- Locate morphine in the left column.
- Find the dose listed for morphine in the IM column. The dose is 10mg. Thus 10mg of morphine IM is an educated guess about the initial dose of morphine IM that would provide the same relief as pethidine 75mg IM.
- Check the list under "Important Characteristics of the Equianalgesic Chart" (see heading on p. 86) and Table 4.10 for any indications that this initial dose should be revised. For example, has the patient been on pethidine so long that it is not being absorbed entirely or has the patient become tolerant to it? If either of these is a possibility, you probably would want to lower the initial dose of morphine 10mg to 7 or 8mg.
- If an analgesic is listed but the dose you are looking for is not the same dose that appears in the IM column, you may still use the list to calculate the initial dose. For example, if a child is receiving pethidine 50mg IM and you wish to switch to morphine IM, you calculate that 50mg is two-thirds of 75mg and that you will need two-thirds of any IM dose listed, e.g. approximately 6.5mg of morphine IM. (NOTE: The IM doses listed in this column are also used for calculating IV doses when switching from one analgesic to another via the IV route or switching from IM to IV; some clinicians regard the IM and IV doses as approximately equal, others suggest that the IV dose equals one-half the IM dose.)

Analgesic	IM Route (mg)†	Oral Route (mg)**	Comments
morphine	10	60 (30)§	Both IM and oral doses of morphine have a duration of action of about 4hr. Sustained-release tablets, rectal suppositories, and preservative-free for spinal analgesia are also available. The oral dose is 3–6 times the IM dose. The lower oral dose is suggested by several clinicians (Lipman, 1980, 1982; Walsh, 1984) and is based on anecdotal evidence, not experimental research (Kaiko, 1986); it may be appropriate for some patients, especially elderly patients with chronic cancer pain. *All IM and oral doses in this chart are considered equivalent to 10mg of IM morphine in analgesic effect.*
buprenorphine	400mcg 300mcg	0.8 800mcg	A narcotic agonist-antagonist that may precipitate withdrawal in patients very physically dependent on narcotics. Dose for the sublingual form is 0.8 mg. Compared with morphine, this drug is longer acting and more likely to produce nausea and vomiting (Bradley, 1984). Respiratory depression is rare but serious because it is not readily reversed by naloxone.
codeine	130	200	Relatively more toxic in high doses than morphine, causing more nausea and vomiting and considerable constipation. The oral dose is about 1.5 times the IM dose.
dextromoramide	— (equivalent to 10mg morphine)	5	Provides intense analgesia, but short duration of action (1–2 hrs) makes it inappropriate for regular administration. Sub-lingual administration gives rapid effect, making it suitable for breakthrough pain or for use prior to painful procedures. Available as 5mg and 10mg tablets.
diamorphine	3	10	Somewhat shorter acting than morphine, 2–4 hours. No advantage over morphine when given orally, or intravenously, but very great solubility offers considerable benefits when given by subcutaneous injection. Potency ratios in the literature vary considerably, 3:1 represents a suitable starting point.
dihydrocodeine	50	60	Roughly equipotent with codeine. May be used in place of codeine in patients with head injuries. Available as 30mg tablets (and 60mg, 90mg, 120mg sustained release). If analgesia is inadequate, it is preferable to reduce dosage interval (i.e. from 4–6 hrly to 2–3 hrly) rather than doubling dose to 60mg. Available as syrup 10mg/5ml. Injection is a Controlled Drug.
dipipanone	—	20	Available only as 10mg dose combined with cyclizine 30mg, which may cause sedation when given regularly, and limits total daily dose, as maximum daily dose of cyclizine is 150mg.
fentanyl	50mcg	—	Most common use is for anaesthesia, given IV. Onset of action when given IM is about 15min; duration of action, about 90min. Analgesic effect is not significantly increased by droperidol (Jaffe and Martin, 1985). Has been used as a substitute for high-dose IV morphine in terminally ill patients when morphine caused excitation. Used IV in neonates and for brief procedures.
methadone	10	20	Longer acting than morphine when given in repeated, regular doses. Careful titration required because drug accumulates; both dose and interval must be adjusted. Onset with oral dose occurs within 1hr. Because drug accumulates, analgesic effect may increase with repeated doses. Initial oral dose is twice the IM dose. Not widely used due to problems of accumulation.
methotrimeprazine	20	—	A phenothiazine (non-narcotic) drug. Duration of action is 4–5hr. Common adverse effect is hypotension; not recommended for ambulatory patients, as it is very sedative. (McGee and Alexander, 1979). Not widely used in the UK as an analgesic, more often for its sedative actions.
nalbuphine	10 (20)	—	A narcotic agonist-antagonist that may produce withdrawal in patients physically dependent on narcotics. Longer acting and less likely to cause hypotension than morphine. In doses above 10mg/70kg, it causes no additional respiratory depression (Romagnoli and Keats, 1980; Vernier and Schmidt, 1985), so patient may be started on a high dose.

Analgesic	IM Route (mg)†	Oral Route (mg)**	Comments
nefopam	20	60	Medium strength analgesic, unrelated to opioids or NSAIDs. Oral dose up to 90mg t.d.s. Anti-cholinergic side-effect profile, and does not tend to constipate. Probably acts at a CNS level by interfering with re-uptake of neurotransmitters.
oxycodone	—	—	Available as 30mg suppositories only. Roughly equipotent with morphine, but longer acting. May be given every 12–24hr. Useful in terminal care for providing background analgesia e.g. during the night.
pentazocine	60	180	Narcotic agonist-antagonist that may produce withdrawal in patients physically dependent on narcotics. Could produce psychotomimetic effects. The oral dose is 3 times the IV dose. Use not recommended.
pethidine	75	300	Shorter acting (2–4hr) than morphine. Watch for toxic effects on the central nervous system (CNS) caused by accumulation of the active metabolite nor-pethidine, which produces neuroexcitability. Use with caution in patients with renal disease. Because of the risk to the CNS, oral doses greater than 300mg are not recommended. Since nor-pethidine has a long half-life (15hr or longer), decreasing the dose in patients exhibiting a toxic reaction may increase CNS excitability, causing seizures. Effects of nor-pethidine are increased (not reversed) by naloxone (Kaiko et al, 1983). The oral dose is 4 times the IM dose.
propoxyphene HCl	—	500	For mild to moderate pain unrelieved by non-narcotics. Never give as much as 500mg orally, only low oral doses (65–130mg) are recommended.

The equianalgesic doses in this chart are based primarily on recommendations of the Analgesic Study Section, Sloan-kettering Institute for Cancer Research, New York, based on double-blind analgesic research (Houde, 1979). This format is adapted from McCaffery,M: A practical, portable chart of equianalgesic doses. *Nursing,* **17**:56–57, Aug 1987.

† Based on clinical experience, many consider the IM and IV dose equianalgesic (Portenoy, 1987). However, some recommend using 1/2 the IM dose for the IV dose (American Pain Society, 1987).

** Initial oral doses are usually lower than those listed here, especially for mild to moderate pain.

§ Values in parentheses refer to differences of opinion among clinicians.

A guide to using the equianalgesic chart

Equianalgesic means **approximately** the same pain relief. Onset, peak effect, and duration of analgesia for each drug often differ and may also vary with individual people.

Variability among individuals may be due to differences in absorption, organ dysfunction, or tolerance to one narcotic and not to another.

An equianalgesic chart is a guideline. The individual patient's response must be observed. Doses and intervals between doses are then titrated according to the individual's response.

Dosages in this chart are not necessarily starting doses. They suggest the ratio for comparing the analgesia of one drug with another.

Based on clinical experience, the IV dose is approximately the same as the IM dose. Dose adjustments are then made according to the individual's response. Some clinicians suggest approximately 1/2 the IM dose equals the IV dose.

Table references

American Pain Society: *Principles of Analgesic Use in the Treatment of Acute Pain and Chronic Cancer Pain: a concise guide to medical practice,* The Society, Washington DC, 1987.

Beaver,W: Management of cancer pain with parental medication. *JAMA,* **244**:2653–2657, Dec 12,1980.

Bradley,J: A comparison of morphine and buprenorphine for analgesia after abdominal surgery, *Anaesth Intens Care,* **12**:303–310, Nov 1984.

Buprenorphine, *Med Lett Drugs Ther,* **28**:56, May 23, 1986.

Houde, RW: Systemic analgesics and related drugs: narcotics analgesics. In Bonica,JJ, and Ventafridda, V, eds: *Advances in Pain Research and Therapy,* vol. 2, pp. 263–273, Raven Press, New York, 1979.

Jaffe, J, and Martin, W: Opioid analgesics and antagonists. In Gilman,A, et al, eds: *The Pharmacological Basis of Therapeutics,* ed. 7, pp. 491–531, Macmillan Publishing Co., New York, 1985.

Kaiko,R, Controversy in the management of chronic cancer pain: therapeutic equivalents of IM and PO morphine. *J Pain Sympt Manag,* **1**:42–45, Winter 1986.

Kaiko, R, et al: Central nervous system excitatory effects of pethidine in cancer patients. *Ann Neurol,* **13**:180–185, Feb 1983.

Kantor, T, et al: Adverse effects on commonly ordered oral narcotics. *J Clin Pharmacol,* **21**:1–8, Jan 1981.

Lipman,A: Comment on pain cocktail article. *Drug Intell Clin Pharm,* **16**:332, Apr 1982.

Lipman,A: Drug therapy in cancer pain. *Cancer Nursing,* **3**:39–46, Feb 1980.

McGee,J, and Alexander, M: Phenothiazine analgesia - fact or fantasy? *Am J Hosp Pharm,* **36**:633–640, May 1979

Narcotic agonists and analgesics. In *Facts and Comparisons: Drug Information,* 242b, JB Lippincott Co., Philadelphia, 1986.

Portenoy,RK: Continuous intravenous infusion of opioid drugs, *Med Clin North Am,* **71**:233–241, Mar 1987.

Romagnoli,A and Keats,A: Ceiling effect for respiratory depression by nalbuphine, *Clin Pharmacol Ther,* **27**:478–485, Apr 1980.

Vernier,V, and Scmidt, W: The preclinical pharmacology of nalbuphine. In Gomez, Q, ed: *Nalbuphine as a component of surgical anaesthesia,* pp. 1–9, Excerpta Medica, Princeton, NJ, 1985.

Walsh,T: Oral morphine in chronic cancer pain. *Pain,* **18**:1–11,Jan 1984.

Table 4.10 Equianalgesic Chart: Approximate Equivalent Doses of IM and Oral Analgesics for Moderate and Severe Pain

3. *Oral Route (mg)* column lists the doses of analgesics by the oral route that are approximately equal to each other in their ability to relieve pain. Any dose in this column would be a reasonable initial dose to use to substitute for any other dose of analgesic in the same column or any dose in the IM column.

For example, if you wished to switch a patient from a dose of codeine 90mg oral to an oral dose of morphine, you would follow these steps:
- Locate codeine in the left column.
- Find the dose listed for codeine in the oral column. In this case the dose listed is 200mg, but you wish to switch from only 90mg, approximately one-half the listed dose. Thus to substitute for the oral codeine, you will need only one-half of whatever oral or IM dose you find in this table.
- Locate morphine in the left column.
- Find the dose listed for morphine in the oral column. The dose is 16mg. Since you need only one-half of this dose, your initial estimate would be about 8–10mg of oral morphine.
- Check the list under "Important Characteristics of the Equianalgesic Chart" (next column) and Table 4.10 for any indications that this initial dose should be revised. For example, if the patient has been on several doses of codeine daily for several weeks, the patient may be tolerant to codeine. Since cross-tolerance is not complete, you probably would lower your initial estimate for the morphine dose to 5mg orally.

As a further example, if you wished to switch a patient from pethidine 75mg IM to a dose of oral morphine that would relieve the same amount of pain, you would follow steps similar to those above and find that the initial dose of morphine is 9.5mg, which is 10mg in practical terms because of how the drug is supplied, e.g. tablets of 1 mg.

4. The *Comments* column mentions various considerations pertinent to the specific analgesic, in particular any differences from the standard of comparison (morphine). Comments may include information about onset, duration of action, accumulation of the analgesic or its active metabolites, the ratio for converting IM to oral, and special formulations such as sustained release.

Important characteristics of the equianalgesic chart

1. The doses in this chart are based on recognized clinical research and are those recommended by the Analgesic Study Section, Sloan Kettering Institute for Cancer Research, New York; and by Regnard, C and Tempest, S: Approximate oral opioid equivalents. In *A Guide to Symptom Relief in Advanced Cancer,* ed. 3, Manchester, Haigh and Hochland Ltd., 1992, p. 12.

2. The table is to be used only as a guide when tailoring drug and dosage for individual patients. The individual patient's response must be observed. Dose, time interval, route, and choice of drug are then adjusted according to the individual's response.

3. The doses in the table are not necessarily starting doses. They suggest the *ratio* to use when calculating doses.

4. The conversion factor for calculating the oral dose needed to substitute for the IM dose is written where applicable in the comments column for each drug. For example, in the comments about morphine, the statement "oral dose is 2 times the IM dose" allows an easy, quick reference for calculating route or dose changes.

5. Based on *clinical* experience an hourly equianalgesic IV narcotic dose is approximately the same as the IM dose (Portenoy, 1987a). If 10mg morphine IM every 4 hrs controls pain and the patient is switched to IV morphine, the initial 4-hourly dose would be 10mg IV or 2.5mg per hour. Other authors suggest that one-half the IM dose gives an equivalent IV dose (Foley, 1982; Yasko, 1983). Controlled studies are needed for this route of administration.

6. All the IM and oral doses listed in the chart are considered equivalent and are compared with the analgesic standard, 10mg of IM morphine. For example, by referring to the oral and IM columns in the equianalgesic chart (Table 4.10), we see the following: diamorphine 3mg IM is equivalent to methadone 20mg oral, and dextromoramide 5mg oral is equivalent to pethidine 75mg IM. Further, these are all approximately equal to each other.

KEY POINT: The initial calculation of an analgesic dose is merely an educated guess. Individualizing the dose, time interval, route, choice of drug, and then monitoring the person's response are vital steps to the effective use of analgesics.

7. Two oral morphine doses are listed as being equivalent to 10mg IM morphine: 60mg and 30mg. The 30mg oral dose is widely used in clinical practice; however, it is not supported by research (refer to comments column next to morphine in Table 4.10 for references). Although it is disconcerting to see this degree of controversy regarding the oral dose of morphine, remember that all doses in the chart are merely educated guesses. When a dose is given, it is immediately titrated up or down according to the patient's response.

8. References are listed within the chart so that when nurses discuss this information with doctors and other health-care team members, their suggestions are supported by appropriate, accessible data.

9. Several factors are considered when changing drugs or route of administration. Although the equianalgesic chart serves as an accurate guideline, there are additional factors to consider when switching from one narcotic to another or when changing the route of medication, for example from IM to oral or oral to IV. Some of the potential problems that may alter the doses suggested in the equianalgesic chart include those listed in Table 4.11.

10. The Equianalgesic Chart can be photocopied from pp. 84–85 and distributed to all key clinical areas and colleagues.

Potential Problems	Possible Solutions
1. Calculating oral dose if incomplete absorption of IM dose.	1. Consider decreasing the amount of the oral dose needed for equal analgesia.
2. Differences in the absorption of oral dose. Example: Mr P's first dose of morphine 30mg orally resulted in sedation with pain relief.	2. The initial dose may need to be adjusted up or down. Approach: Mr P's dose of oral morphine was decreased by 5mg. Pain rating remained between 2 and 3 on 0–10 scale, and sedation decreased. Patient observed for further adjustments.
3. Organ dysfunction.	3. A shorter-acting narcotic or a lower dose may be needed. This may be especially true in the elderly or anyone with poor kidney and liver clearance. Methadone is poorly tolerated by many elderly patients since a general decrease in organ function may lead to a cumulative effect. Analgesia may increase with repeated doses, and metabolites causing side effects are not readily eliminated.
4. Switching narcotics after tolerance to analgesia has developed.	4. Tolerance often develops with repeated administration of a narcotic, but tolerance may not be present to the same extent with a new narcotic, i.e. cross-tolerance tends not to be complete. Therefore to avoid too many side effects, start with a lower equianalgesic dose and adjust up or down according to the patient's response.

Table 4.11 Considerations when Switching Drugs or Routes

> **KEY POINT:** Nurses have a key role in suggesting analgesic titration. Therefore it is important that they are active in educating colleagues about the effective use of an equianalgesic chart.

Know the pharmacology of the specific narcotics

Knowledge of basic pharmacology is essential if initial prescriptions and subsequent changes are to relieve pain as quickly, effectively and safely as possible. Pharmacological facts that guide decision-making include knowing that differences between narcotics determine which one is selected.

Selection of a narcotic

Morphine is the standard strong narcotic for severe acute pain and chronic cancer pain (World Health Organization: *Cancer Pain Relief*, Geneva, WHO, 1986). Reasons for choosing a narcotic other than morphine may include the following:

1. Patient or family member has had a good prior experience with another narcotic or insists on using previous narcotic.
2. The individual patient experiences unacceptable side effects from morphine. For example, some patients may have continued problems with nausea and vomiting despite an aggressive anti-emetic regime.
3. A strong narcotic is needed in a high concentration and limited volume. For example, parenteral administration may be needed for a cachectic patient. Diamorphine can be prepared by the pharmacist in concentrations of more than 100mg/ml. This would be particularly useful for high doses of continuous SC infusions. The solubility of morphine is approximately 62.5mg/ml (Drug Information, 1987) and is usually mixed in concentrations no greater than 50mg/ml. Not only can more milligrams of diamorphine than morphine be concentrated in each millilitre, but each milligram of diamorphine provides approximately 2–3 times more pain relief than each milligram of morphine. For example, the equianalgesic chart (Table 4.10) shows that 3–5mg of IM diamorphine equals 10mg IM of morphine.

4. When rapid absorption and quicker onset of action are needed by the parenteral or spinal route. Methadone, pethidine, and fentanyl are more lipid-soluble than morphine and are therefore more quickly absorbed into the spinal system. Fentanyl given IM or IV has a more rapid onset than other narcotics and it might be more desirable as premedication for a brief painful procedure, e.g. bone marrow aspiration. It only has, however, a short duration of action.
5. The need for a drug of longer duration of action. Methadone and sustained-release morphine provide a longer duration of action than morphine. A longer interval between doses may be desirable, e.g. to allow the patient to sleep through the night uninterrupted and for children and young adults who tend to metabolize narcotics rapidly. This group of drugs is discussed below.

Narcotics of long duration. Oral narcotics that provide a long duration of action are methadone and sustained-release morphine (Wilkes, 1984; Hanks et al, 1987). They may be especially appropriate for the person with chronic pain who is (1) inconvenienced by a 3–4 hour regime with the short-acting narcotics, i.e. pethidine, morphine, and diamorphine, or (2) overwhelmed by the numbers or frequency of tablets prescribed.

Because their cumulative analgesic effect could be even more pronounced, methadone and sustained-release morphine should be used with caution in the elderly (see Chapter 9 for elaboration) and in those patients with liver dysfunction.

Narcotics of long duration, i.e. methadone and sustained-release morphine, should not be escalated rapidly. Therefore a short-acting narcotic, or "rescue" analgesic, is often given along with the long-acting narcotic, either on a regular basis while the long-acting narcotic is being gradually increased or PRN for sudden increases in pain (breakthrough pain).

Specifics about sustained-release morphine tablets. Sustained-release morphine formulations have a long duration of action, i.e. 8–12 hours, without the cumulative effects of methadone. Side effects are essentially the same as those seen with the regular immediate-release morphine.

Suggestions for converting to sustained-release morphine. Several approaches may be used. A common approach is to stabilize the patient's pain on oral immediate-release morphine before beginning the sustained-release preparation. To do this:

- Use an equianalgesic table to convert the present total 24-hour narcotic intake to an equianalgesic dose of oral immediate-release morphine. (See p. 109 for guidelines for changing from IM or IV to oral.)
- Give immediate-release morphine 4-hourly, adjusting dose and interval as needed according to the individual's response.
- When good pain control is achieved on immediate-release morphine, calculate the total 24-hour dose and divide into 2 doses 12-hourly for sustained-release morphine. Although theoretically the initial calculation should work for most patients, it may not always. Be prepared to adjust the dose up or down depending on the individual patient's response. While 12-hour intervals are appropriate for many patients' pain, even after dose adjustments, some patients may need to take sustained-release morphine at 8-hour intervals.

Remember: With any change in narcotic the patient must be observed closely and changes made in dose and interval according to the individual's response.

Other important aspects of using sustained-release morphine are:
- Use a rescue analgesic, or short-acting narcotic, e.g. immediate-release morphine, for breakthrough pain, pain that occurs between dosing intervals. To calculate the rescue dose of immediate-release morphine, consider what the 4-hourly dose would be if the patient were using immediate-release morphine. For example, if the patient is taking sustained-release morphine 120mg 12-hourly, the four hourly dose is 40 mg. A rescue dose is usually 50–100% of this.
- Sustained-release morphine formulations are not appropriate for PRN dosing, or incidental or break-through pain. They have a slow onset and potentially longer duration of action than the incidental or breakthrough pain.

- A patient may initially receive only 8 hours of relief or may need additional doses of short-acting morphine in between. Increasing the dose may allow a 12-hour interval and no need for PRN rescue doses. However, do not escalate a long-acting narcotic rapidly. Use rescue doses of short duration while the sustained-release dose is gradually increased.
- Sustained-release morphine should not be given more frequently than 8-hourly.
- For patients who have difficulty swallowing, choose the formulation with the smaller-size tablet. Consider sustained-release liquid formulations which have recently become available.
- Do not break, crush, or allow patient to chew sustained-release tablets. If patient has problems swallowing tablets or has an N-G tube, use a liquid morphine preparation.

Methadone is less sedating than morphine and has a longer period of action. In prolonged use, methadone should not be administered more often than twice daily, to avoid the risk of accumulation and opioid overdosage. Methadone is not commonly used in the United Kingdom for pain relief.

Potential problems with pethidine

Although pethidine is one of the most frequently prescribed IM narcotics, several characteristics of this drug make its popularity questionable. Compared with other parenteral narcotics, pethidine is:

a. Shorter acting (Beaver, 1980). Although there are no studies to document how short acting pethidine is, the authors and many other clinicians find that it often lasts only 2–3 hours (Jaffe and Martin, 1985; Marks and Sachar, 1973; Westring, 1974). Others disagree (Foley, 1987). Research does show that duration of action may be even shorter in younger people. The younger the patient, the shorter the duration of action tends to be (Kaiko, 1980). Smokers may also experience a short duration of action (Jick, 1974).

b. Irritating to tissue, with the potential for severe muscle tissue fibrosis with frequent injections (Beaver, 1980; Jaffe and Martin, 1985) and must be given IM, not SC.

c. Responsible for neuropsychiatric effects, such as disorientation, bizarre feelings, and hallucinations. These occur frequently with parenteral pethidine, while they occur less frequently with morphine (Miller and Jick, 1978).

d. More toxic, due to the accumulation of an active metabolite, nor-pethidine, which is a CNS stimulant (Kaiko et al, 1983; Szeto et al, 1977).

e. Prescribed in inadequate oral doses, resulting in poor analgesia. An oral dose of 300mg is needed to provide the equianalgesic effect of 75mg IM but is not recommended due to greater amounts of nor-pethidine that would result. *Remember that pethidine 50mg oral is about equivalent to the analgesic effect of 650mg aspirin* (refer to the equianalgesic chart, Table 4.4). The result is often poor pain control with the oral route of administration, as oral pethidine is not well absorbed.

Based on the above data, when pethidine IM is chosen to relieve pain the result is that a neurotoxic, irritating substance with neuropsychiatric effects must be administered frequently for analgesia. *Clearly there is limited use for this drug as an analgesic for ongoing pain.* In fact in two recent publications on analgesic drug therapy, pethidine is listed as "not recommended" in the equianalgesic charts (American Pain Society, 1987, p. 4; Foley and Inturrisi, 1987, p. 214).

Cause, symptoms, and treatment of pethidine-induced toxicity. This discussion concerns toxicity, not side effects. The side effects of pethidine are those that occur with most other narcotics: respiratory depression, sedation, and hypotension. The probable cause of pethidine-induced toxicity is the accumulation of nor-pethidine, an active metabolite of pethidine. Nor-pethidine is a CNS stimulant, whereas pethidine is a CNS depressant. If nor-pethidine accumulates, symptoms of neurotoxicity occur and increase in the following order:

• Shaky feelings.
• Hand tremors.
• Twitches.
• Multifocal myoclonus (muscle jerks).
• Grand mal seizures (Kaiko et al, 1983).

Patients at risk of accumulating nor-pethidine. Patients most at risk of accumulating nor-pethidine and developing toxic symptoms are probably those who are exposed to any one of the following:

• Six days or longer on pethidine with daily doses of 300mg, e.g. 50mg given six times in 24 hours, or 75mg given four times in 24 hours, or more (Kaiko et al, 1983). However, there are unpublished reports of seizures following one dose.

• High, frequent doses to relieve pain of any type, e.g. sickle cell crisis, cancer, terminal illness, or pancreatitis. One study reported a total of 14 instances of grand mal seizures in 7 patients with sickle cell disease who received pethidine (Tang et al, 1980).

• Renal dysfunction (Kaiko et al, 1983; Szeto et al, 1977). However, patients with normal renal function are also at risk (Mauro et al, 1986). In one study of 67 patients, 5 patients who showed severe pethidine toxicity with myoclonus and seizures had no evidence of renal problems (Kaiko et al, 1983).

Nursing interventions related to pethidine-induced toxicity. Unfortunately, pethidine is a most frequently prescribed parenteral narcotic. Nursing responsibilities related to patients for whom pethidine is prescribed are outlined below. A knowledge of research-based literature, e.g. Kaiko et al, 1983 will be useful to support your care.

1. Patients already receiving pethidine:

   a. Be alert to early signs of neurotoxicity, e.g. tremors, twitching, or jerking, or patient's report of being awakened by involuntary jerking movements.

   b. Inform the doctor should any of these symptoms occur.

   c. Obtain copy of the Kaiko et al article to document your concern.

   d. Be aware that the following facts will influence decisions on management:

      • It takes about 5 half-lives for a drug to be eliminated from the body.

      • Pethidine is a CNS depressant with a half-life of about 3 hours.

      • Nor-pethidine is a CNS stimulant with a half-life of about 15 hours or more. Therefore avoid simply decreasing the pethidine since the CNS depressant will leave the body much sooner than the CNS stimulant, leaving the patient at risk of increasing neuro-excitation, including seizures.

- Naloxone, a narcotic antagonist, will eliminate pethidine but not nor-pethidine. If these were given, symptoms of neuro-excitation would worsen and a seizure might occur.

  e. An equianalgesic dose of another pure narcotic agonist may be continued at the same dose for about 3 days to allow time for nor-pethidine to be eliminated from the body.

  f. A CNS depressant may be added to prevent seizures until nor-pethidine has been eliminated.

2. Patients who are at risk of accumulating nor-pethidine but who have not yet received pethidine:

  a. Be alert to those situations that place the patient at risk of accumulating nor-pethidine:
    - High, frequent doses.
    - Renal dysfunction.
    - Prolonged narcotic treatment, e.g. 6 days or longer.

  b. Suggest that pethidine not be given and that another narcotic agonist, e.g. morphine, or narcotic agonist-antagonist, e.g. buphrenorphine, be used.

Alternatives to IM pethidine. The following drugs are less irritating to the tissue, longer acting, and less toxic:
- Morphine IM or SC.
- Diamorphine IM or SC.

Mixed agonist-antagonist narcotics

Drugs in this group are called "agonists" because they bind to opioid receptors to produce analgesia, and "antagonists" because they also partially reverse the effects of pure narcotic agonists (i.e. morphine, pethidine). Refer to Chapter 3 for discussion of these analgesics and the clinical application of the multiple opioid receptor theory.
- Nalbuphine IM, IV (not widely used in the UK).
- Buprenorphine IM, IV, sublingual.
- Pentazocine IM, IV, oral (no longer widely used in the UK).

Buprenorphine is also a narcotic agonist-antagonist, but it is unlike the others in this group. It does not antagonize at the mu site except at very high doses or in very physically dependent persons. Also, although respiratory depression is rare with this drug, it is the only one in which narcotic-induced respiratory depression cannot be completely reversed by naloxone.

Some confusion about the narcotic agonist-antagonists exists because government regulations often do not classify them as narcotics, or controlled substances. However, pharmacologically they are narcotics, or opioids.

Potential problems with narcotic agonist-antagonists. If the narcotic antagonist property of buprenorphine is not understood, it may cause the following difficulties.

It may precipitate withdrawal in a person who has been on pure narcotic agonists for a week or more. After a course of narcotic agonists, the person may become physically dependent, i.e. if the narcotic is abruptly discontinued, the person experiences withdrawal. Narcotics with an antagonist property may precipitate withdrawal by abruptly blocking the action of the pure agonist. Therefore narcotic agonist-antagonists must be used with caution after a person has been on pure narcotics for a week or longer. A physically dependent person may be carefully switched from a narcotic agonist to an agonist-antagonist, but it may take up to 10 days or longer of small, daily decreases in the agonist accompanied by small, daily additions of the agonist-antagonist.

Given along with pure narcotics, they may eventually antagonize analgesia from the pure narcotics. Initially, giving the two narcotic groups together may be additive, and it is difficult to predict when the agonist-antagonist will begin to reverse analgesia of the agonist. Early in narcotic therapy, a decision should be made about which group of narcotics will be used. A person can be switched from a narcotic agonist-antagonist to a narcotic agonist without much difficulty, except for some possible initial decrease in analgesia until the agonist-antagonist is excreted.

Benefits of the narcotic agonist-antagonists. All three of the narcotic agonist-antagonists (buprenorphine, nalbuphine, and pentazocine) have a ceiling on the amount of respiratory depression they cause. Beyond a certain dose, additional respiratory depression does not occur. Therefore an increase in dose usually results in more pain relief without more respiratory depression. There is, however, a ceiling to their analgesic effects too.

However, nalbuphine appears to be the drug of choice if limited respiratory depression is desired when high doses are needed for pain relief. As mentioned above, buprenorphine-induced respiratory depression, although rare, is not completely reversed with naloxone. Further, high doses of pentazocine are likely to cause psychotomimetic effects. By contrast, respiratory depression from nalbuphine can be reversed by naloxone, and psychotomimetic effects are rare, although sedation occurs. Situations in which nalbuphine is recommended include the following:

- Post-operative narcotic-induced respiratory depression. The strong antagonist effect of nalbuphine can be used to reverse unwanted side effects of pure narcotics, particularly respiratory depression, without reducing analgesia. (The other narcotic agonist-antagonists do not seem to have a strong enough antagonist effect at the mu site to be used in this manner. For an explanation of the mu, kappa, and sigma opioid receptor sites, see p. 49). To reverse respiratory depression from a pure narcotic agonist, the usual adult dose of nalbuphine is 2–3mg IV every 2–3 minutes up to 9mg (Magruder, Delaney and Difazio, 1982).
- Post-operative pain relief. There is a ceiling on the amount of respiratory depression beyond a dose of 10–20mg IM, and it is supportive of blood pressure.
- Wound/burn debridement. Up to 1mg/kg can be given without significant risk of respiratory depression or psychotomimetic effects.

Summary of important pharmacological facts

Important pharmacological facts summarized here include reminders about choice of strong narcotic, avoidance of pethidine, and use of narcotic agonist-antagonists. These are reflected in the patient example on this page.

Although morphine, diamorphine and methadone are equally capable of relieving severe pain, morphine is usually the drug of choice. It is available for administration via more routes than the others, including IV, IM, rectal, oral, and spinal. It is also formulated in sustained-release tablets, permitting a long interval between doses without the potential problems posed by the cumulative effects of the longer-acting narcotics, e.g. methadone. However, morphine is not always the drug of choice. Diamorphine may be a better choice than morphine when high doses are required SC or IV, since diamorphine can be prepared in higher concentrations than morphine.

Unfortunately, a most frequently prescribed injectable narcotic is pethidine. There is great risk of toxicity from accumulation of its active metabolite, nor-pethidine.

Narcotic agonist-antagonists have the advantage of a ceiling on respiratory depression. Currently, three are marketed in Great Britain, buprenorphine, nalbuphine, and pentazocine (although nalbuphine and pentazocine are not widely used). Because buprenorphine, nalbuphine, and pentazocine partially antagonize the effects of pure narcotic agonists, they must be used with caution when pure narcotic agonists are being given. These three narcotic agonist-antagonists may reverse the analgesia of pure narcotic agonists, or they may precipitate withdrawal-like symptoms in the patient who has become physically dependent. Physical dependence may occur after a pure narcotic agonist has been administered for a week or longer.

The following patient example illustrates application of the above summary.

Patient Example

Mr F., 61 years old, is terminally ill with metastatic cancer and is being cared for at home. Until yesterday his pain was well controlled with codeine 30mg and paracetamol 500mg (Tylex) plus 500mg paracetamol every 4 hours, with an occasional additional Tylex, especially at bedtime so he could sleep through the night without waking with pain. Increasing the codeine dose might relieve his pain, but there is usually a ceiling to the analgesia that can be obtained by increasing codeine doses, and at high doses codeine often causes nausea and is very constipating. He already takes daily medication to prevent constipation. Further, with progressive disease his pain probably will continue to escalate and soon require even stronger analgesia.

Now is the time to switch to a narcotic that may be used for the remainder of his life—a strong narcotic that can be given orally, with the flexibility of other routes if needed, and with at least a 4-hour duration of action. Following are the reasons for considering or eliminating specific narcotics:

- Pethidine is ruled out mainly because prolonged use increases the risk of pethidine-induced CNS excitability from accumulation of nor-pethidine. It is short acting and also irritating to the tissues if IM or SC routes must be used. For these reasons pethidine is not recommended for chronic cancer pain.

- Narcotic agonist-antagonists, e.g. nalbuphine and buprenorphine are ruled out since the patient probably has developed physical dependence from prolonged use of narcotics, and these drugs could precipitate withdrawal. Only buprenorphine is available in a non-injectable formulation (i.e. sublingual tablet), but nausea and dysphoria may be a problem.
- Choice is narrowed to the following strong narcotics: morphine, diamorphine, methadone.
- Methadone is longer acting than morphine and diamorphine but is not available rectally. The main reason for not selecting methadone is that its long duration of action is due to accumulation, and patients with organ dysfunction due to age or disease (both are possibilities with this patient) may have difficulty eliminating metabolites that cause side effects.
- Morphine and diamorphine are available for all routes of administration and do not accumulate but are relatively short acting.
- Morphine is available in a sustained-release oral formulation that results in a long duration of action without accumulation of metabolites. The sustained-release formulation is a significant reason for choosing morphine over diamorphine.

Decision: Paracetamol 1g 4-hourly is continued, and the patient is begun on sustained-release morphine tablets every 12 hours. The initial dose is calculated by:

1. The total daily dose of codeine (6–7 doses/day × 30mg = 180–210mg/day),
2. Converted to morphine equivalent (200mg codeine oral = 30mg morphine sulphate oral for elderly patient with cancer pain; 180–210mg codeine orally = about 30mg morphine sulphate orally), and
3. Divided into two doses, i.e. 15 mg MST Continus every 12 hours.

The rescue analgesic can be Tylex since the patient has some left and is familiar with its effects, but he must be reminded that it contains paracetamol.

The patient starts at 6:00 p.m. with Tylex plus 500mg paracetamol as usual plus his first dose of MST Continus 15mg. The reason for giving Tylex at the same time as the initial dose of Continus is that initial onset of analgesia for Continus is about 4 hours, so the Tylex will cover the patient until MST takes effect. Other co-adjuvant therapy, e.g. NSAIDs central-acting drugs, will also be considered for appropriate presenting symptoms.

The appropriate route of administration

Adjust the route of drug administration according to the individual patient's needs. These needs would include such considerations as convenience, side effects, and onset of analgesia.

It is also important to consider the method of delivery for a route. Patient-controlled analgesia (PCA) is a method that usually refers to the patient's self-administration of IV boluses of narcotic using a special infusion pump. However, a broader and more useful definition includes all drug routes that allow the patient to be in control.

Therefore PCA evolves into a concept that includes the patient's self-administration of any analgesic drugs and other forms of pain relief by a method that considers safety as well as the patient's ability and willingness to control any or all of the following (McCaffery, 1987b):

- Stopping and starting an on-going form of analgesia.
- Increasing or decreasing the ongoing amount.
- Initiating an occasional increase in relief above the ongoing amount.

The concept of PCA should be applied to all routes of administration, including oral, IV, SC, and spinal routes.

Oral route

The oral route has these advantages:

- Convenient and easy to administer.
- Allows mobility and independence.

Indications for the oral route

- Mild to severe pain.
- If patient can swallow.
- If nausea and vomiting can be controlled.

Misconception: Moderate or severe pain will only be controlled with IM, SC or IV routes of administration.
Correction: Oral narcotics can relieve severe pain if the appropriate drug is chosen, if the doses are high enough and if a preventive approach is used.

Guidelines and recommendations for oral route

Two *guidelines* for controlling moderate to severe pain with oral narcotics are:

1. Use a preventive approach to stay on top of the pain. This is especially important because the onset of oral analgesia is slower than that of IM or IV medication, with the peak effect normally occurring approximately 1.5–2 hours after dosing.
2. Use high enough doses (refer to equianalgesic chart on pp. 84–85). Typically, health-care professionals are accustomed to giving oral narcotics for the relief of mild or moderate pain; therefore they are afraid of the high oral doses needed for severe pain. Re-education is vital and must emphasize equianalgesic doses and the ratio of drug needed depending on the route.

Recommendations for using the oral route include:

- Tablets are usually the first option for administration.
- Liquid may be considered if there is difficulty swallowing or if titration involves very small amounts.
- Use a pain continuous assessment sheet (discussed on pp. 37–41) to determine safety and effectiveness of analgesics. Adjust dose up or down depending on these findings.

Method of administration: oral PCA. In the home setting, the patient and family commonly control administration of oral narcotics and non-narcotics. While patient control of oral analgesics in the hospital is far less common, it has shown good results. For example, hospitalized patients 1–4 days postoperative were given their own supply of 25 capsules of Co-codamol. They kept this medication at the bedside and charted what they self-administered on a hospital medication sheet. The 26 patients who agreed to self-administer experienced no loss of capsules, no overdosage, and no significant difference in number of Co-codamol taken compared with patients given medication by the nurses; all stated they would prefer to self-administer again (Jones, 1987).

In another report, patients and the health-care team on a postnatal unit expressed satisfaction with a 5-year programme of self-administered pain medication and other routinely prescribed drugs (Anderson and Poole, 1983).

Intramuscular route

Although the intramuscular (IM) route is frequently used for most types of postoperative pain, it is often ineffective for self-administering patients as well as others with severe acute pain such as sickle cell crisis.

Disadvantages of the IM route are:

- IM injections are painful to receive.
- Suitable injection sites may be lacking.
- The patient is usually dependent on someone else for pain relief.
- Preparation and administration are time-consuming. This may prolong the interval between doses, allowing pain to return.
- Repeated injections are impractical for prolonged pain.
- In the immediate postoperative period, absorption of IM narcotics may be especially poor. In one study, pethidine 100mg IM given in the first 4 hours postoperatively provided no pain relief in 8 of 10 patients. Blood concentrations of pethidine showed that absorption was poor at this time, probably due to decreased peripheral circulation (Austin et al, 1980).

Variability in absorption poses a specific danger in the postoperative period when an IM dose is repeated. For instance, as a result of poor absorption, the first IM dose may not provide pain relief for the patient. The dose may be repeated. As circulation improves, the initial dose may be absorbed just as the second dose is taking effect. The result may be a patient who is in pain just before the second dose, and who afterwards is more likely to be sedated or have respiratory depression.

- On an ongoing basis, drug absorption is highly variable and dependent on the following factors: blood flow at the injection site, muscle activity, and the choice of site for injection (Lukacsko, 1987). To promote optimal absorption, the nurse should look for healthy muscle mass that is not painful to the touch, e.g. abscesses, sloughing tissue, or degenerated tissue as in the inactive elderly or emaciated patient. Avoid paralysed muscles, e.g. below level of spinal cord injury, or those that are not exercised, e.g. with bedridden patients.

Appropriate Site for Injections. The four choices of site for injections are the deltoid, ventrogluteal, dorsogluteal, and vastus lateralis muscles.

- Whilst the deltoid site has more rapid absorption, it is small and can only take 0.5ml or less in volume once fully developed.
- The ventrogluteal site is probably the most comfortable and safe, but appears to be least used by nurses.
- The dorsogluteal site is the most commonly used and is safe and effective providing it is fully developed.

- The vastus lateralis site is recommended for large volumes, i.e. up to 5ml providing there is no muscle wasting. (Ref. Pagliaro, A.M. and Pagliaro L.A.: *Pharmacologic Aspects of Nursing*, The C.V. Mosby Co., St Louis 1986.).

Recommendations regarding the IM route

As popular as the IM route is, it is not the ideal one. Recommendations concerning the IM route are:

1. IM is appropriate in the following situations, *only if* IV access is impractical or impossible:
   - Premedication before painful procedures.
   - Bolus dose to get rapid control of the pain, before beginning or resuming prescribed oral doses.
2. If the patient is NBM (nil by mouth) and the IV route is not an option as an alternative to IM injections in your setting, few good choices are left. However, the following suggestions may help maximize the effectiveness of the IM method of administration:
   - For quicker absorption consider the deltoid instead of the gluteal sites. Even if the deltoid muscle is developed enough to be an appropriate site, the volume or choice of medication may need to be changed.

     Pethidine should not be given in the deltoid. It causes local irritation, and frequent injections can cause severe fibrosis of muscle tissue (Jaffe and Martin, 1985). If pethidine is used, request a change to an equianalgesic dose of morphine so that the deltoid may be used.

     Anti-emetics prescribed in combination with a narcotic may cause the volume to be too great to inject into the deltoid, as well as cause local irritation. If so, you can request that the IM anti-emetic be changed to a suppository or transdermal patch; however, the effectiveness of this delivery system may be questionable (Ferris *et al*, 1991; Semple *et al*, 1992).
   - If the deltoid muscle is not an appropriate site for an individual patient and the pain continues to be uncontrolled, talk with the doctor again about switching to the IV route, or consider the rectal, sublingual, or buccal route.

Rectal route

The rectal route is often overlooked, probably because it tends to be socially embarrassing. However, patients often prefer it to the IM route once they discover how much easier and less painful it is.

Indications for rectal route. The rectal route is desirable when oral medication is not tolerated. Narcotic suppositories such as morphine or oxycodone should be considered instead of IM, SC or IV injections in patients with the following problems:

- Unable to take oral medication because of nausea, vomiting, or difficulty swallowing. In the home, the need to switch back and forth between oral and rectal route can be anticipated and planned for, thereby preventing readmission to the hospital.
- Unconscious with end-stage disease.
- Fear of injections, especially a child.

Limitations of rectal route. The usefulness of the rectal route is limited by:

- Physical conditions that would make this route inappropriate, such as diarrhoea, anal fissures, or low platelet count.
- The dose of narcotic available commercially.

Calculation of dosage for rectal route. There are limited studies on the absorption, distribution, metabolism, and excretion of rectally administered narcotics. The studies that have been done involve a limited number of patients and show wide variations in absorption and plasma concentrations (Ellison and Lewis, 1984; Westerling et al, 1982).

Dosing for this route is mostly based on clinical experience, not on research. In fact there is a lack of controlled studies establishing the equianalgesic doses for oral and rectal routes.

Clinical experience suggests that the dose used by mouth is the same dose recommended for initial rectal administration (Twycross and Lack, 1983), e.g. morphine suppository 20mg rectally 4 hourly may be given initially for pain that was controlled with 20mg oral morphine. Then watch the patient's response, increasing or decreasing the dose. The principle of careful titration and frequent observation of the individual's response is the only way to safely administer a narcotic, regardless of route or dose.

Recommendations for the rectal route

• Anticipate initial patient resistance to this route. Encourage patient to try this route at least once. Establish reason and spend time with patient exploring other options. The patient is usually willing to try it once the reasons have been explained.

• Use the rectal route as an alternative route when oral analgesics cannot be taken, e.g. because of vomiting.

• Instruct patient/family in method of administering the suppository (Pagliaro, 1986).

• Use a flow sheet to assess effectiveness and safety of the suppository.

Sublingual and buccal routes

Regarding these two routes there are mostly anecdotal reports (Hirsh, 1984; Pitorak and Kraus, 1987; Wallace, 1987; Whitman, 1984). Very little research is available (Bell et al, 1985; Cefali et al, 1991; Ellis et al, 1982; Manara et al, 1990; Pannuti et al, 1982; Simpson et al, 1989). Pending more research and clinical experience, we view the sublingual and buccal routes as temporary alternatives until the patient can be stabilized on another route.

Definition:
• Sublingual—tablet or liquid is placed under the tongue.
• Buccal—tablet is placed between: upper lip and gum, *or* cheek and gum.

Both routes have the potential advantage of avoiding the "first-pass" effect seen with the oral route (Payne, 1987a), provided the patient does not inadvertently swallow. A drug taken orally passes from the GI tract to the liver where it can be extensively metabolized, leaving a minimal amount of active drug available to reach the general circulation. The result is that less of the drug circulates, and less of its effect is seen.

The buccal route does not stimulate salivation and may be better tolerated than the sublingual route (Bell *et al*, 1985).

Disadvantages of sublingual compared with buccal are that unpleasant taste may be a problem and salivation can be promoted causing swallowing of the drug, thereby defeating the purpose of this route.

Indications for sublingual and buccal routes. Both routes are suggested for chronic cancer pain (Pitorak and Kraus, 1987; Whitman, 1984) and in one study the buccal route effectively relieved postoperative pain (Bell et al, 1985). Indications for buccal or sublingual are:
• Oral route impossible: difficulty swallowing; vomiting; bowel obstruction; NG tube.
• Parenteral route temporarily impractical.

Recommendations for sublingual and buccal routes. Although more controlled studies are needed for conclusive answers to the considerations listed below (Wilkie, 1987), experience from anecdotal reports is presented here as a guideline:
• Which formulation—tablets or liquid?

Some prefer tablets over the liquid pain medication because there is less chance of swallowing them (Pitorak and Kraus, 1987).

Others recommend liquid, i.e. morphine solution, as an effective and safe formulation for an SL analgesic (Wallace, 1987).

In the UK, phenazocine and dextromoramide are the two drugs most commonly given by the sublingual route. Further developments in availability may eventually promote the choice of sublingual or buccal route over oral.
• Which route—sublingual or buccal?

Rate and extent of delivery to the general circulation (bioavailability) of buccal morphine is reported to be 40–50% greater than for IM morphine (Bell et al, 1985). However, this was reported in only one study and contrasts with the bioavailability of sublingual liquid morphine, which is less than 10% of that after IM injection (Payne, 1987a).

The buccal route poses less of a problem with swallowing and unpleasant taste.
• Withhold other oral intake to ensure absorption.

After sublingual administration, withhold food, fluids, or other medications for 5–15 minutes (Pitorak and Kraus, 1987; Wallace, 1987).

Narcotic infusion: IV and SC routes

The IV route provides the most rapid onset of analgesia with the shortest duration of action. Analgesic effects can be felt within 6 to 10 minutes, but the duration of analgesia from a bolus dose may be as little as 45 minutes to 1 hour. Therefore with an IV bolus the patient experiences immediate relief but it diminishes quickly. For the vast majority of patients, prescriptions for an IV bolus 3–4 hourly will result in the return of pain long before the next dose is given.

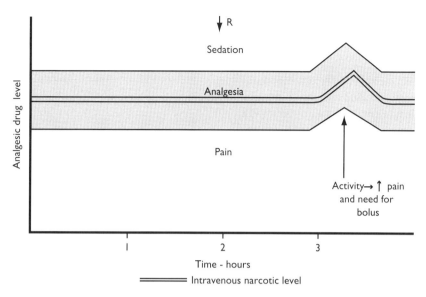

Fig. 4.4 Illustration of the value of continuous IV narcotic infusion to maintain a steady level of analgesia for on-going, relatively stable pain, and the value of a patient-controlled bolus to provide increased analgesia for increased incidental pain. Refer to Fig. 4.1 for explanation of this diagram.

In contrast, a continuous infusion of narcotic, either SC or IV, maintains a constant level of pain relief by delivering a continuous dose into the bloodstream. Figure 4.4 illustrates this concept.

It is common to administer single or separate injections or continuous infusions of medication via the SC route. Continuous infusion of narcotic is often used for prolonged pain in ambulatory patients at home, in part because of the ease with which the route can be accessed.

> **KEY POINT:** IV boluses are appropriate for rapid control of severe pain and for establishing the hourly dose for IV continuous infusion. Continuous infusion is appropriate for a steady level of analgesia to maintain control of pain.

Indications for the use of IV or SC narcotic infusion. For on-going pain, IV or SC infusion is an option that should be considered. However, it should be recognized that the use of continuous IV background narcotic infusions in conjunction with IV boluses, e.g. in PCA, is no longer advocated in the UK. (Royal College of Surgeons,

1990). Indications for the use of IV or SC narcotic infusion are:

- Oral route is unmanageable, i.e. nausea, GI obstruction, difficulty swallowing or breathing.
- Regular oral or rectal routes provide inadequate analgesia. *Note:* First be sure that doses by these routes are high enough and frequent enough.
- Immediate relief is needed. Extreme anxiety from unrelieved pain can increase a person's perception of pain or make pain intolerable, which in turn promotes a cycle of increased anxiety and pain. By providing analgesia *quickly*, continuous infusions break this cycle and eliminate the fearful anticipation of pain.

Misconceptions associated with IV/SC narcotic infusion. Fears and misconceptions associated with the administration of IV/SC narcotics can prevent this route from being considered and used effectively.

Misconception: IV/SC narcotic infusion is only to be used for the patient who is dying.
Correction: This route may be appropriate for postoperative pain (Rutter et al, 1980), pain in severe burns (Wermeling et al, 1986), sickle cell crisis (Cole et al, 1986; Ives and Guerra, 1987), and acute pancreatitis.

Avoid limiting the use of IV/SC infusion to certain diseases or to end-stage conditions only. Instead assess each individual pain situation and apply "the indications for use" discussed above as guidelines.

Misconception: Once the patient is on IV/SC narcotics, a return to oral is difficult and unlikely.
Correction: Controlling a person's pain with IV/SC infusion does not interfere with switching back to the oral route when the pain is stabilized (Wright, 1981).

Not knowing how to change from IV/SC continuous infusion to the oral route may be another reason why the latter route is not readily considered for situations where the pain will decrease.

Changing to another route can be successful if equianalgesic doses are used and the person's individual response is assessed using a flow sheet. Guidelines for changing routes are discussed on p. 109.

Misconception: IV/SC infusion may enhance a patient's chance of becoming addicted.
Correction: There is no evidence to support this statement.

Research shows that addiction rarely occurs in people who are taking narcotics for the relief of pain (Porter and Jicks, 1980). In fact the overwhelming majority of patients stop taking narcotics when the pain stops (see pp. 76–77). For example, no evidence of addictive behaviour was observed in 76 episodes of sickle cell vaso-occlusive crisis in 38 children and adolescents treated via continuous IV infusion (Cole et al, 1986).

Recommendations for IV or SC infusion. Following are guidelines for safe and effective use of infusions of narcotics IV or SC (Bruera et al, 1987a; Coyle et al, 1986; McGuire and Wright, 1984; Payne, 1987a; Portenoy, 1987a):

1. Choice of narcotic is usually morphine. However, diamorphine may be used for continuous SC infusion when a high concentration of drug in a volume is needed.

At present there are no studies comparing the effectiveness and side effects of various narcotics administered by infusion. Pethidine should be avoided especially in the SC route because of its irritation to tissue and its toxicity. Prolonged use or high doses of pethidine may result in CNS excitation and dysphoria (Kaiko et al, 1983) (see pp. 89–91 for further discussion). This toxicity is particularly important to note for the treatment of sickle cell crisis pain for which pethidine is unfortunately frequently used (Tang et al, 1980).

It is suggested that infusions with drugs having a long half-life,* i.e. methadone, may result in delayed side effects as plasma levels of the drug can continue to increase long after pain relief is reached. Therefore infusion with drugs with a short half-life, i.e. morphine or diamorphine, is preferred especially for debilitated or elderly patients who have difficulty eliminating a drug (Bruera et al, 1987a; Portenoy, 1987a).

2. Calculate the appropriate concentration of drug to fluid. For continuous IV infusion, approximately 60ml/hr or less of fluid is appropriate for most adults. For instance, 1mg morphine per 5ml may be appropriate if the patient is receiving 4–6mg morphine/hr; this would be 20–30ml/hr. However, this concentration would result in too much fluid, 500ml/hr, for a patient receiving 100mg morphine/hr.

For continuous SC infusion, the volume of fluid absorbed without irritation into the SC tissue is limited (Coyle et al, 1986). When a patient is cachectic and the tissue is unable to absorb much volume, increasing the narcotic concentration can provide small volumes of fluid for effective absorption. Morphine and diamorphine can both be reconstituted at even higher concentrations than those commercially available; morphine can be reconstituted at 50mg/ml; diamorphine in concentrations of more than 100mg/ml. Refer to p. 101 for further discussion of fluid volume as it pertains to site irritation in continuous SC infusion.

3. Increases or decreases in dosage are made in terms of percentages (%) instead of a fixed number of milligrams. Percentages allow adjustments to be in proportion to the original dose and can be widely applied regardless of the dose.

For example, is an increase of 5mg/hr of morphine appropriate? It may be appropriate for a patient receiving continuous infusion at 20mg/hr. However, for the patient receiving an infusion at 150mg/hr, this increase is only a small percentage of the dose and may have little analgesic effect. Instead, a guideline that

---

*Half-life: The time it takes a drug to fall to half of its plasma concentration. It takes approximately five half-lives for a drug to be completely eliminated from the body.

suggests increasing morphine by 20%, for example, is preferred to stating the number of milligrams. This promotes proportionate titrations regardless of the route.

4. Use a pain continuous assessment sheet (blank form on p. 38) to determine safety and effectiveness of dosage (example on p. 39). A flow sheet provides data in a format that allows quick scanning for the patient's respiratory function and pain rating. It can be a particularly helpful tool to all members of the health-care team when fear and concern result in hesitancy to try a specific drug, route or dosage.

Dosages may vary widely. Most of the time, patients with severe pain obtain relief from "usual" or initial, "recommended" doses, but the literature clearly shows that pain control in some patients requires titrating up to unusually high doses. Examples of high doses follow:

High doses for continuous IV infusions:
- 4–480mg/hr morphine equivalent (Portenoy et al, 1986).
- 440mg/hr morphine (Lo and Coleman, 1986).
- 80mg/hr morphine in a child (Miser et al, 1980).
- 1568mg/hr morphine in teenager alert and talking with family (Miser et al, 1986).

High doses for continuous SC infusions:
- 3.5–97mg/hr morphine (Coyle et al, 1986).
- 15mg/hr morphine (Campbell et al, 1983).

5. The actual amount by which a dose is increased or decreased is determined by finding a dose that relieves pain to the patient's satisfaction with minimal side effects. This is done by using a flow sheet and looking at the following patient responses in consecutive order:

- First, respiratory function, usually rate.
- Second, pain rating, e.g. on 0–10 scale (0 = no pain, 10 = worst pain).
- Third, based on the above information, determine whether to increase or decrease the number of milligrams of analgesic and at what percentage, e.g. 10%, 50%, 100%.

Because patients' responses to analgesics are so individual, there are no easy formulas that give the "right percentage." However general guidelines for increases might be 10% if pain is almost controlled, 50% if pain is partially controlled, and 100% if there is no pain relief. No matter what percentage is chosen, it is vital to assess this adjustment immediately. Document the patient's response in the flow sheet so that further increases or decreases can be made without the patient enduring long painful periods between titrations. If a conservative dose increase is chosen, e.g. from 10% to 20%, for a patient who is rating pain at 8 on a 0–10 scale, realize that you will probably need to (1) increase at more frequent intervals than if you began with a more liberal dose, (2) anticipate that the total percentage increase may be 50% to 100%.

6. In the general guidelines or policy for continuous infusion, avoid a specific respiratory rate at which the infusion should be stopped or altered, e.g. do not specify "If respirations are below 14/min, stop the infusion."

Each patient's average respiration rate is different, so it is not appropriate to state a set rate in a written procedure that applies to all patients. Instead the health-care team decides for *each individual situation* at which respiration rate the infusion rate is changed.

7. If possible, treat respiratory depression by decreasing the infusion flow rate instead of using naloxone. If not titrated slowly, naloxone reverses all analgesia and can result in total return of pain. Of course, treatment of respiratory depression must be individualized in every case.

Calculation of initial doses for IV narcotic infusion. Each individual patient's response to a dose of medication is highly variable. Therefore the guidelines below are suggested as a *starting point* to determine hourly infusion rates (Lukacsko, 1987; McCaffery, 1987b). Adjustments can then be made after the onset (within 10 minutes) or peak effect (within 20 minutes) based on the patient's pain rating and an evaluation of side effects.

Hourly infusion rate. Use the equianalgesic chart, Table 4.10.

• **PO to IV using same narcotic.** For the patient who has been on an oral narcotic that can be used IV:

a. Calculate the 24-hour oral narcotic dose.
b. Convert this 24-hour dose to the equivalent IM dose using the equianalgesic chart. Based on clinical experience, many consider the IM and IV dose to be equianalgesic (Portenoy, 1987a). However, some recommend using half the IM dose for the IV dose (American Pain Society, 1987; Foley, 1982). To date,

there is no research comparing equivalencies of IV doses with other parenteral routes.

c. Divide by 24 to arrive at the hourly IV continuous infusion dose and set the infusion accordingly.

Note: This conversion method is intended to provide the *same analgesia* as with the original narcotic. If the patient was not comfortable with the original dose, then increase the dose estimated for IV infusion. Remember, the equianalgesic chart is only a *guideline*. So the initial dose is always an educated guess. The vital step in this process is *consistent assessment* with titrations made up or down according to the patient's pain rating and respiratory status.

• **IM to IV using same narcotic**. If the patient has been on intermittent IM or SC narcotic and the same narcotic can be given IV:

a. Calculate the 24-hour IM/SC dose.

b. Divide by 24 to obtain the hourly IV continuous infusion dose and set the infusion accordingly.

• **Oral, IM, SC to IV using a different narcotic.** If the patient is changed to a different narcotic when switching from oral, IM, SC to IV continuous infusion, use the equianalgesic chart to:

a. Calculate the total 24-hour dose of the present narcotic and convert it to a 24-hour IV dose of the new narcotic.

b. Start with one-half or two-thirds of the calculated 24-hour IV dose. This is recommended because tolerance may have developed with the previous narcotic, but it may not be totally present when a new narcotic is started. This approach avoids possible overdose with the new narcotic. Be prepared to increase the dose quickly if this lower equianalgesic dose is not effective or to decrease it if it is too much.

• **Continuous IV infusion if no previous narcotic.** If the patient has not been on any narcotics:

a. In an adult, start with a bolus of morphine 2–5mg IV or diamorphine 1–2.5mg IV. Repeat bolus every 10 minutes until pain is controlled unless respiratory rate drops to an unacceptable level.

b. Calculate the cumulative bolus doses/hr and immediately start the hourly rate of infusion based on this number.

Calculation of initial doses for SC narcotic infusion.
Each individual patient's response to narcotics is highly variable; therefore the guidelines below are suggested as a starting point for SC infusion.

• To calculate the initial doses for infusion, follow the same guidelines as for IV infusion (see p. 98). However, unlike the IV route there is no debate about SC doses being equianalgesic with IM doses. Also, some clinicians suggest an initial bolus dose equivalent to 2 hours of the infusion rate (Bruera et al, 1987a).

Since the onset of analgesia is much longer for SC doses than for IV, escalating doses by the SC route takes considerably longer. For example, if morphine 5mg is given IV, the analgesic effect will be known in about 10 minutes. However, if morphine 5mg is given SC, the analgesic effect may not occur for 60 minutes or longer.

Special considerations regarding SC narcotic infusion

This route can deliver a continuous infusion of narcotic into the SC tissue using a portable infusion pump. It offers an alternative to IV infusion for ambulatory patients. However, for *rapid* control of severe pain where frequent boluses and/or changes in dose are needed, SC continuous infusion may not be the route of choice. Instead, the IV route provides immediate onset of action and is ideal in this instance. SC continuous infusion is particularly useful for prolonged administration when a parenteral route other than IV is needed.

The *advantages* of using SC continuous infusion are (Bruera et al, 1987a; Coyle et al, 1986; Payne, 1987a):

• Avoids repetitive IM or SC injections.

• Avoids need for IV access. This is particularly helpful in home-care situations, or for situations involving adults or children in whom it is difficult to maintain chronic IV access.

• Provides a continuous level of analgesia.

• Promotes patient mobility. A portable infusion pump allows patients to ambulate and go about their daily activities.

• Is less frightening for the health-care team, patients, and families. Unlike IV continuous infusion, this route does not involve needles inserted directly into veins resulting in almost immediate absorption of the drug. Patients and families readily learn insertion of an SC needle.

Although one disadvantage may be the slower onset of action when compared with the IV route, the *primary disadvantage* is a limitation to the amount of fluid the SC tissue can absorb. If rapidly escalating doses are needed and require large volumes of fluid, this route is often discontinued because the tissue cannot absorb the volume. At this time there is no research that addresses the ideal volume of fluid to use for effective absorption. One clinical report noted local irritation when volumes greater than 1ml/hr were used (Coyle et al, 1986). Another noted that a volume up to 10ml/hr could be administered without irritation or pain at the site of infusion (Bruera et al, 1987a).

Following are *recommendations* for initiating and maintaining the SC continuous infusion route (Bruera et al, 1987a; Coyle et al, 1986):

• Selecting site for SC continuous infusion. Any SC site can be used on a rotating basis. The abdomen, subclavicular area, and the anterior chest wall are areas to consider first since they allow free movement of the patient's arms and legs. In one study of 17 children, the injection site was the thigh (Miser et al, 1983).

• Rotating sites for SC continuous infusion. The infusion site should be inspected regularly for signs of irritation, i.e. swelling, redness, leakage from the site, and the site changed if needed. The patient or family member can, for example, be instructed to inspect the site in the morning before dressing and in the evening when undressing for bed.

• One study of 45 patients with a total of 119 SC insertions for continuous infusion of narcotics reported that the frequency with which sites needed to be changed varied from 1 to 29 days (Brenneis et al, 1986). Other than this there are no controlled studies examining frequency of site changes, but descriptive reports include site changes every 48 hours (Campbell et al, 1983; Sheehan and Sauerbier, 1986); every 24–48 hours (Miser et al, 1983); every 7 days unless symptomatic, then as often as needed (Coyle et al, 1986); and only when showing signs of irritation at the site (Moss, 1986).

Coyle et al (1986) reported increased irritation at the infusion site when the volume of fluid required was greater than 1ml/hr. In those instances, changing the needle site daily to an opposite side of the body was an effective preventive measure.

• Handling breakthrough pain. If breakthrough pain occurs despite dose adjustments, poor absorption at that particular site may be the problem. Changing the infusion site may re-establish analgesia without increasing the dosage (Coyle et al, 1986).

• Increasing patient/family willingness to maintain SC continuous infusion. This is a vital factor to evaluate before considering the continuous SC route. Instructions on pump management and site care along with a contact person to call for help can ease some of the initial anxiety.

• Reassuring patient and family. Explain that another route can be substituted at any time if this one does not work.

Spinal route*

Narcotics for spinal analgesia are presently administered in two ways: (1) into the epidural space and (2) into the subarachnoid space (Figure 4.5). In the past, these routes have most commonly been used to administer anaesthetics for regional anaesthesia, e.g. a spinal anaesthetic.

Analgesia by the spinal route is the result of the drug's direct effect on the opioid receptors in the spinal cord, rather than supraspinally in the brain.

When systemic narcotics, i.e. oral or parenteral, are given, CNS side effects may be seen such as sedation and disorientation. The hope with spinal narcotic administration is that the drug will remain only at the spinal level and not ascend supraspinally (above the spine) to brain centres responsible for central side effects. Even though it is now known that small amounts of spinal narcotics do reach these supraspinal levels, fewer side effects are seen with this route than with the systemic administration of narcotics.

Purpose and limitations of this section on spinal route. "Few areas of clinical research have exploded into practice as rapidly as this method [spinal analgesia] of providing pain relief" (Rawal and Sjostrand, 1986, p. 43). Unfortunately, there are still many unanswered

*The authors would like to thank Judith A. Paice, RN, MS, Assistant Professor and Acting Coordinator, Oncology Graduate Program, College of Nursing, Rush University; Oncology Clinical Nurse Specialist, Rush Presbyterian-St. Luke's Medical Center, Chicago, Illinois, for her review of the spinal route section, helpful comments, and for supplying the Patient Example.

Fig. 4.5 Catheter placement for epidural and intrathecal routes for administration of analgesia.
Adapted from Moulin, DE, and Coyle, N: Spinal opioid analgesics and local anaesthetics in the management of chronic cancer pain. *J Pain*, 1: 79–86, Spring 1986.

questions as to the role of spinal analgesia for acute and chronic pain. However, nurses everywhere are finding themselves monitoring these patients and in some instances administering the analgesic dose.

Because this route of administration is still in its developmental stages, there is simply not enough information to present specific guidelines similar to those presented for the other routes already discussed. We will present general findings to date that will enable the nurse to monitor a patient for safety and effectiveness of the spinal analgesic.

KEY POINT: The spinal route of administration is to be approached with caution. Many aspects about its safety and efficacy are not yet known. At this time, its role should be questioned for patients who obtain effective pain relief from systemic analgesics, e.g. oral, IV, SC.

Possible indications for the use of spinal route
It is vital to understand that more research is needed to define specific indications for using the spinal route to relieve pain. The spinal route has been used for both acute and chronic pain in the following situations:
- Postoperative pain following thoracic, orthopaedic, and abdominal surgery (Leib and Hurtig, 1985; Ozuna and Snyder, 1987; Rawal and Sjostrand, 1986; Stenseth et al, 1985).
- Multiple trauma pain (Rawal and Tandon, 1985).
- Malignant pain (Moulin and Coyle, 1986; Payne, 1987a and b; Penn and Paice, 1987).
- Chronic non-malignant pain as a result of low back conditions, multiple sclerosis, arachnoiditis, herpes zoster, and severe osteoporosis (Auld et al, 1985; Dallas et al, 1987; Penn and Paice, 1987).

It is suggested that the spinal route may be particularly helpful for patients in the following circumstances:

- Acute pain *if*:

  Mobility and full lung expansion immediately postoperatively are particularly important.

  There is compromised pulmonary function.

- Chronic cancer pain *if* (Moulin and Coyle, 1986; Payne, 1987a):

  Pain is unresponsive to pharmacologic approaches that have included aggressive titrations and combinations of narcotics, non-narcotic analgesics, and adjuvant analgesics.

  Pain is poorly controlled with systemic narcotics, e.g. oral, IV, SC, because of dose limiting side effects, e.g. sedation.

  Pain is located bilateral or midline below the midthoracic level, e.g. sacral or perineal pain.

The spinal route is *contra-indicated* in the following situations:

- Bleeding disorder or clotting deficiency.
- Spinal abnormality or obstruction.
- Local skin infection or CNS infection.
- Lack of personnel to provide continuous monitoring in hospital, or lack of patient/family willingness or resources to continue safe care for this route at home.

Analgesia by the spinal route has several potential advantages for postoperative and chronic cancer pain. For analgesia following orthopaedic surgery, Lanz et al (1982) found that the spinal route had the following advantages:

- Pain was of shorter duration and less severe.
- Alertness was heightened.
- Post-operative feeling of well-being was noted.
- Additional need for analgesia and sedation was less.

For cancer pain, longer-lasting analgesia was seen without sedation in patients with dose-limiting responses to systemic drugs (Caballero et al, 1986; Coombs et al, 1984; Malone et al, 1985; Penn and Paice, 1987). The patients were:

- More alert.
- Less depressed.
- Able to resume daily activities when possible.
- Able to be cared for at home.

The long duration of analgesia, e.g. 16 hours or longer after spinal morphine, may also be an advantage. This is in comparison to a range of 3–12 hours for systemic administration, e.g. every 3–4 hours for most oral and IM narcotics and up to 12 hours for sustained-release oral morphine.

Important considerations in choosing spinal route. In spite of favourable results observed with spinal analgesia, it is still important to consider, is this an appropriate route? To answer this question, one must be aware that there is a critical lack of knowledge, research, and clinical experience concerning the spinal route. More information is needed to identify types of pain effectively treated via this route, which drug should be used, and whether it should be administered epidurally or intrathecally. In addition, use of the spinal route requires careful monitoring for an extended period of time after administration to detect potentially life-threatening respiratory depression. Other side effects also occur, but the incidence varies widely. Tolerance to analgesia may develop rapidly via this route, and contamination of the route is obviously extremely dangerous. Following is a discussion of problems and unanswered questions regarding the spinal route.

1. Knowledge about this route is still inadequate. Further clinical studies are needed to address the following controversial issues regarding appropriate selection of patients, drugs, and route (epidural or intrathecal).

a. Which patients and/or types of pain are appropriately treated? While numerous reports document the effectiveness of spinal analgesia for acute and chronic pain, criteria for patients most likely to benefit from this route have not been clearly identified.

In the treatment of labour and delivery pain, the spinal route is controversial (Rawal and Sjostrand, 1986). However, spinal analgesia following caesarean section appears to be effective (Cohen and Woods, 1983; Rimar, 1986). It seems especially appropriate for the breast-feeding mother so that analgesics in the breast milk are avoided.

In the treatment of cancer pain, few definitive criteria exist for patient selection. The spinal route appears to be successful in relieving pain from gynaecological and colorectal tumours. Tumour infiltration of bone seems to be more likely to respond to spinal analgesics than deafferentation pain where there is tumour infiltration of nerve (Moulin and Coyle, 1986).

b. What is the most effective drug for spinal analgesia? Although many narcotics have been tried successfully, morphine is the most researched and the most widely used. However, its properties may not make it the ideal drug for spinal analgesia (Cousins and Mather, 1984; Moulin and Coyle, 1986).

The degree to which a drug is lipid-soluble will directly affect its onset and duration of action. Morphine is the least lipid-soluble; therefore it slowly moves into the spinal cord and blood vessels and may linger in the cerebrospinal fluid. The result is:

• A tendency for morphine to ascend to the brainstem centers responsible for central side effects (Moulin and Coyle, 1986). This may be less of a problem with very small doses given by continuous infusion.

• Delay in the onset of analgesia of 30–60 minutes, and a prolonged duration of action of 12–24 hours (Yaksh, 1981). Continuous infusions of spinal morphine circumvent the problem of delayed onset of analgesia.

The issue of ascension to the brainstem and delayed onset of action may not be as important for chronic continuous infusion via the spinal route. Very small doses of narcotic in a continuous spinal infusion do not appear to ascend supraspinally to the same degree as large doses.

Fentanyl is highly lipid-soluble; pethidine follows closely. Therefore each has a quick analgesic onset but a short duration if given by bolus.

Although the "best" drugs have not yet been identified, ideally they would have a segmental action of analgesia, without migration to the brainstem via the cerebrospinal fluid or systemic circulation (Moulin and Coyle, 1986; Payne, 1987b).

c. Which route is indicated? Intrathecal or epidural administration? Figure 4.5 shows the placement of the catheter tip in relation to the spinal cord for intrathecal and epidural analgesia. Understanding the very different process of distribution via the intrathecal or epidural approach helps explain the difference in the size of dose between the two routes. Although this process is not totally understood, the following pathways are suggested (Cousins and Mather, 1984; Moulin and Coyle, 1986):

• After intrathecal administration, and once in the cerebrospinal fluid, the drug moves gradually upward while diffusing into the spinal cord several centimeters away from the catheter tip. A small amount is also absorbed into surrounding blood vessels.

• After epidural administration, there are several factors that complicate drug distribution. The thick barrier of the dura mater may limit drug diffusion to the cerebrospinal fluid. At the same time, drug uptake into the general circulation and the cerebral venous system may be potentiated by the vast blood supply of the epidural space. Therefore it may be possible for a moderate to large portion of the drug to access the brainstem centers where central side effects are seen.

The variables in these two routes help to explain that the intrathecal dose is smaller than that needed for the epidural dose. Some suggest that the intrathecal route requires about one-tenth of the epidural dose for comparable analgesia (Lukacsko, 1987; Moulin and Coyle, 1986). However, there are no studies to support this. Morgan (1989) provides a comprehensive discussion of this topic.

How this dose compares to the 24-hour equianalgesic dose systemically is also unknown. Some suggest that the 24-hour epidural dose is about one-tenth that required IV or IM per 24 hours; the 24-hour intrathecal dose, about one one-hundredth that required IV or IM per 24 hours (Lukacsko, 1987). Again, while these ratios are cited in the literature, there are presently no controlled studies to support these figures.

The larger the volume of drug injected, the greater the chance of spread to the brainstem where central side effects can occur (Moulin and Coyle, 1986).

2. Careful monitoring is needed following spinal analgesia. Respiratory depression is a potentially life-threatening side effect of this route. Significant respiratory depression, however, has been reported mostly in acute postoperative pain and in patients who are narcotic naive, i.e. lacking tolerance because of no recent narcotic administration (see p. 107 for further discussion of respiratory depression following spinal analgesia).

3. The rapid development of tolerance may be a major limiting factor to the more widespread use of

spinal analgesia for chronic pain. Although the mechanism of tolerance is not yet fully understood (see p. 79 for discussion of tolerance), there is some cross-tolerance between narcotics administered spinally and those administered systemically (Yaksh, 1981). In general, patients who require high doses of systemic narcotics will eventually require high spinal doses to achieve pain relief.

As the dose increases, central side effects may occur, thereby limiting the effectiveness of this route. With dose escalation, there is also the concern that eventually a dose too high in concentration or volume will be needed. Preservative-free solutions are highly recommended for the spinal route but can be difficult to obtain commercially in high concentrations.

Further research is needed to clarify the extent and rate at which tolerance develops. In one study, 43 patients receiving intrathecal morphine by an implanted pump for 6 months or longer did not show evidence of rapid tolerance and its related problems. Of the 35 patients with cancer pain, the majority did need two or more times the initial spinal dose over the course of their treatment. This did not result in any central side effects that limited analgesic effectiveness. Only 2 of the 43 patients developed the need for drug dosages that were beyond the pump capabilities (Penn and Paice, 1987).

Another study involved 43 patients with non-malignant pain receiving spinal morphine for up to 2 years. Tolerance appeared to develop, but in many patients the increased dose was due instead to technical problems with the catheter (Auld et al, 1985).

4. Incidence of side effects varies widely and may not occur in all patients. Pruritus, urinary retention, and nausea and vomiting are the most common and will be discussed here. Respiratory depression is also a side effect and is discussed on p. 107.

a. Although the mechanism is unknown, the characteristics of pruritus are that it (Payne, 1987b):
- Is not dose related and occurs after acute and chronic spinal administration.
- May occur after epidural or intrathecal route.
- May continue for the duration of analgesia. However, some report that in patients receiving continuous morphine infusion, pruritus resolves in 48–72 hours (Penn et al, 1984).
- Usually occurs in the face and palate.

- Is not related to preservative in the drug solution.
- Is frequent in pregnant women.
- May worsen with co-administration of steroids.
- May be severe enough to limit therapy.
- May not be relieved with an antihistamine, i.e. diphenhydramine hydrochloride (Benadryl), although there is disagreement over this.
- May be reversed with naloxone.

b. The characteristics of *urinary retention* are that it (Payne, 1987b):
- May be a direct effect of the narcotic on the spinal cord which results in altered bladder tone.
- Occurs mostly in elderly males or in people with pre-existing bladder disorders.
- Seems to have a higher incidence in the post-operative period and in pregnant women.
- Has occurred as long as 18 hours after spinal administration and with epidural doses as low as 3–4mg.

c. *Nausea and vomiting* may occur in patients with cancer, obstetric, and postoperative pain treated with spinal analgesia. However, tolerance to this side effect develops rapidly (Yaksh, 1981).

5. Serious complications from contamination. While this is a problem with IM, IV, or SC routes, the complications are much more dangerous if the spinal route is contaminated. The potential for contamination is greater in chronic external catheter use than in implanted systems.

Recommendations for the spinal route. Clinical reports and associated research are varied and inconclusive regarding guidelines for the spinal route. Therefore this section will not discuss specific protocols and calculation of doses.

Instead, we will present recommendations that promote your effective delivery of spinal analgesia and safe monitoring of its effects. Because of the direct access of the spinal route, the pain continuous assessment sheet (p. 38) is a vital tool to monitor the patient's safety and level of comfort.

General guidelines for nursing care of patients receiving narcotics via the spinal route are:

1. Identify the method of narcotic delivery by the spinal route. This varies for acute and chronic pain. Possibilities are:

a. Single bolus. To control acute post-operative pain, the patient may receive one bolus dose in the operating theatre, and there may be no further access to the spinal route since additional doses are not needed.

b. External catheter. For control of prolonged pain and sometimes for postoperative or brief pain, a catheter is placed intrathecally or epidurally to allow the administration of narcotics by:

• Single or intermittent boluses. May be used to control acute or chronic pain. However, this method is not ideal. With intermittent injections, the patient may be subjected to peaks of potent analgesia followed by valleys of pain when the dose wears off.

• Continuous infusion. This method avoids the peaks and valleys and provides a constant level of pain control. It is primarily used in chronic prolonged pain. However, it is certainly appropriate for acute pain because it not only avoids peaks and valleys, but also it limits the total volume delivered at one time. The larger the volume of drug injected, the greater the chance of spread to the brainstem where central side effects can occur.

c. Implanted port or reservoir. A catheter into the epidural or intrathecal space is tunnelled under the skin and attaches to a port or reservoir which is implanted subcutaneously. These devices may be accessed for individual boluses or continuous infusion.

d. Implanted infusion pump. These devices are implanted in SC pockets in the abdomen and provide continuous infusion for a constant level of pain relief. However, because of the cost of the device and the need for a major surgical procedure, this method requires careful patient selection. Patients who might be considered appropriate candidates include those with (Paice, 1986 and 1987; Penn and Paice, 1987):

• Life expectancy of greater than a few months.
• Pain below the mid-cervical dermatome.
• Pain unsuccessfully treated with an aggressive regime of analgesic therapy.
• Pain inappropriate for neurosurgical procedures.

2. Assess family/patient willingness and resources to care for chronic delivery of spinal analgesia. Each of the external delivery systems for spinal analgesia requires that the patient or family be willing and able to care for the system and administer the narcotic safely.

3. Limit the concentration of morphine. Morphine may be concentrated at no more than 50 mg/ml. If higher concentrations are used, morphine will not stay in solution and will precipitate. This may limit the dose of spinal morphine that can be given. Although there is controversy over the necessity of preservative-free morphine, many recommend it because some of the preservative agents are neurotoxic.

4. Increase or decrease the dose in terms of percentages instead of a fixed number of milligrams. Percentage adjustments keep dosage changes in proportion to the original dose and can be more widely applied regardless of the dose. See p. 98 for an example of this concept.

5. Use a pain continuous assessment sheet to determine safety and effectiveness of dosage (see form on p. 38). The sheet provides information in an easily read format that allows quick scanning for such responses as respiratory depression or unrelieved pain. This assessment form is particularly vital in assessing safety and efficacy of analgesia with spinal narcotics. It can be a helpful tool to all members of the health-care team when fear and concern result in hesitancy to try a particular drug, route, or dosage.

Dosages for this route will vary depending on whether the patient is narcotic naive, e.g. a post-operative patient, or whether the patient has been on a long-term course of narcotics, e.g. a patient with cancer pain (see a discussion of tolerance to analgesia on p. 79).

• An initial bolus dose of morphine for the patient who is narcotic naive can range from 5 to 10mg epidurally, 0.5mg to 2mg intrathecally.
• A total dosage range of epidural morphine 4–18mg is reported following thoracic, abdominal, urological, or orthopaedic surgery in over 1000 patients (Stenseth et al, 1985).
• For cancer pain:

Continuous intrathecal doses of up to 100mg/day (Penn and Paice, 1987).

Continuous epidural doses of up to 90mg/day (Caballero et al, 1986).

6. Be aware of the wide variety of analgesic onset and duration of spinal narcotics.

a. The usual onset of pain relief from a spinal narcotic varies greatly depending on what drug is used:

• Approximately 5 minutes for lipophilic drugs, e.g. pethidine or methadone (Jacobson, 1984).
• Approximately 30–60 minutes for morphine, a hydrophilic drug (Yaksh, 1981).

Knowledge of these variations will serve as a guide to assess the individual patient for a repetition of bolus doses.

b. The interval between bolus doses involves considering the wide variability in duration of action among the spinal narcotics. The following have been reported (Yaksh, 1981):

• For epidural analgesia: the duration can be from 4 to 36 hours with morphine administration, 4 to 18 hours with pethidine, and is 4 hours with fentanyl.

• For intrathecal analgesia: duration can be 12–24 hours following morphine and pethidine.

KEY POINT: For spinal analgesia, due to limited research and clinical experience, individual assessment of onset, duration, and side effects in each situation is essential.

7. The actual amount by which a dose is increased or decreased is determined by finding a dose that relieves pain to the patient's satisfaction with minimal side effects. This is done by using a flow sheet and looking at the following patient responses in consecutive order:

• First, respiratory function, usually rate.
• Second, pain rating on a 0–10 scale.
• Third, based on the above information, determine whether to increase or decrease the number of milligrams of analgesic and at what percentage, e.g. 10%, 50% or 100%.

Because patients' responses to analgesics are so individual, there are no easy formulas that give the "right percentage." No matter what percentage is chosen, it is vital to assess this adjustment based on the drug used and its onset of spinal analgesia. Document the patient's response on the flow sheet so that further increases or decreases can be made without the patient enduring long painful periods between titrations. If a conservative dose increase is chosen, e.g. 10–20%, for a patient who is rating pain at 8 on a 0–10 scale, realize that you will probably need to go higher in percentage increases, e.g. 50–100%, and at more frequent intervals than if you began with a more liberal percentage increase.

8. Close monitoring of respiratory depression is required.

a. Characteristics of respiratory depression include the following (Leib and Hurtig, 1985; Payne, 1987b):

• Onset is variable. An *early* onset, within 1 to 2 hours, may be related to uptake of the drug by the systemic vasculature with shunting to the brain, *or* a *late* onset, within 4 to 24 hours, may be as a result of drug distribution in the cerebrospinal fluid with uptake by the receptors in the respiratory centre.

• It seems to be more common with hydrophilic (water-soluble) drugs, e.g. morphine, as opposed to lipophilic drugs, e.g. pethidine.

• Life-threatening respiratory depression has been seen mostly in the post-operative setting with narcotic naive patients. It is rarely seen with treatment of chronic cancer pain since most of these patients have been on systemic narcotics long enough to develop tolerance to life-threatening side effects.

b. Factors for the nurse to be aware of that can predispose to respiratory depression include (Cousins and Mather, 1984):

• Advanced age.
• Hydrophilic (water-soluble) narcotics, e.g. morphine.
• Marked changes in thoracic–abdominal pressure, including mechanical ventilation or "grunting" respiration associated with pain.
• Narcotic naive or non-tolerant patient.
• Simultaneous administration of narcotics or other CNS depressants by systemic routes.

Because of the increased chances of respiratory depression when additional systemic narcotics or sedatives are used, protocols for spinal therapy state that these additional drugs will not be used unless approved in writing by, and usually given by, the anaesthetist. If they are used, extra-careful monitoring is advised.

The only exception to this may be in cancer pain when concurrent drugs that contribute to analgesia are often administered systemically without the danger of decreased respiration.

c. In the acute care setting, there is current disagreement about the use of apnoea monitors or ear oximeters vs. the nurse personally observing the patient's respiratory function every 30 minutes. However, no one disagrees with the importance of consistent, careful monitoring in whatever form for this patient population. Careful monitoring of respiratory function should not only include assessment of respiratory rate, but also assessment of (Leib and Hurtig, 1985):

- Respiratory volume.
- Quality of respiratory effort.
- Skin colour.
- Auscultation of chest.
- Arterial blood gas analysis.
- Apnoeic spells.

The health-care team establishes acceptable limits to these respiratory functions for each patient. Documentation in the flow sheet under respiration would include additional categories to reflect this, e.g. blood gas results and duration of apnoea.

Naloxone IM or IV effectively reverses respiratory depression related to spinal analgesia. Because some of the spinal narcotic enters the general circulation and acts at the level of the brain, naloxone will also reverse some analgesia. Reversal with naloxone may require multiple, repeated doses since its duration is shorter than the analgesic, i.e. duration of naloxone may be as short as 30 minutes.

9. Further research is needed before definitive recommendations for the spinal route can be made. Continuing research will offer the nurse new and more specific guidelines and will certainly explore the following unanswered questions (Moulin and Coyle, 1986; Payne, 1987a):

- What are the optimal narcotics for spinal analgesia?
- What are equianalgesic doses of epidural and intrathecal narcotics in comparison to oral and parenteral routes?
- For chronic pain, what are appropriate indications for effective use of spinal route?
- How can development of tolerance to analgesia be delayed or handled in chronic spinal administration of analgesics?
- What is the role and approach to spinally administered non-narcotics, e.g. clonidine, bupivacaine?

Patient Example

A 45-year-old woman diagnosed with adenocarcinoma of the rectum was treated surgically with resection of the rectum and the formation of a colostomy. Due to the advanced stage of her disease at presentation, she was also treated with chemotherapy and radiotherapy. She received intermittent co-dydramol for mild pain.

After 6 months the patient developed severe pain in the rectal vault. Radiographic examination revealed a large tumour in that region as well as metastatic disease to the liver and abdomen. The patient was placed on trials of codeine, immediate-release morphine, and sustained-release morphine. She was unable to tolerate these agents due to severe nausea and sedation. Due to the midline nature of the pain, local blocks and neurosurgical procedures were not appropriate.

An epidural catheter was placed in the lumbar region and tunnelled under the skin so that the exit site was several inches away from the midline of the back. An infusion was started at 2ml/hr of 0.1mg/ml preservative-free morphine via an accurate volumetric-type pump. After titrating the dosage to 20mg morphine/24hr the patient received excellent analgesia. At this point an ambulatory infusion pump was attached and filled with 1.0mg preservative-free morphine/ml. The patient and her family were taught how to manage the pump. A district nurse was consulted to ensure pain management continued in the patient's home.

After receiving excellent relief for over 3 months the patient experienced severe pain one evening. Her daughter noticed that the catheter had become dislodged. The pain clinic staff reinserted the catheter, and the patient returned to her previous level of analgesia. After 1 month the husband noticed redness and drainage at the insertion site. The patient complained of pain upon palpation of the site. The doctor ordered antibiotics, removed the catheter, cultured the tip, and reinserted a new catheter after establishing that the infection was only superficial and had not extended into the CNS. However, after several weeks this catheter also became dislodged.

Due to these significant problems and the patient's excellent response on epidural narcotics, an implanted pump was inserted to provide continuous analgesia. Excellent relief was obtained with 35mg morphine/day intrathecally. The device required refilling every 3 weeks. This was done either in the outpatient clinic or at home (Paice, 1988a).

Method of administration: PCA by the IV, SC, or spinal route

The ideal way to administer IV, SC, spinal, or any form of analgesia is by a method that allows the patient control of pain; for example, a patient-controlled pump that allows the patient to self-administer the required analgesia to control sudden increases of pain, e.g. from movement or coughing, and/or breakthrough pain in addition to the primary pain.

The technology of pumps is a constantly changing field. Examples of options or features that may need to be considered in choosing an appropriate pump for the individual patient or clinical setting are:

- Complexity and expense of operation, e.g. cost of pump, cost of any cartridges to reload, ease of operating and teaching patient, and ease of reloading.
- Alarms for malfunction, low battery, or low residual volume.
- Size and portability. For the ambulatory patient it is important to have a small, portable pump, a frequently desirable feature for patients with continuous SC narcotic infusion.
- Ability to convert easily from IV pole to wearable pump.
- Continuous hourly infusion option for specific cases, e.g. cancer pain.
- Boluses with or without a continuous infusion.
- Wide range of possible volume of bolus dose.
- Range of possible volumes infused per hour, e.g. from 0.5ml to 99ml or more. Very large doses are sometimes needed for the IV route and very small doses for the SC and spinal routes.
- Range of possible lockout intervals, e.g. 5–90 minutes.
- Stored retrievable information, e.g. total dose per hour, per 4 hours, or per 24 hours, number of attempts to administer bolus vs. number of boluses given.
- Information on display panel, e.g. alarm messages, amount delivered.
- Allow patient various combinations of control, e.g. stop/start plus initiate bolus.

Changing from one route to another

Changing the route of narcotic administration has the highest potential for undermedicating patients. To avoid problems and to make this transition as smooth as possible, the following guidelines are suggested:

1. Calculate the dose of narcotic for the new route using the equianalgesic chart (Table 4.10). Remember this chart is a guideline for *initial* doses. The dose required varies from one patient to another. Use a continuous assessment sheet (p. 38) to assess the patient's comfort frequently and increase or decrease the dose according to the individual's response.

2. Educate the patient about the differences in this new route, especially when changing from IM or IV to oral. With oral narcotics, he/she will not experience the same fast onset of pain relief as with the IM or IV route;

however, the duration of oral medication is often longer. Explain that it may take a few days of adjustment to determine the most effective dose and interval.

3. Anticipate anxiety and possible doubts from the patient that the new route, especially the oral route, can control the severity of the pain. The patient may never have been given strong oral narcotics in adequate doses, or a previous attempt to switch routes may have failed. Reassure the patient that you will check with him/her frequently. If the route is oral, also make reassurances that an IM or IV dose can always be given if immediate pain control is needed. Let the patient know he/she will not be abandoned on this new route and made to "grin and bear it."

Guidelines for changing from IM or IV to oral. This change must be handled with care to prevent return of unnecessary pain, loss of faith in the idea, abandonment of the attempt to titrate onto oral analgesics, and to minimize nausea and vomiting. Although it is possible to discontinue all IM or IV analgesics at once and give an amount orally that is estimated to be equianalgesic, there is significant potential for under- or over-dosing. It is important to remember that the parenteral route may need to be continued in conjunction with the new oral dose for a period of time to allow the oral dose to reach therapeutic efficacy.

Use a flow sheet to implement the following guidelines for changing from IM or IV to oral narcotic/non-narcotic analgesia:

1. Assess the pain relief obtained from the current IM or IV narcotic before making a change.

2. Select a non-narcotic and administer it on a regular schedule.

3. Select an oral narcotic and use the equianalgesic chart (pp. 84–85) to calculate the approximate total dose needed to replace the current dose of IM or IV narcotic.* Consider a lower estimate if a non-narcotic analgesic is added.

4. Assess the effectiveness of these analgesics, i.e. the non-narcotic, the decreased dose of IM or IV narcotic, and the oral narcotic dose calculated to replace the amount omitted from the IM or IV dose.

5. Adjust the oral narcotic dose up or down depending on the person's response.

---

*Based on clinical experience, many consider the IM and IV doses to be equianalgesic (Portenoy, 1987a). However, some recommend using one-half the IM dose for the IV dose (American Pain Society, 1987; Foley, 1982).

> **KEY POINT:** In converting routes of medication, calculate equianalgesic doses using the chart as a guideline. Initial doses may not be effective. Therefore it is vital to consistently assess, titrate, and evaluate so that dose adjustments up or down can be made until the most effective dose is found.

Side effects of narcotics

Regardless of route, narcotics given regularly will result in side effects. The more common ones are constipation, nausea and vomiting, and sedation. They must be anticipated, and if they occur, they must be treated on a regular, preventive basis. However, these symptoms are not always due to narcotics. Assess patients for other causes. This is particularly important in the person with cancer in whom symptoms may be related to treatment, advancing disease, or a condition unrelated to the cancer.

Constipation caused by narcotics

The *mechanism* underlying constipation caused by narcotics is the binding of narcotics to receptor sites in the gastro-intestinal tract. The result is decreased motility and delayed passage of gastric contents. Poor fluid intake, inadequate diet, and a lack of exercise intensify the problem.

The majority of people taking narcotics regularly will become constipated. Anticipate this and check prescriptions. If a narcotic is prescribed, a stool softener–stimulant should automatically be included. If constipation is not controlled, it can become as problematic as the pain itself.

> **KEY POINT:** Use a *preventive, regular,* and *aggressive* approach to avoid constipation. The need to treat constipation usually means a failure to prevent it.

Points to remember in managing narcotic-induced constipation are:
- The goal is a bowel movement at least every 2–3 days, except of course for the patient who is NBM or not taking fluids by mouth.
- Ask about the patient's usual bowel habits and methods used to control irregularity.

- Explain that the methods the patient usually uses probably will not be sufficient. A more aggressive approach is needed. However, the patient's preferences are incorporated into bowel care as much as possible.
- Frequent small liquid stools or faecal incontinence could mean impaction. Do a rectal examination to check.
- If fluid intake is decreased, avoid bulk laxatives, e.g. ispaghula, because their effectiveness depends on a sufficient intake of fluids.
- Encourage a large intake of water each day.
- Encourage foods and liquids that have helped the patient have bowel movements in the past. These might include foods rich in dietary fibre such as beans, carrots, bran-containing cereals, and liquids such as prune juice or hot lemon water.

Table 4.12 shows a list of preparations and their specific actions.

No magic formula exists for preventing or treating constipation. Each individual reacts differently. Monitoring the patient's initial response to medication and then making adjustments up or down accordingly is essential. See patient/family teaching point (*Common side effects of narcotics*, Appendix) concerning constipation caused by narcotics.

Nausea and vomiting caused by narcotics

The mechanism underlying narcotic-induced nausea and vomiting is complicated. Narcotics may cause nausea in three different ways:
1. Stimulation of the chemoreceptor trigger zone in the brain.
2. Inhibitory effect on GI motility.
3. Stimulation of the vestibular nerve (which carries the impulses for balance).

Points to remember in managing narcotic-induced nausea and vomiting are:
- Nausea may occur when a narcotic regime is first begun, but it usually subsides after several days. If it does not subside or is not controlled with anti-emetics, consider changing to a different narcotic.
- Nausea is often automatically blamed on narcotics. There may be other reasons, e.g. hypercalcaemia, copious sputum, uncontrolled pain, or medications for conditions other than pain.

Medication	Suggested Beginning Dose	Usual Range of Dosage
1. Begin with one of the combined stool softener and mild peristaltic stimulants: e.g. danthron* 25mg poloxamer '188' 200mg in 5ml (co-danthromer) or	5–10ml	
docusate sodium 60mg plus danthron 50mg (co-danthrusate)	1 capsule nocté	1–3 capsules nocté
2. If no bowel movement in any 48-hr period, add one to two of the following: senna 187mg bisacodyl Milk of Magnesia Lactulose (3.35g in 5ml)	1–2 tablets nocté 10–15mg nocté (oral) 30–60ml nocté 15–30ml daily	2 tablets nocté to 4 tablets tds 5mg nocté to 15mg tds 30–60ml qds or bd up to 60ml daily
3. If no bowel movement by 72 hr, perform rectal examination to rule out impaction. If no impaction, go to no. 4. If impaction, go to no. 5.		
4. If no impaction, try one of the following: bisacodyl suppository magnesium sulphate mixture sodium picosulphate	10mg 10ml 2-hrly 5–15ml	
5. If impaction: Manually disempact if stool is soft enough If not, soften with glycerin suppository or oil retention enema, then disempact manually Follow up with phosphate enema until clear Increase daily bowel regimen		

Adapted from Levy, MH: Pain management in advanced cancer. *Semin Oncol,* 12:404, 1985.

* Compounds containing danthron are licensed only for treatment of analgesic-induced constipation in the terminally ill, constipation in the elderly, cardiac failure, and coronary thrombosis.

Table 4.12 Bowel Regimen to Prevent Narcotic-Induced Constipation.*

- The principle of good anti-nausea therapy is to *add* anti-emetics that work at different levels. That is, continue the original anti-emetic and add another that is effective at a different level.

Examples of drugs available for nausea and vomiting and their specific actions are summarized in Table 4.13.

Anti-emetics	Usual Range of Dosage
Start with:	
prochlorperazine	5mg 4-hrly to 20mg 6-hrly orally, 12.5mg 6-hrly IM
	Rectal 5–25mg 6-hrly
haloperidol	1.5mg daily orally
	1mg daily IM
If there is a component of motion sickness and patient is ambulatory, *add*:	
cyclizine	50mg 8-hrly orally
	IM 50mg 8-hrly
If above is ineffective *add*:	
metoclopramide	IV start with 10mg every 6hr and increase as needed.
	10mg 6-hrly orally
Less commonly used anti-emetics:	
hyoscine hydrobromide	0.3–0.6mg every 4hr orally or sublingually
	Transdermal patch, usually behind ear: replace every 3 days

Table 4.13 A Sample Regimen for Narcotic-Induced Nausea.

> **KEY POINT:** To treat narcotic-induced nausea, apply the same approach that is used to effectively treat pain, *preventive and regular*.

Patient Example

Mrs M. is just back from surgery. After two doses of morphine 10mg IM 3-hourly, she rates her pain at 4 on a 0–10 scale (0 = no pain, 10 = worst pain). She states that she is feeling nauseated. The nurse notes that Mrs M. becomes very anxious and holds her breath whenever she moves. Morphine 15mg is given and pain is now rated at 2, however, some nausea is still present. Prochlorperazine 25mg suppository is given and controls Mrs M.'s nausea.

Sometimes phenothiazines are given parenterally as anti-emetics. A common misconception is that they will provide added analgesia. In fact there are no data to support the frequent use of phenothiazines, e.g. prochlorperazine and chlorpromazine, solely as potentiators of the analgesia of narcotics (McGee and Alexander, 1979). They may, however, be useful additions to the narcotics if nausea and vomiting are present.

See patient/family teaching point (*Common side effects of narcotics,* Appendix) concerning nausea and vomiting caused by narcotics.

Sedation caused by narcotics

The mechanism underlying narcotic-induced sedation is partly due to the narcotic's direct depressant effect on the CNS. However, total exhaustion from unrelieved pain is also a factor that can contribute to sedation once the pain is controlled.

Points to remember in managing narcotic-induced sedation are:

- Sleep deprivation resulting from unrelieved pain may be the main reason for signs of sedation. As long as respiratory function is stable and the person can be aroused, continue with the regime.
- Sedation may occur when a narcotic regime is first begun or when there is a significant dosage increase. It usually decreases in 1–3 days, partly due to the patient developing tolerance to sedation.
- If sedation continues after 3 days and is unacceptable to the patient, consider lowering the narcotic dose and adding NSAIDs to boost analgesia without sedative side effects. The key here is to be able to lower the dose without decreasing pain relief. If this is not effective, consider changing to another narcotic.

- Sedation may be due to other factors, e.g. undiagnosed organic pathology, drugs other than narcotics, or psychological causes. Unfortunately the narcotic is often blamed before these other factors are explored.
- Sedation can occur without adequate pain relief. That is, a person might barely be able to stay awake while rating the pain at 8 on a 0–10 scale. *Do not doubt the patient in this situation*. Side effects of the narcotic have outweighed the beneficial analgesic effects. Alternatives to this must be explored, e.g. lowering the dose, changing to another narcotic, or changing to the spinal route of administration.

See patient/family teaching point in the Appendix concerning sedation caused by narcotics.

> **KEY POINT:** A patient can be both sedated and in pain. Do not confuse sedation with analgesia.

The following two examples of sedation illustrate different causes and approaches.

Patient Example

Mrs A. had widespread bone metastasis from end-stage breast cancer.

Pain medication: Morphine 120mg orally 4-hourly aspirin 600mg qds.

Mrs A. had been on this regime for about 2 weeks with pain relief rated at 3 on a 0–10 scale. The family noticed that she became hard to arouse and would fall back to sleep immediately after speaking. The doctor attributed the sedation to the morphine. However, the nurse could document on the flow sheet that although Mrs A. was sedated, her respiratory rate remained stable at 18–20, so she was in no physiological danger. Further exploration showed that she had hypercalcaemia. This was treated and the sedation subsided.

Patient Example

Mr W., 22 years old, had haemophilia and was hospitalized to manage increased bleeding and to control severe pain from spontaneous haemorrhage into several muscles and joints. Upon admission he stated that his pain had been at 7 and 8 during the last 3 days in spite of oral codeine and paracetamol and that he had not slept for at least 2 nights. Respirations were shallow at 20–24/min. Cold compresses were applied to the bleeding sites to help control both pain and bleeding. Diamorphine IV was started with a 1mg bolus and titrated up every 15 minutes to relieve pain. He was also receiving blood components IV. Within 1 hour he received a total of 4mg of diamorphine. After the last bolus his respirations were 12/min and deeper, he rated his pain at 2, and said he was comfortable. A continuous infusion of IV diamorphine was started at 4mg/hr. After 30 minutes the patient was sleeping and respirations remained about the same, 10–12/min. Sleep and inactivity tend to further lower respiratory rate, but this is not necessarily a concern if respirations are regular and deep and no cyanosis is noted. The patient slept for the next 8 hours, but he was coherent when he was aroused and continued to rate his pain at 2. When pain has been uncontrolled for a few days, it is not unusual for the patient to sleep for as long as 24 hours after pain is relieved. Sleep is not the same as sedation and is not an indication that the narcotic dose should be lowered. As long as the patient ventilates sufficiently, sleep does not indicate potential undesirable side effects.

Health professionals' and families' concerns can be addressed with re-education and the use of a pain continuous assessment sheet or daily diary (see p. 38) to allay fears. In the Appendix is a patient/family teaching point regarding narcotic side effects.

Adjuvant analgesics and medications

These drugs were originally intended for treatment of conditions other than pain. Most continue to be used in that manner, but they may also relieve pain in specific situations. Drugs that are not classified pharmacologically as analgesics but are used alone or in combination with narcotics to relieve pain are known as *adjuvant analgesics* or co-analgesics. Other medications often used to treat symptoms that commonly accompany pain, e.g. sleep disturbance, are referred to here simply as adjuvant medications. Table 4.14 summarizes some of the *adjuvant analgesics* and medications helpful for certain problems.

The appropriate use of these drugs is dependent on careful assessment of each individual person and thesymptoms. Specifically, adjuvant analgesics are appropriate when a pain syndrome does not respond to narcotics, e.g. phantom limb pain, causalgia, or post-herpetic neuralgia. Adjuvant medications are appropriate when there is a component to the pain that

Problem	Examples of Drugs Helpful for Problem	Usual Initial Oral Dosage
Various types of pain, eg. dull aching, neuropathic pain	*Tricyclic antidepressants:*	
	amitriptyline	10–25mg/day
	doxepin	10–25mg/day
	imipramine	25mg/day
	desipramine	25mg/day
Lancinating neuropathic pain	*Anticonvulsants:*	
	phenytoin	300mg/day
	carbamazepine	100mg/day
	sodium valproate	15mg/kg/day divided into b.d. or t.d.s.
Muscle spasm	*Antispasmodic Agents:*	
	baclofen	5mg t.d.s.
	orphenadrine	100mg b.d.
Pain resulting from : Spinal cord compression	*Corticosteroids:* dexamethasone	100mg IV followed by a maintenance oral dose
Tumour infiltration of peripheral nerve or plexus	dexamethasone	4–24mg/day
Sleep disturbance	*Tricyclic antidepressants:*	
	amitriptyline	25mg/day
	doxepin	50mg/day
	Antihistamine:	
	hydroxyzine	10–25mg/day
Anxiety	*Benzodiazepines:*	
	diazepam	2–5mg
	Antihistamine (when there is a component of pain and nausea in addition to anxiety):	
	hydroxyzine	25–100mg q.d.s.
	Tricyclic antidepressants (when there are signs of agitation, insomnia, and depression in addition to anxiety):	
	amitriptyline	25mg nocté
	doxepin	50mg nocté
Psychosis (euphoria, paranoia, hallucinations) or delirium (acute onset of agitation, altered attention span, fluctuating level of consciousness)	*Anti-psychotic medication:* haloperidol	0.5–1mg (0.25–0.5mg IM)
Depression not caused by unrelieved pain	Various antidepressants including tricyclics	Higher than that required to relieve pain.

Table references:
American Pain society : *Principles of Analgesic Use in the Treatment of Acute Pain and Chronic Cancer Pain : a concise guide to medical practice,* Washington D.C., The Society; 1987.
Foley, KM : Adjuvant analgesic drugs in cancer pain management. In Aronoff, GM, ed : Evaluation and Treatment of Chronic Pain, pp. 425–434, Baltimore, 1985, Urban and Schwartzenberg.
Holland, JC : Managing depression in the patient with cancer. *CA–Cancer J Clinic,* **37**:366–371, Nov-Dec 1987.
Massie, MJ, and Holland, JC : the cancer patient with pain : psychiatric complications and their management. *Med Clin North Am,* **71**:243–258, Mar 1987.
Pagliaro, AM, and Pagliaro, LA : *Pharmacologic Aspects of Nursing,* St Louis, 1986, The CV Mosby Company.
Plezia, PM, and Linford, J : Innovative approaches to refractory pain, *Hosp Ther* **10**:25–42, Oct 1985.

Table 4.14 Selected Adjuvant Analgesics and Medications.

analgesics alone cannot address, e.g. depression, sleeplessness, anxiety, or agitation. There may be considerable overlap with these drugs, i.e. one drug such as an antidepressant may serve dual purposes.

The use of an adjuvant drug in the following situation illustrates how a medication may not only relieve pain but also address a dimension of comfort that the narcotic alone could not.

Patient Example

Mr W. rates his pain at 4 on a 0–10 scale. Frequent awakenings during the night and a feeling of nervousness are what he describes as most bothersome at the present time. The narcotic and non-steroidal anti-inflammatory combination have been adjusted as carefully as possible. Mr W. wants a better overall level of comfort. The nurse in this situation suggests adding a tricyclic antidepressant to help with the sleep disturbance. With amitriptyline 25 mg nocté, the nervous feelings stop and Mr W. sleeps through the night. He rates his general comfort at night at 1–2 on a 0–10 scale.

> **KEY POINT:** Adjuvant analgesics and other medications are not a substitute for adequate doses of narcotic and non-narcotic analgesics. Aggressive titration of analgesics to control pain comes first. Then, if additional symptoms remain, adjuvant analgesics or medications can be added.

Indications for adjuvant analgesics

Adjuvant analgesics characteristically do one of two things: enhance the effects of narcotics or non-narcotic analgesics or have analgesic properties of their own. Examples of situations in which adjuvant analgesics may be appropriate are:

• Desire for analgesia in addition to or instead of narcotic or non-narcotic analgesics, e.g. when narcotic or non-narcotic use is limited by side effects or when they do not provide adequate relief, e.g. in neuropathic pain.

• Sleepless nights with increased anxiety and pain. These symptoms may improve with sub-therapeutic doses (10–50mg per day) of tricyclic antidepressants such as amitriptyline.

• Sharp, shooting or lancinating pain, e.g. trigeminal neuralgia, may respond to anticonvulsants such as carbamazepine.

• Dull aching or burning pain, e.g. post-herpetic neuralgia or diabetic neuropathy, may respond to tricyclic antidepressants such as amitriptyline.

• Pain from bone metastasis or nerve compression may respond to corticosteroids, such as dexamethasone or prednisolone.

Disadvantages of adjuvant analgesics

While adjuvant analgesics are a logical consideration in the management of pain, it is important to realize that their role and guidelines for use are still being established. For drugs such as phenytoin and carbamazepine, clinical trials have documented their analgesic effect in the treatment of trigeminal neuralgia (Swerdlow, 1984). However, for the use of antidepressants in cancer pain, clinical experience rather than research provides the guidelines.

Examples of possible limitations or disadvantages of relieving pain with adjuvant analgesics are:

• Very little research has been done on these drugs, so guidelines are minimal and results are unpredictable.

• Health-care team members tend to be under-educated about the new uses of these drugs for pain relief, and they are misinformed about so-called "potentiators" of narcotic analgesia, which often only sedate without contributing to pain relief.

• All have the potential for causing various undesirable side effects.

• Pain relief is not always immediate, and the full effect of some of these drugs may not occur until after days or weeks of regular administration.

• Patients may fail to have prescriptions made up or to adhere to a medication regime because pain relief is not immediate or because of a misunderstanding about why the drug is prescribed. Many of the adjuvant analgesics are called tranquillizers or antidepressants, and this may cause patients to believe their pain is discounted and that they are being treated for anxiety or depression only.

Types of adjuvant analgesics

Antidepressants for relief of various types of pain

Antidepressants can affect the perception of pain and mood. The antidepressants most widely used as analgesics seem to be the tricyclics: amitriptyline, doxepin, imipramine (Stauffer, 1987). These drugs appear to have analgesic activity that is thought to be separate from their antidepressant actions (Spiegel et al, 1983). Although the exact mechanisms are still not known, it is thought that they (1) block the re-uptake of brain serotonin (5HT), thereby increasing the availability of serotonin and blocking pain transmission; and (2) decrease the perception of pain by inhibiting the enzyme which breaks down encephalin (Hendler, 1984).

> **KEY POINT:** Anxiety and depression rarely cause pain. Anxiety and depression do make pain more difficult to handle. Brief pain often causes anxiety. Prolonged pain often causes depression. When anxiety or depression is caused by pain, it should be treated by relieving the pain, usually with narcotics and non-narcotics.

When antidepressants are not needed in patients with pain for the sole purpose of decreasing depression, they may be used at sub-therapeutic doses for:
• Relief of anxiety.
• Bedtime sedation.
• Analgesia.

The first two effects are discussed later in the adjuvant medication section. The analgesic effects can be seen in the following pain syndromes which all respond to antidepressants: headache, arthritis, low back pain, diabetic neuropathy, postherpetic neuralgia, and cancer pain (Max et al, 1987; Stauffer, 1987). Usually the analgesic effects are seen at lower doses (often 25–150mg/day for amitriptyline) than the antidepressant effects (American Pain Society, 1987).

Enhancement of the analgesia of morphine post-operatively has been noted with the tricyclic desipramine, if taken for 1 week prior to surgery (Levine, 1986). Also there is evidence that amitriptyline may increase the bioavailability (the rate and extent of delivery of a drug to the general circulation) of morphine in cancer patients (Ventafridda et al, 1987).

Doses must be titrated to effect, starting low and increasing upward. For depression and chronic non-malignant pain, doses tend to begin at 50mg/day and can increase up to 200mg/day. However, patients with chronic cancer pain require much lower doses beginning with 25mg/day and increasing by 25mg every 1–2 days until the desired effect is reached

(Massie and Holland, 1987). Starting with an even lower dose of 10mg/day may be wise if the patient is elderly, severely ill, or has a cardiac problem.

Many patients may not have their prescriptions made up or may take it only a few times. The primary reasons are:

1. The assumption that a prescription for an antidepressant means that their pain is being discounted or that it is due mainly to depression.

2. The delay in feeling the benefits from the medication: sometimes 7–10 days for analgesia; 14–21 days for antidepressant effects. However, the sedative effect occurs within 1 to 2 hours, and insomnia may be relieved with the first dose if it is high enough.

Guidelines for titrating tricyclic antidepressants for analgesia include:
• Give the total daily dose 1–3 hours before bedtime.
• Start with a low dose, e.g. 10–25mg.
• Increase gradually over a few weeks.
• Final dose for analgesia is usually 75–150mg or less if patient cannot tolerate a higher dose.
• Encourage patient to continue at this dose for 1–3 weeks before deciding whether it works.

The patient teaching form in the Appendix may be helpful to explain these important points about antidepressant medication for pain.

Anticonvulsants for relief of lancinating pain

Typically this kind of pain begins and ends suddenly and repeatedly occurs in the same area. It is described by patients as "shock-like," "shooting," or "like lightning" and may be accompanied by muscle spasm. These are descriptions of neuropathic pain, i.e. pain that is a result of injury to the nerve tissue. This pain is characteristic of trigeminal neuralgia, post-herpetic neuralgia, diabetic neuropathy, and traumatic neuralgias.

Anticonvulsant drugs, phenytoin and carbamazepine, are particularly useful for lancinating pain (Swerdlow, 1984). Their mechanism of action is suppression of abnormal nerve firings that occur as a result of nerve tissue injury (Plezia and Linford, 1985). For a detailed review of anticonvulsants see Swerdlow (1984); for a detailed review of treatment of neuropathic pain see Maciewicz et al (1985).

While it is generally agreed that carbamazepine is the drug of choice for trigeminal neuralgia pain

(American Pain Society, 1987; Swerdlow, 1984), there are conflicting opinions about the choice of drugs for other neuropathic pain syndromes. For many patients, shooting pain has an additional dimension of burning or aching. Some have found that anticonvulsant therapy is not effective in controlling this component of the pain (Foley, 1985a; Swerdlow, 1984).

Muscle relaxants for relief of muscle spasm

These can occur as a result of anxiety-related muscle tension, arthritis, vertebral disc protrusions, or a pain-producing process such as a compressed nerve, or bone metastasis.

Muscle relaxants may be helpful in this situation. baclofen and diazepam are two effective antispasmodic agents. Although baclofen and diazepam are considered comparable in effect, baclofen is preferred due to its fewer sedative effects. Further it may be more helpful for intermittent, painful flexor spasms (Aronoff and Evans, 1985). It is also being used successfully alone and in combination with carbamazepine in the treatment of neuralgias (Fromm et al, 1984). Abrupt withdrawal of baclofen should be avoided because it can result in temporary hallucinations and a rebound in the number and severity of spasms (Aronoff and Evans, 1985).

Corticosteroids for relief of various types of cancer pain

For many years corticosteroids have been widely recognized as effective in relieving cancer pain, particularly bone pain or pain related to nerve or spinal cord compression. Many anecdotal reports suggest that steroids relieve this type of pain and reduce the amount of narcotic needed (American Pain Society, 1987; Ettinger and Portenoy, 1988; Foley 1985a); however, there is little additional research on this topic (Marshall, 1984; Naldi et al, 1990).

In 1985, a controlled study was reported regarding the analgesic effects of steroids in cancer pain. A randomized double-blind crossover study compared placebo with methylprednisolone 16mg orally twice daily to establish its ability to relieve pain in patients with end-stage cancer. Those patients who received methylprednisolone for 5 days demonstrated a significant reduction in both pain and analgesic use (Bruera et al, 1985). Additional research is needed to explore the effective dose, the consequences of long-term use, and the differences among the various steroids.

Available data suggest that even with chronic administration of steroids the incidence of serious toxicity is low (Ettinger and Portenoy, 1988). Although possible side effects include peptic ulcer, GI haemorrhage, systemic oedema, and weight gain, in most cases, the effects of providing comfort for patients with a short life expectancy outweigh the potential risks.

Other Possible Adjuvant Analgesics

Caffeine. Adding doses of caffeine to aspirin or paracetamol seems to increase analgesia for conditions such as post-partum uterine cramping, episiotomy pain, dental pain, and headaches. When aspirin or paracetamol was given without caffeine, the doses had to be about 40% larger to obtain the same degree of pain relief as was obtained when the analgesics were given in combination with caffeine (Laska et al, 1984; Beaver, 1984a). On a long-term basis, adding caffeine to each 650mg daily dose of aspirin or paracetamol is felt to be safer than repeatedly giving larger doses without the caffeine.

An effective dose must contain 100–200mg of caffeine. Examples of sources of caffeine are tea, coffee, cola, and Pro-Plus tablets. A large cup of automatic filter coffee contains 181mg of caffeine; percolated coffee, 125mg; instant coffee, 75mg; and strong tea, 80mg (National Headache Foundation, 1987-1988).

Alcohol. Researchers have found that alcohol in non-intoxicating quantities may be an effective adjunct to other analgesic modalities. Apparently the increase in pain tolerance that results from two ordinary cocktails (ethyl alcohol 100% 2mg/kg) is comparable to that obtained from about 10mg morphine SC (0.17mg/kg) (Woodrow and Eltherington, 1988).

Beverages containing alcohol are actually nonprescription medications. Rarely do people consider that they are taking a drug when they drink alcohol socially, but in fact alcohol is usually consumed for its drug effects, not because of its taste or nutritional value.

Of all the effects that alcohol may have, those most relevant to the patient with pain usually are its tranquillizing, sedating, and/or analgesic effects. Years ago, alcohol in 5–10% solution was administered intravenously drip to relieve mild to moderate pain. Taken orally it may have a similar analgesic effect in some people (Cutter, O'Farrell, Whitehouse, and Dentch, 1986). A moderate amount of alcohol, well below that causing inebriation, does not cause respiratory depression and has been recommended for pain relief in patients in whom respiratory depression from narcotics may be a problem, e.g. the elderly (Halpern and Bonica, 1976).

In selected patients, alcohol may be safely combined with narcotics and non-narcotics. Caution the patient about the probability of an additive sedative effect when it is given with narcotics and about the possibility of alcohol increasing gastro-intestinal upset or irritation.

Adjuvant medications for symptoms accompanying pain

Adjuvant medications that are effective for patients with pain are listed in Table 4.14. Clinical signs and symptoms that the nurse might assess as part of a patient's pain are listed below with a discussion of the corresponding adjuvant medication that is indicated.

Sleep disturbance

This can include not being able to fall asleep, frequent awakenings throughout the night, early morning awakenings without being able to go back to sleep, or simply not feeling well-rested after a night's sleep.

Important questions to ask before adding medication for sleep:

1. Is the pain controlled? Unrelieved pain can interrupt every part of a person's life. If the pain is not controlled, refer to the previous sections in this chapter on narcotics and non-narcotic analgesics and Chapters 5–6 for non-pharmacological approaches.
2. Is the sleep disturbance a problem that began with the pain or has it been a lifelong occurrence? Other issues may need to be assessed if this has been a lifelong problem. It may not be possible to change these now.
3. Does the patient consider the sleep disturbance to be a problem?

Sleep disturbance is a common symptom in patients with pain. If the pain is controlled and the sleep disturbance continues, one of the following three groups of drugs might be helpful: tricyclic anti-depressant, antihistamine, or temporary use of a short-acting hypnotic. These are discussed below (refer to Table 4.14, for specific pharmacological information).

1. Tricyclic antidepressant. The sedative effects of an antidepressant have a useful hypnotic effect if the total daily dose is given 1–3 hours before bedtime. The initial drugs of choice are amitriptyline and doxepin at dosages of 10–75mg per day to normalize sleep patterns and possibly provide pain relief. Begin with a low dose and increase gradually over a few weeks. These dosages are much lower than those used to treat depression.

One pain specialist suggests amitriptyline as the first-line sleeping medication in patients with cancer pain (Foley, 1985a).

2. Short-acting hypnotic. Although a hypnotic agent can relieve "simple" insomnia, the routine use of this class of drugs is not recommended (American Pain Society, 1987; Foley, 1985a). If a hypnotic is used, one with a short half-life is suggested,* e.g. temazepam with a half-life of 5–12 hours as opposed to nitrazepam with a half-life of 20-48 hours.

NOTE: It is acceptable to give a sleeping pill or anti-depressant *at the same time* as the usual dose of narcotic. As with any medication, the individual's response must consistently be evaluated and adjustments made accordingly.

Anxiety

Anxiety is a common symptom in patients with pain. Efforts to deal with this symptom should focus first on relieving the pain with analgesics. When this is accomplished, the anxiety often subsides.

Anxiety may be acute or chronic. Acute anxiety may relate to the treatment of an underlying condition, e.g. procedures or surgery, while awaiting diagnosis or test results. Chronic anxiety may have existed before the medical condition and may be exacerbated by it. Relaxation therapy and distraction techniques (Chapter 6) can be helpful.

If the pain is controlled but anxiety still remains, the classes of drugs that can be useful are the benzodiazepines, antipsychotics, antihistamines, and antidepressants (Massie and Holland, 1987). Refer to Table 4.14 for pharmacological specifics.

*Half-life is the time it takes the drug to fall to one half its concentration in the bloodstream. The longer the half-life, the longer the effects from the drug.

INDIVIDUALIZED NURSING CARE PLAN*

Patient Who May Benefit from Individualized Pharmacological Approach to Pain Control

Patient Description: Mrs C., 53 years old, is bedridden at home due to extensive bone metastases in the thoracic and cervical spine, and right and left ribs from breast cancer. During the initial home visit, the nurse reports to the doctor the following pain assessment so that they can plan an effective analgesic regime: Mrs C. rates her neck, back, and rib pain at 9 on a 0–10 scale (0 = no pain; 10 = worst pain). When she tries to turn in bed, pain becomes "unbearable." The best the pain has been in the last 2 days is 7, when she lies totally still. She takes morphine 10mg orally irregularly and tries to hold off as long as possible between doses. She has been unable to sleep for the past 2 nights because of the pain, and she insists on remaining at home. Her husband supports her decision. The nurse suggests a 50–100% increase in morphine until Mrs C. is comfortable. Then she suggests regular dosing of morphine, a non-steroidal anti-inflammatory medication, and in anticipation of constipation, a stool softener/stimulant combination. The doctor agrees with this plan and prescribes diclofenac 50mg t.d.s. and co-danthrusate capsules 1–2 b.d..

Assessment Outcomes	Potential Nursing	Planning/Intervention	Evaluation/Expected Problems
• Complete Initial Pain Assessment tool (p. 32) and give priority to determining: location of pain, pain intensity, what helps pain or what makes it worse. • Determine ability to use 0–10 scale to rate pain. • Establish what number on 0–10 scale is acceptable. • Determine pain rating and duration of pain relief after oral morphine. • Determine knowledge about use of non-narcotic analgesics in combination with narcotics for added effectiveness.	Pain in back, neck, and ribs related to bone metastases as a result of breast cancer	• Use a preventive approach: diclofenac 50mg t.d.s. regularly and morphine probably 4-hrly regularly. • Begin with 100% increase in oral morphine and one dose of oral diclofenac. • Monitor and document pain rating and side effects on Pain Continuous Assessment Sheet (p. 38) (using 0–10 scale at least every 2hr) by phone call or home visit during the first 24hr. If pain is uncontrolled, calculate additional doses of morphine that can be given in between the regular 4-hourly dose for breakthrough pain and instruct patient/husband on administration. Then if pain is controlled, monitor and document at least twice a day for 48hr, then at every home visit.	Patient reports her pain is at or below the acceptable rating for her pain with side effects absent or acceptable.
		• When pain is controlled, calculate the total 24-hour dose of oral morphine from increases and implement this dose regularly. • Teach patient/husband how to use Daily Diary (Appendix) and to document every 2hr during first 24hr, then about every 4hr: patient's pain rating on 0–10 scale, analgesics given, and any difficulty arousing patient. • Report to doctor if analgesic regime does not decrease pain rating to an acceptable level for patient.	Patient/husband maintains Daily Diary and shares this with nurse via telephone or during home visit.
• Determine patient/husband's fears or misconceptions about addiction or narcotics losing their effectiveness.		• Initiate discussion about fears concerning narcotics, e.g. fears about addiction. If needed, review following patient/family teaching points: Preventive Approach with Pain Medication (Appendix) Instructions for Home Use of Non-narcotic Analgesics (Appendix)	Patient/husband demonstrate understanding of importance of preventive, regular dosing of narcotic and non-narcotic analgesic by documenting their administration in Daily Diary.
• Sleep assessed above in relation to pain.	Sleep pattern disturbance related to unrelieved pain	Implement the above measures for pain relief which will ultimately help sleep disturbance.	As pain decreases, sleep increases.

continued

*Although there are many additional diagnoses and interventions for this patient situation, the care plan is limited to the nurse's initial active role in the multidisciplinary approach to pharmacological control of pain.

INDIVIDUALIZED NURSING CARE PLAN—cont'd.			
Patient Who May Benefit from Individualized Pharmacological Approach for Pain Control—cont'd.			
Assessment	**Potential Nursing Problems**	**Planning/Intervention**	**Evaluation/ Expected Outcomes**
• Determine measures that have helped constipation in the past, i.e. laxatives, foods, liquids.	Constipation related to regular narcotic regime and no physical activity	• Use preventive approach: begin with co-danthrusate capsules b.d. • If no bowel movement in any 48-hr period, obtain prescription for laxative and increase co-danthrusate. • Monitor and document frequency of bowel movements at each home visit. • Review following patient/family teaching point: Common Narcotic Side Effects Related to Narcotic Use: Constipation Caused by Narcotics (Appendix).	Patient reports daily use of bowel regime with a bowel movement at least every 2 days.

1. Benzodiazepines. This class of drugs has no analgesic properties and does not result in additive analgesia when combined with a narcotic (Foley, 1985a). It is suggested that their usefulness in patients with pain is limited to situations in which severe anxiety is the principal and disabling symptom. Diazepam is still one of the most commonly used drugs.

The severity of the anxiety, the patient's hepatic and respiratory status, and the use of other medications are all factors in determining the starting dose. Refer to Table 4.14 for a listing of initial dosages.

2. Antipsychotic medication. Haloperidol can be beneficial for patients showing signs of psychosis (euphoria, fears, paranoia, or hallucinations) or delirium (acute onset of agitation, impaired cognitive function, altered attention span, or a fluctuating level of consciousness).

Although it has been suggested that haloperidol is useful as an adjuvant analgesic in cancer pain (Breivik and Rennemo, 1982), presently its main role in cancer pain is the management of acute psychosis (Massie and Holland, 1987).

Haloperidol is chosen over other antipsychotics because of its low incidence of orthostatic hypotension and anticholinergic effects.

3. Antihistamines. Although not as effective for severe anxiety as the other classes of drugs mentioned in this section, hydroxyzine can be helpful when there are additional dimensions to anxiety such as pain and nausea (Foley, 1985a).

4. Antidepressants. Usually these are not used for symptoms of anxiety alone. However, when there are signs of depression, agitation, and insomnia, tricyclic antidepressants with sedating effects, e.g. amitriptyline or doxepin, can be helpful (Massie and Holland, 1987).

Depression

Depression can affect a person's ability to handle pain. The clinical picture of depression includes insomnia, anorexia, fatigue, and weight loss. In the person with cancer or other prolonged illnesses these may be signs of pain or the disease process itself. Therefore the identification of depression in these patients must depend on psychological symptoms such as feelings of sadness, anxiety, helplessness, worthlessness, guilt, loss of self-esteem, and thoughts of "wishing for death" (Massie and Holland, 1987).

Differentiating between the cause and effect within the cycle of pain-depression-insomnia-anxiety is difficult. The important point for the nurse to realize is that early assessment of the presence of this cycle is vital so that active treatment can begin. If depression has been a prolonged symptom predating the pain or medical problem, then a psychiatrist or psychologist may be helpful to consult for a supportive plan of care or appropriate psychotropic medication.

REFERENCES AND SELECTED READINGS

Aguwa, CN, and Olusanya, OA: Analgesic prescribing for severe pain studied. *Drug Intell Clin Pharm*, **12**:556, Sept 1978.

Amadio, P, and Cummings, DM: Nonsteroidal anti-inflammatory agents: an update. *Am Fam Physic*, **34**:147–154, 1986.

American Pain Society: *Principles of Analgesic Use in the Treatment of Acute Pain and Chronic Cancer Pain: a concise guide to medical practice*, Washington D.C., The Society, 1987.

Anderson, AB, Haynes, PJ, Fraser, IS, and Turnbull, AC: Trial of prostaglandin-synthetase inhibitors in primary dysmenorrhea. *Lancet*, **1**:345–348, 1978.

Anderson, K, and Poole, C: Self-administered medication on a postpartum unit. *Am J Nurs*, **83**:1178–1180, Aug 1983.

Angell, J: The quality of mercy. *N Engl J Med*, **306**:98–99, Jan 14, 1982.

Aronoff, GM, and Evans, WO: Pharmacological management of chronic pain. In Aronoff, GM, ed.: Evaluation and *Treatment of Chronic Pain*, pp. 435–449, Baltimore, 1985, Urban and Schwartzenberg.

Auld, AW, Maki-Jokela, A, and Murdock, DM: Intraspinal narcotic analgesia in the treatment of chronic pain. *Spine*, **10**:777–781, 1985.

Austin, KL, Stapleton, JV, and Mather, LE: Multiple intramuscular injections: a major source of variability in analgesic response to pethidine. *Pain*, **8**:47–62, 1980.

Baggerly, J: Epidural catheters for pain management: the nurse's role. *J Neurosci Nurs*, **18**:290–295, Oct 1986.

Ballantyne, J, Loach, AB, and Carr, DB: Itching after epidural and spinal opiates. *Pain*, **33**:149–160, 1988.

Barkas, G, and Duafala, M: Advances in cancer pain management: a review of patient-controlled analgesia. *J Pain Sympt Manag*, **3**:150–160, Summer 1988.

Beaver, WT: Management of cancer pain with parenteral medication. *JAMA*, **244**:2653–2657, Dec 12, 1980.

Beaver, WT: Aspirin and acetaminophen as constituents of analgesic combinations. *Arch Intern Med*, **141**:293–300, Feb 23, 1981.

Beaver, WT: Caffeine revisited. *JAMA*, **251**:1732–1733, 1984a.

Beaver, WT: Combination analgesics. *Am J Med*, **77**(3A): 38–53, Sept 10, 1984b.

Beaver, WT, and Feise, GA: Comparison of the analgesic effects of morphine, hydroxyzine, and their combination in patients with postoperative pain. In Bonica, JJ, and Albe-Fessard, D, eds: *Advances in Pain Research and Therapy*, pp. 553-557, vol. 1, New York, 1976, Raven Press.

Bell, MDD, Mishra, P, Waldon, BD, et al: Buccal morphine – a new route for analgesia? *Lancet*, **1**:71–73, Jan 12, 1985

Belville, JW, Dorey, F, Capparell, D, et al: Analgesic effects of hydroxyzine compared to morphine in man. *J Clin Pharmacol*, **19**:290–296, May-June 1979.

Bernstein, J: Anti-inflammatories for migraine. *Aches & Pains*, **3**:32–37, Mar 1982.

Blumenkopf, B: Combination analgesic-antispasmodic therapy in postoperative pain. *Spine*, **12**:384–387, May 1987.

Botney, M, and Fields, HL: Amitriptyline potentiates morphine analgesia by a direct action on the central nervous system. *Ann Neurol*, **13**:160–164, Feb 1983.

Breivik, H, and Rennemo, F: Clinical evaluation of combined treatment with methadone and psychotropic drugs in cancer patients. *Acta Anaesthesiol Scand*, (Suppl.) 74:135-140, 1982.

Brena, SF: Drugs and pain: use and misuse. In Brena, SF, and Chapman, SL, eds: *Management of Patients with Chronic Pain*, pp 121–310, New York, 1983, Raven Press.

Brenneis, C, Michaud, M, Bruera, E, et al: Local toxicity during subcutaneous infusion of narcotics: a prospective study. In *Proceedings of the VI World Congress on the Care of the Terminally Ill*, Montreal, Sept 1986.

Brook-Williams, P: Morphine suppositories for intractable pain. *Can Med Assoc J*, **126**:14, Jan 1982.

Brozovic, M, Davies, SC, and Yardumian, A: Pain relief in sickle cell crises. *Lancet*, **2**:624–625, 1986.

Bruera, E, Brennels, C, and MacDonald, RN: Continuous SC infusion of narcotics for the treatment of cancer pain: an update. *Cancer Treat Rep*, **71**:953–957, Oct 1987a.

Bruera, E, Chadwick, S, Brennels, C, et al: Methylphenidate associated with narcotics for the treatment of cancer pain. *Cancer Treat Rep*, **71**:67–70, Jan 1987b.

Bruera, E, Roca, E, Cedaro, L, et al: Action of oral methylprednisolone in terminal cancer patients: a prospective randomized double blind study. *Cancer Treat Rep*, **69**:751–754, 1985.

Burns Stewart, SM: Controlling pain with epidural narcotics: nursing implications. *Crit Care Nurs*, **6**:50–56, May-June 1986.

Caballero, GA, Ausman, RK, and Himes, J: Epidural morphine by continuous infusion with an external pump for pain management in oncology patients. *Am Surg*, **52**:402–405, 1986.

Cancer Pain Relief, Geneva, World Health Organization, 1986.

Catalano, RB: Pharmacologic management in the treatment of cancer pain. In McGuire, DB, and Yarboro, CH, eds: *Cancer Pain Management*, pp. 151–201, Grune & Stratton, Orlando, 1987.

Charap, AD: The knowledge, attitudes and experience of medical personnel treating pain in the terminally ill. *Mt Sinai J Med*, **45**:561–580, July-Aug 1978.

Cefali EA, Bell, WE, Miller, LG, et al: The bioavailability of a novel buprenorphine buccal delivery system. *Drug Information*, 1173–1178, 1991.

Clark, BE: Considerations in pain management of the hospice patient. *Am J Hospice Care*, **1**:23-27, Fall 1984.

Cleeland, CS: Barriers to the management of cancer pain, *Oncology* (Suppl.) **1**:19–26, Apr 1987.

Cohen, F: Postsurgical pain relief: patient's status and

nurses' medication choices. *Pain,* **9**:265–274, 1980.

Cohen, SE, and Woods, WA: The role of epidural morphine in the post-cesarean patient: efficacy and effects of bonding. *Anesthesiology,* **58**:500–504, 1983.

Cole, T, Sprinkle, R, Smith, S, and Buchanan, G: Intravenous narcotic therapy for children with severe sickle cell pain crisis. *Am J Dis Child,* **140**:1255–1259, Dec 1986.

Coombs, DW, Maurer, LH, Saunders, RL, and Gaylor, M: Outcomes and complications for continuous intraspinal narcotic analgesia for cancer pain control. *J Clin Oncol,* **2**:1414–1420, Dec 1984.

Cousins, MJ, and Mather, LE: Intrathecal and epidural administration of opioids. *Anesthesiology,* **61**:276–310, 1984.

Coyle, N, Mauskop, A, Maggard, J, and Foley, KM: Continuous subcutaneous infusions of opiates in cancer patients with pain. *Oncol Nurs Forum,* **13**:53–57, July-Aug 1986.

Cutter, HSG, O'Farrell, TJ, Whitehouse, J, and Dentch, GM: Pain changes among men from before to after drinking: effects of expectancy set and dose manipulations with alcohol and tonic as mediated by prior experience with alcohol. *Int J Addict,* **21**:937–945, 1986.

Dallas, TL, Lin, RL, Wu, W, and Wolskee, P: Epidural morphine and methylprednisolone for low-back pain. *Anesthesiology,* **67**:408–411, Sept 1987.

Dawood, MY: Dysmenorrhea and prostaglandins: pharmacological and therapeutic consideration. *Drugs,* **22**:42–56, 1981.

Dingfelder, JR: Primary dysmenorrhea treatment with prostaglandin inhibitors: a review. *Am J Obstet Gynecol,* **140**:874–879, 1981.

Dionne, RA, and Cooper, SA: Evaluation of preoperative ibuprofen for post-operative pain after removal of third molars. *Oral Surg,* **45**:851–856, June 1978.

Drug Information, American Hospital Formulary Service, p. 979, Maryland, American Society of Hospital Pharmacists, 1987.

Dundee, JW, Love, WJ, and Moore, J: Alterations in response to somatic pain associated with XV: further studies with phenothiazine derivatives and similar drugs. *Br J Anaesthesiol,* **35**:597–609, 1963.

Dundee, JW, and Moore, J: The myth of phenothiazine potentiation. *Anaesthesiology,* **16**:95–96, 1961.

Enck, RE: The role of continuous intravenous and subcutaneous narcotic infusions in pain management. *Am J Hospice Care,* **4**:43–45, Nov-Dec 1987.

Ellis, R, Haines, D, Shah, R, et al: Pain relief after abdominal surgery—a comparison of IM morphine, sublingual buprenorphine and self-administered IV pethidine. *Br J Anaesthesiol,* **54**:421–427, 1982.

Ellison, NM, and Lewis, GO: Plasma concentrations following single doses of morphine sulfate in oral solution and rectal suppository. *Clin Pharm,* **3**:614–617, Nov-Dec 1984.

Ettinger, AB, and Portenoy, RK: The use of corticosteroids in the treatment of symptoms associated with cancer. *J Pain Sympt Manag,* **3**:99–103, Spring 1988.

Farley, HF, Joyce, N, Long, B, and Roberts, R: Will that IM needle reach the muscle? *Am J Nurs,* **86**:1327–1331, Dec 1986.

Feighner, JP, Aden, GC, Fabre, LF, et al: Comparison of alprazolam, imipramine, and placebo in the treatment of depression. JAMA, **249**:3057–3064, 1983.

Feldman, HR: Practice makes perfect but research makes a difference. Nursing, **17**:47, Mar 1987.

Ferrel, BR, and Schneider, C: Experience and management of cancer pain at home. *Cancer Nurs,* **11**:84–90, 1988.

Ferrel, BR, Wenzl, C, and Wisdom, C: Evolution and evaluation of a pain management team. *Oncol Nurs Forum,* **15**:285–289, 1988.

Ferris, FD, Kerr, IG, Stone, M et al: Transdermal scopolamine use in the control of narcotic induced nausea. *J Pain Symp Management,* **6**(6):389–393, 1991.

Flower, RJ, Moncada, S, and Vane, JR: Drug therapy of inflammation, pp. 674–715. In Gilman, AG, et al, eds: Goodman and Gilman's *The Pharmacological Basis of Therapeutics,* ed. 7, Macmillan Publishing Co., New York, 1985.

Foley, KM: The practical use of narcotic analgesics. *Med Clin North Am,* **66**:1091–1104, 1982.

Foley, KM: Adjuvant analgesic drugs in cancer pain management. In Aronoff, GM, ed: *Evaluation and Treatment of Chronic Pain,* pp. 425–434, Urban and Schwartzenberg, Baltimore, 1985a.

Foley, KM: The treatment of cancer pain. *N Engl J Med,* **313**:84–95, July 11, 1985b.

Foley, KM: Current controversies in opioid therapy. In Foley, K, and Inturrisi, C, eds: *Advances in Pain Research and Therapy,* vol 8, Opioid analgesics in the management of clinical pain, pp. 3–11, Raven Press, New York, 1986.

Foley, KM: Author's reply. *CA Cancer J Clinic,* **37**:376–377, Nov 1987.

Foley, KM, and Inturrisi, CE: Analgesic drug therapy in cancer pain: principles and practice, *Med Clin North Am* **71**:207–232, Mar 1987.

Foley, KM, and Rogers, A: The management of cancer pain. *The Rational Use of Analgesics in the Management of Cancer Pain,* vol. 2, Hoffmann-La Roche, Inc., Nutley, NJ, 1981.

Forrest, WH: Tranquilizer-narcotic combinations in management of acute pain: rationale and history. In *Considerations in Management of Acute Pain,* pp. 14–16, HP Publishing Co., New York, 1977.

Forrest, WH, Brown, BW, Brown, CR, et al: Dextroamphetamine with morphine for treatment of postoperative pain. *N Engl J Med,* **296**:712–715, 1977.

Frank, RM: Pain management and the appropriate use of analgesics. *Cancer Nurs,* **3**:155–157, Apr 1980.

Fromm, GH, Terrence, CF, and Chatha, AS: Baclofen in the treatment of trigeminal neuralgia: double-blind study and long-term follow up. *Ann Neurol,* **15**:240–244, 1984.

Fultz, J, Senay, E, Pray, B, and Thornton, W: When a narcotic addict is hospitalized. *Am J Nurs*, **80**:478–481, Mar 1980.

Gold, MS, Redmond, E, and Kleber, HD: Noradrenergic hyperactivity in opiate withdrawal. *Am J Psychiatry*, **136**:100 102, Jan 1979.

Goudie, TA, Allan, MWB, Longsdale, M, et al: Continuous subcutaneous infusion of morphine for postoperative pain relief. *Anaesthesia*, **40**:1086–1092, 1985.

Grabinski, PY, Kaiko, RF, Rogers, AG, and Houde, RW: Plasma levels and analgesia following deltoid and gluteal injections of methadone and morphine. *J Clin Pharmacol*, **23**:48–55, 1983.

Greenberg, HS, Taren, J, Ensminger, WD, et al: Benefit from and tolerance to continuous intrathecal infusion of morphine for intractable cancer pain. *J Neurosurg*, **57**:360–364, 1982.

Grossman, SA, and Sheidler, VR: Skills of medical students and house officers in prescribing narcotic medication. *J Med Ed*, **60**:552–557, July 1985.

Grossman, SA, Sheidler, VR: An aid to prescribing narcotics for the relief of cancer pain. *World Health Forum*, **8**:525–529, 1987.

Guthrie, SK: Pharmacologic interventions for the treatment of opioid dependence and withdrawal. *Ann Pharmacother*, **24**:721–733, 1990.

Halpern, LM, and Bonica, JJ: Analgesics. In Modell, W, ed: *Drugs of Choice*, pp. 195–232, The CV Mosby Co., St. Louis, 1976.

Heidrich, G, Slavic-Svircev, V, Kaiko, R: Efficacy and quality of ibuprofen and acetaminophen and codeine analgesia. *Pain*, **22**:385–397, 1985.

Hanks, GW, Twycross, RG, Bliss, JM: Controlled release morphine tablets — a double-blind trial in patients with advanced cancer. *Anaesthesia*, **42**:840–844, 1987.

Hendler, N: Depression caused by chronic pain. *J Clin Psychiatry*, **45** (3, sec 2):30–36, 1984.

Hill, CS: Patients in pain—case reports. *Primary Care & Cancer* **6**:43–48, Sept 1986.

Hill, CS, Jr.: Don't be `spooked' into giving naloxone inappropriately, *Primary Care & Cancer* **7**:31–34, March 1987.

Hirsh, JD: Sublingual morphine sulfate in chronic pain management, *Clin Pharm* **3**:585–586 (letter), Nov-Dec 1984.

Houde, RW: Analgesic effectiveness of the narcotic agonist-antagonist, *Br J Clin Pharmacol* **7**:2975–3085, 1979.

Houde, RW, Wallenstein, SL, and Rogers, A: Clinical pharmacology of analgesics: a method of assaying analgesic effect, *Clin Pharmacol Ther* **1**:163–174, 1960.

Inturrisi, CE: Role of opioid analgesics, *Am J Med* **77**:27–37, Sept 10, 1984.

Inturrisi, CE, and Umans, JG: Pethidine and its active metabolite, norpethidine, *Clin Anaesthesiol* **1**:123–138, Apr 1983.

Ives, TJ, and Guerra, MF: Constant morphine infusion for severe sickle cell crisis pain, *Drug Intell Clin Pharm* **21**:625–626, July-Aug 1987.

Jaffe, JH: Drug addiction and drug abuse. In Gillman, AG, Goodman, LS, Rall, TW, and Murad, F, eds: Goodman and Gillman's *The Pharmacological Basis of Therapeutics*, ed. 7, Macmillan Publishing Co., New York, 1985.

Jaffe, JH, and Martin, WR: Opioid analgesics and antagonists. In Gillman, AG, Goodman, LS, Rall, TW, and Murad, F, eds: *The Pharmacological Basis of Therapeutics*, ed. 7, pp. 532–581, Macmillan Publishing Co., New York, 1985.

Jain, AK, Ryan, JR, McMahon, FG, and Smith, G: Comparison of oral nalbuphine, acetaminophen, and their combination in postoperative pain, *Clin Pharmacol Ther* **39**:295–299, Mar 1986.

Jick, H: Smoking and clinical drug effects, *Med Clin North Am* **58**:1143–1149, Sept 1974.

Jones, L: Patient-controlled oral analgesia, *Orthoped Nurs* **6**: 38–41, Jan-Feb 1987.

Kaiko, RF: Age and morphine analgesia in cancer patients with postoperative pain, *Clin Pharmacol Ther* **28**:823–826, Dec 1980.

Kaiko, RF, Foley, KM, Grabinski, PY, et al: Central nervous system excitatory effects of pethidine in cancer patients, *Ann Neurol* **13**:180–185, 1983.

Kane, NE, Lehman, ME, Dugger, R, Hansen, L, and Jackson, D: Use of patient-controlled analgesia in surgical oncology patients, *Oncol Nurs Forum* **15**:29–32, Jan-Feb 1988.

Kantor, TG: Anti-inflammatory drug therapy for low back pain. In Stanton-Hicks, M, and Boas, R, eds: *Chronic Low Back Pain*, pp. 157–169, Raven Press, New York, 1982.

Kantor, TG: Nonsteroidal anti-inflammatory analgesic agents in management of cancer pain. In *The Management of Cancer Pain* (Monograph), pp. 30–34, Hospital Practice, Summer 1984.

Kay, B, and Krishnan, A: On-demand nalbuphine for post-operative pain relief, *Acta Anaesthesiol Belg* **37**:33–37, 1986.

Keats, AS, Telford, J, and Kurosu, Y: "Potentiation" of pethidine by promethazine, *Anesthesiology* **22**:34–41, Jan-Feb 1961.

Keen, MF: Comparison of intramuscular injection techniques to reduce site discomfort and lesions, *Nurs Res* **35**:207–210, July-Aug 1986.

Kleiman, RL, Lipman, AG, Hare, BD, et al: A comparison of morphine administered by patient-controlled analgesia and regularly scheduled intramuscular injection in severe, postoperative pain, *J Pain Sympt Manag* **3**:15–22, Winter 1988.

Kreek, MJ, Hahn, EF, Schaefer, RA, and Fishman, J: Naloxone, a specific opioid antagonist reverses chronic idiopathic constipation, *Lancet* **1**:261, 1983.

Kruszewski, A, Lang, S, and Johnson, J: Effects of positioning on discomfort from intramuscular injections in the dorsogluteal site, *Nurs Res* **28**:103–105, 1979.

Lanz, E, Theiss, D, Reiss, W, and Sommer, U: Epidural morphine for postoperative analgesia: a double-blind study, *Anesthesiol Analg* **61**:236–240, Mar 1982.

Laska, E, Sunshine, A, Mueller, F, et al: Caffeine as an analgesic adjuvant, *JAMA* **251**:1711–1718, 1984.

Leib, RA, and Hurtig, JB: Epidural and intrathecal narcotics for pain management, *Heart Lung* **14**:164–174, Mar 1985.

Leporati, NC, Chychula, LH, Lo, SL, and Coleman, RR: How you can really help the drug-abusing patient, *Nursing* **12**:46–49, June 1982.

Levine, JD, Gordon, NC, Smith, R, and McBryde, R: Desipramine enhances opiate postoperative analgesia, *Pain* **27**:45–49, 1986.

Levy, MH: Pain management in advanced cancer, *Semin Oncol* **12**:394–410, Dec 1985.

Lim, RKS: Pain mechanisms, *Anesthesiology* **28**:106–110, Jan-Feb 1967.

Lo, SL, and Coleman, RR: Exceptionally high narcotic analgesic requirements in a terminally ill cancer patient, *Clin Pharm* **5**:828–832, Oct 1986.

Lukacsko, P: A guide to the parenteral management of moderate to severe pain, *Hospital Pharm* **22**:361–412, Apr 1987.

Maciewicz, R, Bouckoms, A, and Martin, JB: Drug therapy of neuropathic pain, *Clin J Pain* **1**:39–49, 1985.

Magruder, MR, Delaney, RD, and Difazio, CA: Reversal of narcotic-induced respiratory depression with nalbuphine hydrochloride, *Anesthesiol Rev* **9**:34–37, Apr 1982.

Maguire, LC, Yon, JL, and Miller, E: Prevention of narcotic induced constipation, *N Engl J Med* **305**:1651, 1981.

Malhotra, V, and Artusio, JF: Management of postoperative pain, *Semin Urol* **3**:204–215, Aug 1985.

Malone, BT, Beye, R, and Walker, J: Management of pain in the terminally ill by administration of epidural narcotics, *Cancer* **55**:438–440, Jan 15, 1985.

Manara, AR, Bodenham, AR, Park, GR: Analgesic efficacy of peri-operative buccal morphine, *Br J Anaesth* **64**:551–555, 1990.

Marks, RM, and Sachar, EJ: Undertreatment of medical inpatients with narcotic analgesics, *Ann Intern Med* **78**:173–181, 1973.

Marshall, JG, Walton, RE: The effect of intramuscular injection of steroid on post-treatment endontic pain, *J Endod* **10**:584–588, 1984.

Marx, J: Dysmenorrhea: basic research leads to a rational therapy, *Science* **205**:175–176, July 1979.

Massie, MJ, and Holland, J: The cancer patient with pain: psychiatric complications and their management, *Med Clin North Am* **71**:243–258, Mar 1987.

Mauro, VF, Bonfiglio, MF, and Spunt, AL: Pethidine-induced seizure in a patient without renal dysfunction or sickle cell anemia, *Clin Pharmacol* **5**:837–839, 1986.

Max, MB, Culnane, M, Schafer, SC, et al: Amitriptyline relieves diabetic neuropathy pain in patients with normal or depressed mood, *Neurology* **37**:589–596, Apr 1987.

McCaffery, M: *Nursing Management of the Patient with Pain*, ed. 2, JB Lippincott, New York, 1979.

McCaffery, M: Large doses are safer than you think, *Nurs Life* **1**:41–42, Nov-Dec 1981.

McCaffery, M: Problems with pethidine, *Am J Nurs* **84**:525, Apr 1984.

McCaffery, M: Giving pethidine for pain—should it be so mechanical? *Nursing* **17**:61–64, Apr 1987a.

McCaffery, M: Patient-controlled analgesia: more than a machine, *Nursing* **17**:62–64, Nov 1987b.

McGee, JL, and Alexander, MR: Phenothiazine analgesia—fact or fantasy? *Am J Hosp Pharm* **36**:633–640, May 1979.

McGuire, DB, Barbour, L, Boxler, J, et al: Fixed-interval v. as-needed analgesics in cancer outpatients, *J Pain Sympt Manag* **2**:199–205, Fall 1987.

McGuire, L, and Wright, A: Continuous narcotic infusion: it's not just for cancer patients, *Nursing 84* **14**:50–55, Dec 1984.

McManus, M, and Panzarella, C: The use of dextroamphetamine to counteract sedation for patients on a morphine drip, *J Assoc Pediatr Oncol Nurs* **3**:28–29, 1986.

Miller, RR, and Jick, H: Clinical effects of pethidine in hospitalized medical patients, *J Clin Pharm* **18**:180–189, Apr 1978.

Miser, A, Moore, L, Greene, R, et al: Prospective study of continuous intravenous and subcutaneous morphine infusions for therapy-related or cancer-related pain in children and young adults with cancer, *Clin J Pain* **2**:101–106, 1986.

Miser, AW, Ayesh, D, Broda, E, et al: Use of a patient-controlled device for nitrous oxide administration to control procedure related pain in children and young adults with cancer, *Clin J Pain* **4**:5–10, 1988.

Miser, AW, Davis, DM, Hughes, CS, et al: Continuous subcutaneous infusion of morphine in children with cancer, *Am J Dis Child* **137**:383–385, 1983.

Miser, AW, Miser, JS, and Clark, BS: Continuous intravenous infusion of morphine sulfate for control of severe pain in children with terminal malignancy, *J Pediatr* **96**:930–932, 1980.

Moore, J, and Dundee, JW: Alterations in response to somatic pain associated with anaesthesia v. the effect of promethazine, *Br J Anaesthesiol* **33**:3–8, 1961.

Morgan, JP: American opiophobia: customary underutilization of opioid analgesics, *Adv Alcohol Subst Abuse* **5**:163–173, Fall 1985-Winter 1986.

Moss, H: Subcutaneous continuous infusion narcotics at home, *Oncol Nurs Forum* (suppl) **13**:128, 1986 (abstract).

Moulin, DE, and Coyle, N: Spinal opioid analgesics and local anesthetics in the management of chronic cancer pain, *J Pain Sympt Manag* **1**:79–86, Spring 1986.

Naldi, L, Zucchi A, Brevi A et al: Corticosteroids and post-herpetic neuralgia (letter), *Lancet* **336**:947, 1990.

National Headache Foundation Newsletter, no. **63**:12, Winter 1987–88.

Ozuna, J, and Snyder, G: An experience with epidural morphine in lumbar surgery patients, *J Neurosci Nurs* **19**:235–239, Oct 1987.

Pagliaro, AM: Preparation, administration, and monitoring of medications. In Pagliaro, AM, and Pagliaro, LA, eds: *Pharmacologic Aspects of Nursing*, pp. 30–67, The CV Mosby Co., St. Louis, 1986.

Paice, JA: Intrathecal morphine infusion for intractable cancer pain: a new use for implanted pumps, *Oncol Nurs Forum* **13**:41–47, May-June 1986.

Paice, JA: New delivery systems in pain management, *Nurs Clin North Am* **22**:715–726, 1987.

Paice, JA: Personal communication, 1988a. This clinical example was given to us by Judy Paice, RN, MS, Assistant Professor and Acting Coordinator, Oncology Graduate Program, College of Nursing, Rush University and a doctoral student at the University of Illinois at Chicago. We appreciate her willingness to share this example.

Paice, JA: The phenomenon of analgesic tolerance in cancer pain management, *Oncol Nurs Forum* **15**:455–460, July-Aug 1988b.

Pannuti, F, Rossi, AP, Iafelice, G, et al: Control of chronic pain in very advanced cancer patients with morphine administered by oral, rectal, and sublingual route, *Pharmacol Res Commun* **14**:369–380, 1982.

Parish, K, and Thompson, G: Epidural `port-a-cath', *Austral Nurs J* **17**:44–47, Sept 1987.

Pasternak, GW: Multiple morphine and enkephalin receptors and the relief of pain, *JAMA* **259**:1362–1367, Mar 4, 1988.

Payne, R: Novel routes of opioid administration in the management of cancer pain, *Oncology* **1**(special suppl):10–18, Apr 1987a. Free copies available from Roxanne Laboratories—makers of Roxanol and Roxanol SR.

Payne, R: Role of epidural and intrathecal narcotics and peptides in the management of cancer pain, *Med Clin North Am* **71**:313–327, Mar 1987b.

Penn, RD, and Paice, JA: Chronic intrathecal morphine for intractable pain, *J Neurosurg* **67**:182–186, 1987.

Penn, RD, Paice, JA, Gottschalk, W, and Ivankovich, AD: Cancer pain relief using chronic morphine infusion, *J Neurosurg* **61**:302–306, 1984.

Pfeiffer, FG: Nonsteroidal antiinflammatory drugs. In Pagliaro, AM, and Pagliaro, LA, eds: *Pharmacologic Aspects of Nursing*, pp. 1319–1345, The CV Mosby Co., St Louis, 1986.

Pitorak, EF, and Kraus, JC: Pain control with sublingual morphine, *Am J Hosp Care* **4**:39–41, Mar-Apr 1987.

Plezia, PM, and Linford, J: Innovative approaches to refractory pain, *Hospital Ther* **10**:25–42, Oct 1985.

Portenoy, RK: Continuous infusion of opioid drugs in the treatment of cancer pain: guidelines for use, *J Pain Sympt Manag* **1**:223–228, 1986.

Portenoy, RK: Continuous intravenous infusion of opioid drugs, *Med Clin North Am* **71**:233–241, Mar 1987a.

Portenoy, RK: Drug treatment of pain syndromes, *Semin Neurol* **7**:139–149, June 1987b.

Portenoy, R, Moulin, DE, Rogers, A, et al: Intravenous infusion of opioids in cancer pain: clinical review and guidelines for use, *Cancer Treat Rep* **70**:575–581, 1986.

Porter, J, and Jick, H: Addiction rare in patients treated with narcotics, *N Engl J Med* **302**:123, 1980.

Rawal, N, and Sjostrand, UH: Clinical application of epidural and intrathecal opioids for pain management, *Int Anesthesiol Clin* **24**:43–57, Summer 1986.

Rawal, N, and Tandon, B: Epidural and intrathecal morphine in intensive care units, *Intens Care Med* **11**:129–133, 1985.

Reasbeck, PG, Rice, ML, and Reasbeck, JC: Double-blind controlled trial of indomethacin as an adjunct to narcotic analgesia after major abdominal surgery, *Lancet* **2**:115–118, 1982.

Rickels, A, Feighner, JP, and Smith, WT: Alprazolam, amitriptyline, doxepin, and placebo in the treatment of depression, *Arch Gen Psychiatr* **42**:134–141, 1985.

Rimar, J: Epidural morphine for analgesia following a cesarean, *Matern Child Nurs* **11**:345, Sept-Oct 1985.

Ritter, MA, and Gioe, TJ: The effect of indomethacin on para-articular ectopic ossification following total hip arthroplasty, *Clin Orthop Rel Res* **167**:113–117, July 1982.

Rogers, A: Analgesic consultation: the use of methadone in opioid-tolerant patients, *J Pain Sympt Manag* **3**:45, 1988a.

Rogers, A: Analgesic consultation, *Am J Nurs* **88**:100, Jan 1988b.

Royal College of Surgeons of England College of Anaesthetists: Report of the Working Party; *Pain After Surgery*, Sept. 1990.

Rumore, MM, and Schlicting, DA: Clinical efficacy of antihistaminics as analgesics, *Pain* **25**:7-22, 1986.

Rutter, PC, Murphy, F, and Dudley, HAF: Morphine: controlled trial of different methods of administration for postoperative pain relief, *Brit Med J* **280**:12–13, Jan 5, 1980.

Semple, P, Madej, TH, Wheatley, RG et al: Transdermal hyoscine with patient controlled analgesia, *Anaesthesia* **47**:399–401, 1992.

Sheehan, AP, and Sauerbier, GA: Continuous subcutaneous infusion of morphine, *Oncol Nurs Forum* **13**:92, 1986.

Simpson, KH, Tring, IC, Ellis, FR: An investigation of pre-medication with morphine given by the buccal or intramuscular route, *Br J Clin Pharm* **27**:377–380, 1989.

Slavic-Svircev, V, Kaiko, G, Heidrich, RF, and Rusy, BF: Ibuprofen in the treatment of postoperative pain, *Am J Med* **77**:84–86, July 13, 1984.

Smith, KA: Teaching family members intrathecal morphine administration, *J Neurosci Nurs* **18**:95–97, Apr 1986.

Spiegel, K, Kalb, R, and Pasternak, GW: Analgesic activity of tricyclic antidepressants, *Ann Neurol* **13**:462– 465, 1983.

Sriwatanakul, K, Weis, OF, Alloza, JL, Kelvie, W, Weintraub, M, and Lasagna, L: Analysis of narcotic analgesic usage in the treatment of postoperative pain, *JAMA* **250**:926–929, 1983.

St. Marie, B, and Henrickson, K: Intraspinal narcotic infusions for terminal cancer pain, *J Intravenous Nurs* **11**:161–163, May-June 1988.

Stambaugh, JE, and Sarajian, C: Evaluation of hydroxyzine versus pethidine in the relief of chronic pain due to malignancy. In *Pain Abstracts*, vol. 1, p. 203, International Association for the Study of Pain, Seattle, 1978.

Stambaugh, JE, Jr, and Wainer, IW: Drug interaction: pethidine and chlorpromazine, a toxic combination, *J Clin Pharmacol* **21**:140–146, 1981.

Stapleton, JV, Austin, KL, and Mather, LE: A pharmacokinetic approach to postoperative pain: continuous infusion of pethidine, *Anaesth Intens Care* **7**:25–32, Feb 1979.

Stauffer, JD: Antidepressants and chronic pain, *J Fam Pract* **25**:167–170, Aug 1987.

Stenseth, R, Sellevold, O, and Breivik, H: Epidural morphine for postoperative pain: experience with 1085 patients, *Acta Anaesthesiol Scand* **29**:148–156, 1985.

Stimmel, B: Pain, *Analgesia and Addiction: the Pharmacologic Treatment of Pain*, pp. 294–297, Raven Press, New York, 1983.

Stuart, GJ, Davey, EB, and Wight, SE: Continuous intravenous morphine infusions for terminal pain control: a retrospective review, *Drug Intell Clin Pharm* **20**:968–972, Dec 1986.

Swerdlow, M: Anticonvulsant drugs and chronic pain, *Clin Neuropharmacol* **7**:51–82, 1984.

Szeto, H, Inturrisi, C, Houde, R, et al: Accumulation of norpethidine, an active metabolite of pethidine, in patients with renal failure or cancer, *Ann Intern Med* **86**:738–741, 1977.

Tang, R, Shimomura, SK, and Rotblatt, M: Pethidine-induced seizures in sickle cell patients, *Hosp Formul* **15**:764–772, Oct 1980.

Tejada, IM: Indocin suppository for control of pain in post-thoracic surgery patient, *Oncol Nurs Forum* **13**:87, May-June 1986.

Trotter, JM, Scott, R, Macbeth, FR, et al: Problems of the oncology outpatient: role of the liaison health visitor, *Br Med J* **282**:122–124, Jan 10, 1981.

Twycross, RG: Clinical experience with diamorphine in advanced malignant disease, *Int J Clin Pharmacol* **9**:184–198, 1974.

Twycross, RG, and Lack, SA: *Symptom Control in Far Advanced Cancer*, Pitman, London, 1983.

Twycross, RG: The management of pain in cancer: a guide to drugs and dosages, *Primary Care & Cancer* **8**:15–23, May 1988.

Ventafridda, V, Fochi, C, DeConno, D, et al: Use of non-steroidal anti-inflammatory drugs in the treatment of pain in cancer, *Br J Clin Pharmacol* **10**:3435–3465, 1980.

Ventafridda, V, Ripamonti, C, DeConno, F, et al: Antidepressants increase bioavailability of morphine in cancer patients (letter) *Lancet* **1**:1204, May 23, 1987.

Wallace, J: Morphine sulfate administered sublingually to control chronic pain, *Oncol Nurs Forum* (Practice Corner) **14**:66, Mar-Apr 1987.

Walsh, TD: Common misunderstandings about the use of morphine for chronic pain in advanced cancer, *CA–Cancer J Clinic* **35**:164–169, May-June 1985.

Ward, NG: Tricyclic antidepressants for chronic low-back pain, *Spine* **11**:661–665, Sept 1982.

Washton, AM, Resnick, RB, Geyer, G: Opiate withdrawal using lofexidine, a clonidine analogue with fewer side-effects, *J Clin Psychiatry* **44**:335–337, 1983.

Watt-Watson, JH: Nurses' knowledge of pain issues: a survey, *J Pain Sympt Manag* **2**:207–211, Fall 1987.

Weingart, WA, Sorkness, CA, and Earhart, RH: Analgesia with oral narcotics and added ibuprofen in cancer patients, *Clin Pharm* **4**:53–58, Jan-Feb 1985.

Weinstock, M, et al: Effect of physostigmine on morphineinduced postoperative pain and somnolence, *Br J Anaesthesiol* **54**:429–432, 1982.

Wenzloff, NJ, and Shrimp, L: Therapeutic management of primary dysmenorrhea, *Drug Intell Clin Pharm* **18**:22–26, 1984

Wermeling, DP, Record, KE, and Foster, TS: Patient-controlled high dose morphine therapy in a patient with electrical burns, *Clin Pharm* **5**:832–835, Oct 1986.

Westerling, D, et al: Absorption and bioavailability of rectally administered morphine in women, *Eur J Clin Pharmacol* **23**:5964, 1982.

Westring, EW: Pethidine vs morphine, *JAMA* **230**:1512, Dec 16, 1974.

White, PF: Use of patient-controlled analgesia for management of acute pain, *JAMA* **259**:243–247, Jan 8, 1988.

Whitman, HH: Sublingual morphine, *Am J Nurs* **84**:939, July 1984.

Wilkes, E (ed.): Controlled release morphine tablets are effective in twice daily dosage in cancer pain. In *Advances in Morphine Therapy, the 1983 International Symposium on Pain Control.* Royal Society of Medicine International Congress and Symposium, series no. 64, pp 103–105, 1984.

Wilkie, D: Sublingual efficacy challenged, *Oncol Nurs Forum* **14**:13 (letter) Sept-Oct 1987.

Woodrow, KM, and Eltherington, LG: Feeling no pain, alcohol as an analgesic, *Pain* **32**:159–163, 1988.

Wright, Z: From IV to PO: titrating your patient's pain medication, *Nursing 81* **11**:39–43, July 1981.

Yaksh, TL: Spinal opiate analgesia: characteristics and principles of action, *Pain* **11**:293–346, 1981.

Yasko, JM: *Guidelines for Cancer Care: Symptom Management*, pp. 73–93, Reston Publishing Co., Virginia, 1983.

5

Cutaneous Stimulation

Relevant Patient/Family Teaching Points (see Appendix):
• **Ice Application or Massage for Pain Relief**
• **Massage of Body, Hands or Feet**
• **Pain Relief with Heat? Cold? Both?**

The warmth of the sun, massage by a human hand, and ice or snow (in those climates where it was available) may well have been among the very first pain-relief methods used by primitive man. But today if you had pain somewhere between your lower trunk and upper thighs, would you seek relief by sitting in a basin of cold water or warm water? Research shows that some people tried both with varying results. These and other methods of stimulating the skin, such as vibrators and electric impulses, continue to be widely used in pain control. In fact, some methods of pain relief consist in inflicting pain to relieve pain. But what works for some people and some types of pain does not work for others. Each to his own device.

Ideas about uses of heat, cold, and other methods of cutaneous stimulation are more likely to be derived from our culture and personal experiences than from well-tested, scientific information. In fact, well-controlled research on this topic is scarce and these techniques should not be practised without appropriate prior training.

DEFINITION OF CUTANEOUS STIMULATION

In this chapter the term *cutaneous stimulation* is defined quite simply as *stimulating the skin for the purpose of relieving pain.* The techniques selected, however, will be limited to those that meet the following criteria:

• Non-injurious or very low risk when used properly.
• Usually readily available in the home or hospital setting.
• Require very little expertise to use safely and effectively.

To increase patient acceptance and to avoid the complication of tissue damage, the directions will be to use the techniques at levels of stimulation that are either *comfortable to the patient or only moderately uncomfortable* for a brief time.

The methods of cutaneous stimulation discussed in this chapter are the mild or superficial forms of the following that are readily accessible to the nurse providing appropriate training has been received.
• Superficial massage.
• Pressure/massage.
• Vibration.
• Superficial heat and cold.
• Ice application/massage.
• TENS (transcutaneous electrical nerve stimulation).

All of the above may be used by skilled, prepared nurses or other health professionals, such as physiotherapists, for reasons other than those covered in this chapter. For example, a physiotherapist may use ice massage to facilitate stretching a painful muscle or mobilizing a painful joint, but that use of ice massage is not included here.

IMMEDIATE HELP FOR CUTANEOUS STIMULATION

Time involved. Reading time, 5–10 minutes; implementation time, 5–10 minutes.

Sample situation. The patient is in agony with sudden, unexpected, but fairly well-localized pain. This could be in A&E, in the home, or on a clinical unit in the hospital. The doctor is notified and does not want to order analgesics until the patient is assessed. How can you relieve at least some of the pain without the risk of masking symptoms?

Possible solution. Ask the doctor to authorize the use of local application of heat, cold, or ice until diagnostic procedures begin or assessment is complete. These methods of cutaneous stimulation are almost always available. If the physician says these might be contra-indicated or if there is an open wound, suggest that heat, cold, or ice can be used at a site distant to the pain (see *Do's* below), e.g. on the opposite side of the body. Explain that this may partially over-ride or mask the sensation of pain temporarily and will reassure the patient that something is being done. NOTE: Cold application is not the same as ice application. Cold is applied at a comfortable level of intensity, usually wrapped. In ice application a frozen substance is in direct contact with the skin.

Expected outcome. Patient temporarily experiences partial or complete pain relief.

Do's

1. Assure the patient you know he hurts as much as he says he does, and explain why medications cannot be used at the present time to relieve the pain.
2. Tell the patient what options you have for providing pain relief, e.g. heat, cold, or ice.
3. If there is a choice, tell the patient he can try whichever one has helped him before, but that cold or ice probably has a better chance than heat of relieving the pain.
4. Apply heat, cold, or ice to the site of pain if possible.
5. If the site of pain cannot be used for application, explain that heat, cold, or ice need not be applied to the site of pain. Acknowledge that it probably sounds unlikely but that clinical experience and research have shown the application of heat, cold, or ice to sites distant from the pain sometimes relieves pain, perhaps by distraction. The simple possibilities for sites distant from the pain are:
   - Between pain and the brain.
   - On the other side of, beyond, the pain (e.g. use the hand if the forearm is injured).
   - On the opposite side of the body corresponding to the site of the pain.

NOTE: More than one of the above sites can be used at one time. (For further information regarding sites for application of cold, heat, or ice, see Fig. 5.1 for general recommendations, Figs. 5.2–5.5 for trigger points for musculoskeletal injuries, and Fig. 5.7 for acupuncture points at a distance from the pain site.)

6. If heat or cold is used, encourage the patient to use intermittent stimulation, developing his own rhythm of on and off, perhaps every 5 seconds or every 1–2 minutes.
7. If heat and cold are both allowed, alternate them every few seconds or minutes.
8. If increased sensation of heat or cold is desired, use a moist cloth next to the skin.
9. If ice massage is used, remember:
   - Warn the patient that the sensations are not very comfortable and generally progress from extreme cold to burning, aching, and finally numbness.
   - Ice should be in direct contact with the skin (do not cover with anything waterproof).
   - Ice may be rubbed gently on the skin, avoiding pressure over boney prominences.
   - Provide a cloth to wipe up the water as the ice melts.
   - Discontinue application of ice after 10 minutes or whenever there is shivering, numbness, or skin irritation; skin colour alternates between white and red; or the patient says it is intolerable. If ice must be discontinued at that site, another site may be tried. (For further information, refer to "Ice Application or Massage for Pain Relief", Appendix.)
10. Allow the patient or family to participate as much as they wish.
11. After 5–10 minutes, ask the patient if this has helped. If not, try one or more of the following:
    - Changing sites or using an additional site.
    - Switching to another form of stimulation if it is allowed (e.g., switch from warm to cold application).
    - Use intermittent stimulation. If this has been done, vary the rhythm.
12. Reassure the patient that more effective pain relief probably will be provided once the diagnosis is made.

Don'ts

1. Do not expect or suggest that this will relieve all of the patient's pain.
2. Do not tell the patient he simply must endure the pain until the doctor finds out what is causing it.
3. Do not tell the patient that he is merely frightened or that his pain is not as bad as it seems.
4. Do not tell the patient nothing else can be done to help him.
5. Do not apply heat to a site where there is bleeding or swelling.
6. Do not apply ice for longer than 10 minutes (to avoid tissue damage).
7. If cold completely relieves the pain, do not apply cold for longer than 30 minutes because pain returns much more slowly following cold than heat. You want to avoid pain relief that long outlasts the application of cold since the return of pain may be important in making a medical diagnosis.

In this chapter discussion of cutaneous stimulation will be limited to methods that the nurse in general practice may use for palliative pain relief. Methods that have only a superficial effect on skin and subcutaneous tissues will be covered. Thus superficial heating and cooling will be discussed, but vigorous or deep heating such as ultrasound or diathermy to heat a joint will not be. Nevertheless, remember that even superficial use of cutaneous stimulation has indirect effects on deep, striated muscles and on smooth muscles of visceral organs.

BENEFITS AND LIMITS OF CUTANEOUS STIMULATION

The cutaneous stimulation methods as discussed in this chapter are *not therapeutic or curative*, rather they are palliative, for the purpose of pain relief.

The effects of cutaneous stimulation are variable and unpredictable, but in general the expectation is that pain will be eliminated or the intensity of pain may be decreased, during and/or for varying periods after stimulation. Sometimes cutaneous stimulation is briefly painful, and then pain relief occurs following the stimulation. In some instances the character of the pain may simply change to a sensation that is more acceptable, e.g. a change from sharp to dull.

Some methods of cutaneous stimulation undoubtedly have relaxing or distracting effects in addition to activating mechanisms that actually reduce the intensity of pain. Since cutaneous stimulation involves touching the patient in some way with the intent of helping the patient, it is also possible that the effectiveness of a method may be related to therapeutic touch.

> **KEY POINT:** The major effect of cutaneous stimulation is usually a reduced intensity of pain during stimulation and/or for a period afterwards.

The underlying mechanisms of pain relief from cutaneous stimulation are usually unknown. Broadly speaking, the gate control theory suggests that stimulation of the skin may activate the large-diameter fibres. In turn, that activation may provoke an inhibition of the pain messages carried by the smaller fibres, i.e. close the gate to the transmission of impulses felt as painful. Another possibility is that certain types of cutaneous stimulation may increase levels of endorphins, the body's natural morphine. Some types of cutaneous stimulation, such as vibration or cold application, may cause decreased sensitivity to pain, such as partial or complete anaesthesia or numbness of the skin.

When pharmacologically active substances are applied topically, pain may be relieved because an analgesic or anaesthetic is absorbed through the skin and depresses cutaneous receptors, or because stimulation of cutaneous receptors causes distraction from pain by inducing sensations such as warmth.

Hyperstimulation analgesia, or counter-irritation, is one type of cutaneous stimulation. These terms usually apply to various types of moderate to intense sensory stimulation, such as with cold, heat, rubbing, or pressure. Obviously, at intense levels these stimuli are often painful. This is an example of the phenomenon of one painful stimulus reducing pain caused by another painful stimulus—producing pain to abolish pain. A woman who bites her lip during a labour contraction may explain that biting relieves discomfort from the contraction by acting as a distraction, but the pain relief is very likely due to more complicated events. Brief, moderate pain seems to produce nerve impulses that act as a complex neural inhibitory mechanism leading to relief of more intense, prolonged pain at near or distant sites.

The *potential benefits* of cutaneous stimulation methods as seen in clinical practice can be summarized as:

1. Decrease intensity of pain, sometimes eliminate pain. In some instances the sensation of pain may be changed to a more acceptable sensation, e.g. a change from sharp pain to a feeling of warmth.

2. Relieve muscle spasms secondary to underlying skeletal and joint pathology or nerve root irritation, i.e. interrupt the vicious cycle of muscle spasm, ischaemia, pain, and more muscle spasm.

3. Increase physical activity and ability to engage in therapeutic exercises due to relief of muscle spasm and/or decreased perception of pain.

4. Some patients may report that the cutaneous stimulation distracts them from pain, promotes general relaxation, or decreases anxiety.

5. The onset and duration of pain relief may include the period during stimulation and/or a period following stimulation.

6. Strengthen the nurse-patient relationship and convey caring through socially acceptable physical contact, e.g. touching, especially valuable for someone who is uncomfortable with physical demonstrations of affection or concern.

7. Physical contacts may improve body image, especially for a person who has undergone recent body image disturbances, e.g. mastectomy or amputation of a limb, or long periods of pain. Perception of a comfortable sensation such as warmth may be in marked contrast to constant awareness of pain.

8. Most methods require very little patient participation/activity and are therefore especially appropriate for patients with limited physical or mental energy or for use at bedtime.

9. Some methods, e.g. massage, essential oils or simply application of heat or cold packs, are ideal ways to involve family and friends who feel helpless or want to do something for the patient.

10. Some methods, e.g. application of topical analgesia anaesthetic preparations or pressure on a trigger point, are quickly and easily done by patients, providing them with a sense of control and independence while they continue other activities.

Some *possible limitations or disadvantages* of cutaneous stimulation for pain relief are:

1. Successful cutaneous stimulation may be misunderstood by the patient as meaning that the condition is cured.

2. Some methods may be unacceptable to certain patients because of inherent characteristics of the methods, e.g. the confusing or visible equipment associated with TENS, the odour of topical agents, or the discomfort of ice massage.

3. Massage/pressure, vibration, cold, heat and ice are so ordinary and commonplace that their effectiveness is usually underestimated by both patients and health professionals.

4. In spite of appropriate precautions, tissue damage may accidently occur, e.g. blistering from heat or cold applications.

Pointers on Selecting a Method of Cutaneous Stimulation

- Massage (p. 137). Minimal side effects and contra-indications. Backrubs or body massage can be time consuming and may relieve only mild pain, but pain need not be localized and most patients enjoy this therapy. Modest patients may object to touch or disrobing. Massage of feet and hands may be more accessible, acceptable, and even more effective.

- Pressure, sometimes with massage (p. 138). Massage/pressure to trigger points or acupuncture points may be very effective but is briefly uncomfortable. Initially it requires time to locate the points. But then patients can learn to work on some trigger points on their own.

- Vibration (p. 147). A more vigorous form of massage that may be more effective. Low risk of tissue damage. Check on availability or cost of a vibrator. May be used for trigger points. May be unacceptable due to noise or intensity of stimulation if vibrator is not adjustable. Sometimes this is a less expensive substitute for TENS.

- Heat and cold (p.140). Probably works best for well-localized pain. Both may be done with a minimum of equipment and both should be applied at a comfortable level of intensity. Cold has more advantages than heat. Unwanted side effects, e.g. burns, and contra-indications, e.g. bleeding and swelling, are more frequent with heating than with cooling. When cold relieves pain, it tends to be more effective than heat. However, patients usually prefer heat to cold, and use of cold often requires some persuasion.

- Ice application/massage (p.145). A frozen substance applied to the skin is uncomfortable, but only for a few minutes before numbness occurs. Continuous use for 10 minutes or less. Pain must be well localized. May relieve severe pain. Simple, low-risk technique for brief, painful procedures. Especially effective in obliterating needle stick pain. May be used on trigger points. Sometimes this is a very inexpensive substitute for TENS.

- Menthol (p.139). Refers to menthol-containing substances for application to skin. Intensity increases with amount of menthol; may be uncomfortable at higher concentrations. Odour offensive to some people. Use influenced by culture; more restricted use in America than in other cultures, e.g., Asia. Inexpensive. Once it is applied, it provides continuous stimulation without additional effort. Well-suited for nighttime use.

- TENS (p.149). Compared with above methods, much more expensive, less available, and more time needed to teach nurse and patient, but supported by more research and regarded by many as more "scientific."

5. Mild forms of cutaneous stimulation, such as those covered in this chapter, usually produce milder, more superficial, and less prolonged effects than vigorous types of cutaneous stimulation such as kneading massage (squeezing and movement of deep tissues) or ultrasound for deep heating, e.g. to joint.

NURSING-CARE GUIDELINES FOR SELECTING, DEVELOPING, AND USING CUTANEOUS STIMULATION FOR PAIN RELIEF

These general suggestions are intended to point you in the right direction. You will need to read further in this chapter for specific guidelines about the method selected. The following includes general information about the practical aspects of:

• Selecting the most appropriate type of cutaneous stimulation for the patient and the condition.

• Choosing a site for application.

• Determining duration and frequency of use.

• Modifying the method, e.g. to achieve greater relief or patient acceptability.

For all of the above, the basic approach is trial and error. Because these are physical modalities with well-defined parameters, e.g. measurable temperature ranges, it is tempting to think that we possess fairly precise knowledge about which conditions certain methods should and should not be used for, how often, how long, and where.

> **KEY POINT:** Determining which method to use for the patient, at which site, when, and for how long is mostly a matter of trial and error.

Selection of method

1. Keep in mind availability of method, cost, amount of time required of patient or caregivers, safety and possible side effects, potential effectiveness, contra-indications, and patient acceptability. See the box on the previous page for a brief overview of these points for each method, including pages for further reading.

2. As much as possible, give the patient a choice, especially initially. But keep in mind the following:

• For many types of pain cutaneous stimulation methods can be used interchangeably unless there are contra-indications. For example, contrary to popular opinion, heat and cold can be used interchangeably for many conditions, and cold is often more effective than heat.

• Potentially effective methods may be disregarded because of preconceived ideas about which method can be used for specific types of pain.

• Sensations produced by cutaneous stimulation may be uncomfortable or unacceptable in the absence of pain, but they may be preferable or helpful in the presence of pain.

> **KEY POINT:** Although massage, heat, cold and ice seem ordinary, they may be used to provide very effective pain relief and one may work as well as the other.

Terms Related to Site Selection

Acupuncture point. A point or spot on the body associated with a conceptual (not anatomical) system of meridians. Between 500 and 800 points were identified centuries ago by cultures of the Far East. Some are related to pain syndromes, but others are not. Those related to pain are often located near or in the same place as trigger points.

Contralateral. On the opposite side of the body; opposed to ipsilateral.

Distal. Farthest from the centre of the body; opposed to proximal.

Ipsilateral. On the same side of the body; opposed to contralateral.

Proximal. Nearest the centre of the body; opposed to distal. May be referred to here as "between pain and the brain."

Trigger point. A point or area of hyperirritability in tissue such as myofascia (skeletal muscle and its fascia). When compressed it is tender and may give rise to referred pain, but after stimulation, e.g. with ischaemic pressure, pain may be relieved. Trigger points are often located near or in the same place as acupuncture points.

Selection of site. Trial and error combined with open-mindedness are needed. Following are groups of sites that may be stimulated in an effort to relieve pain (see the box below for definitions of terms used in this section; see Figs. 5.1–5.7 for examples):

- Directly over or around pain. This is usually, but not always, the best site.
- Proximal to pain—"between pain and brain."
- Distal to pain.
- Contralateral to pain.
- Acupuncture point.
- Trigger point.
- Any site distant to the pain.

The *mechanisms* underlying pain relief produced by stimulation of sites distant to pain are not fully understood. Stimulation at one site may produce at least mild effects at distant sites in the body, called the *consensual response*. For example, heat applied to one site increases blood flow in other parts of the body such as the contralateral limb.

Still another explanation for pain relief at a site distant from stimulation is *counter-irritation*, which is thought to produce nerve impulses that act as a complex neural inhibitory mechanism leading to relief of other pain. Surprisingly, spraying ethyl chloride (ice sensation) on the skin of the leg to the point of causing pain significantly reduced pain from electrical stimulation of a tooth filling (Parsons and Goetzl, 1945)—truly a case of inflicting pain to relieve pain, and it demonstrates that stimulation of sites very distant from the inflicted pain can affect pain.

It has also been theorized that the area of the brain responsible for exerting inhibitory control over pain signals may not have an anatomically correct representation of the human body. Not only may certain areas of the body be larger or smaller in the brain's representation than in reality, but also some areas may be close to each other in the brain but not on the actual body. Thus when one area of the body is stimulated, this may be perceived in the brain at a point near a representation of an area anatomically unrelated. However, the strength of the stimulation may spill over into the nearby area and send inhibitory signals to the anatomically unrelated body part.

Stimulation of *acupuncture points and trigger points*, within the area of pain or at a distance from the pain, have long been known to produce pain relief, but the underlying reason is unclear.

What is interesting and of great practical significance is that the locations of acupuncture points for pain and trigger points are similar. Further, both can often be found simply by using the balls of the fingers and thumbs to probe areas within and around the site of pain, asking the patient to identify which

areas beneath the skin are the most sensitive. Sometimes pressure on the area produces or increases the pain. Hopefully, pain will decrease following stimulation of the point with one of the cutaneous stimulation methods, e.g. pressure or moist heat.

Since it is beyond the scope of this book to explain the location of all trigger points or acupuncture points, a few of each have been selected. Figs. 5.2–5.5 illustrate trigger points associated with some common pain problems in the head, neck, and back. Trigger point sites vary from person to person, more so than acupuncture points are often thought to do. Therefore the trigger point illustrations are to be considered as examples, and references cited in this chapter can be followed up if more in-depth knowledge is required.

Some acupuncture points that are distant from the site of pain are illustrated in Fig. 5.6. Traditionally, these points were needled to relieve pain. However, there are more practical approaches to finding and using acupuncture points. Not only can they often be located by probing with the fingers, but research has shown that the site of at least some points is not necessarily a discrete point but is a large area. For example, stimulation of the Hoku point (Fig. 5.7) often relieves dental pain, but so does immersing the entire hand in ice water or stimulating between the fourth and fifth fingers. In this instance the site that can be effectively stimulated may be any point on the entire hand. In other words, stimulation of an acupuncture point may be effective even when the stimulation is not exactly where the point is supposed to be.

> **KEY POINT:** Experiment to find the most effective stimulation site for the patient. It may be at some distance from the pain.

Duration and frequency. Again, this is determined by trial and error in addition to what is convenient and practical. Consider the following:

1. The most frequent period of time suggested for all cutaneous stimulation techniques, except ice application/massage, is 20–30 minutes.
2. To a certain extent, the longer stimulation is used, the longer pain relief will last after the stimulation is stopped.
3. Whenever possible, use the method before pain occurs or increases.

4. If either of the following occur, discontinue the method immediately:
   • Increased pain.
   • Skin irritation.

Modification of method that fails to relieve pain is certainly indicated since the lack of specific guidelines makes cutaneous stimulation largely a matter of trial and error. Modification may include the following considerations:

1. A single, initial failure need not be cause for discarding the technique. Several trials may be warranted.
2. Try changing some characteristics of the specific technique selected, e.g. switch from dry to moist, or reduce pressure or weight of anything touching the skin.
3. Increasing the intensity of stimulation is especially likely to be effective.
4. If modifications of the originally selected technique are not successful, change from one type of cutaneous stimulation to another type, e.g. change from heat to cold or cold to ice. Each cutaneous stimulation technique produces a different sensation from the others.
5. Alternate methods of cutaneous stimulation. This may prevent adaptation to the sensation. Cutaneous stimulation methods may be alternated in several ways:

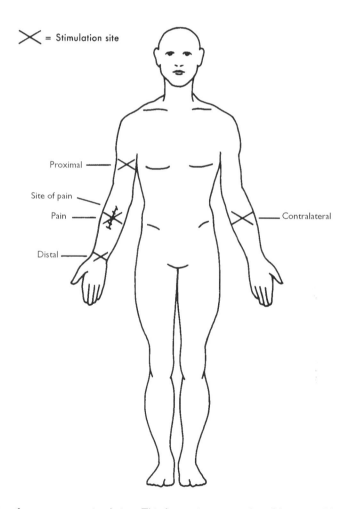

Fig. 5.1 Illustration of sites for cutaneous stimulation. This figure gives examples of four possible sites: site of pain, proximal to pain, distal to pain, and contralateral.

Figs 5.2–5.5 Trigger points and related areas of pain. X, Trigger point; *solid*, region of pain present in almost every patient; *stippling*, region where some but not all patients experience pain. Stimulation of the trigger point(s), e.g. by pressure, should produce the pain pattern shown. The major muscle involved is noted, and comments are made about names given to the conditions and certain characteristics of the pain.

NOTE: Appropriate therapy should be used to treat the condition and reduce the pain, but techniques such as spraying the area with a *vapocoolant* and stretching the muscle are beyond the scope of this book. Temporary relief can be obtained by using the various cutaneous stimulation techniques described in this chapter. Moist heat and ischaemic pressure are most often recommended. Experiment with what works best for the patient.

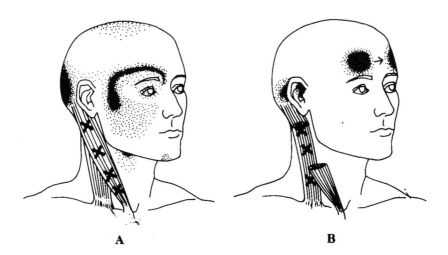

Fig. 5.2 Muscle: sternocleidomastoid. A, Sternal (superficial) division; B, clavicular (deep) division. Comment: tension headache, atypical facial neuralgia, sometimes accompanied by ipsilateral sweating of forehead, tearing and reddening of eye, rhinitis, or visual disturbances; some soreness in neck but no stiffness. Called "whiplash" when muscles are bilaterally involved.

Adapted from Travel, JG, and Simmons, DG: *Myofascial Pain and Dysfunction: the Trigger Point Manual*, Baltimore, 1983, Williams & Wilkins.

Fig. 5.3 Muscle: occipitofrontalis. A, Right frontalis belly; B, left occipitalis belly. Comment: headache; these trigger points respond well to ischaemic pressure easily applied by patient.

Redrawn with permission from Travel, JG, and Simmons, DG: *Myofascial Pain and Dysfunction: the Trigger Point Manual*, p. 291, Baltimore, 1983, Williams & Wilkins.

Fig. 5.4 Muscle: subscapularis. Comment: frozen shoulder; severe pain both at rest and on motion; progressive limitation of arm movement.

Redrawn with permission from Travel, JG, and Simmons, DG: *Myofascial Pain and Dysfunction: the Trigger Point Manual*, p. 411, Baltimore, 1983, Williams & Wilkins.

Fig. 5.5 Muscles: superficial (erector spinae) group of the thoracolumbar paraspinal muscle consisting of iliocostalis thoracis, iliocostalis lumborum, and longissimus thoracis. *T*, Thoracic vertebra; *L*, lumbar vertebra. Comment: back pain or 'lumbago' markedly restricts activity; usually caused by sudden or sustained overload, e.g. when lifting. The patient can learn to apply ischaemic compression to the trigger points in these superficial back muscles by lying on a tennis ball on the floor, moving around until the ball presses on the sensitive point and gradually applying increasing body weight for 1 minute or longer. Moist heat may be applied afterward.

Redrawn with permission from Travel, JG, and Simmons, DG: *Myofascial Pain and Dysfunction: the Trigger Point Manual*, p. 638, Baltimore, 1983, Williams & Wilkins.

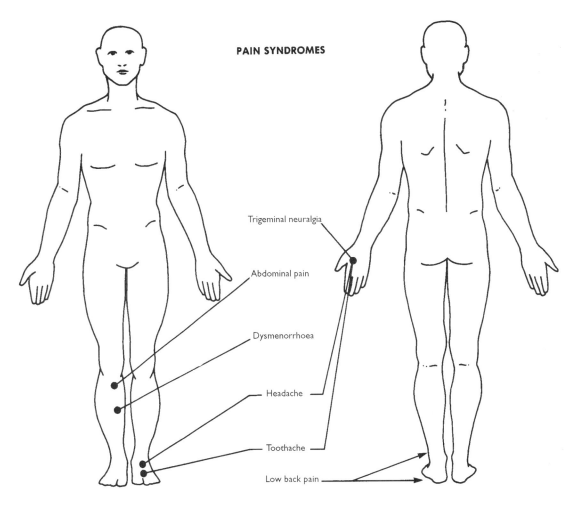

PAIN SYNDROMES

Trigeminal neuralgia

Abdominal pain

Dysmenorrhoea

Headache

Toothache

Low back pain

Fig. 5.6 Basic acupuncture points that are at a distance from the site of pain.
Adapted from Melzack, Stillwell and Fox, 1977, p. 19.

Fig. 5.7 Hoku point, an acupuncture point, stimulated to relieve a variety of conditions, particularly those from the neck up, e.g. headaches and tooth pain. It may be stimulated sufficiently either with ice massage to the skin over the point or by pressure with the thumb against the second metacarpal bone.

- Choose two or more different methods and use each at different times, e.g. moist heat in the morning and topical analgesic/anaesthetic preparation at night.
- Rhythmically alternating between two different methods every few seconds or minutes can be very effective, e.g. pressure to a trigger point for 15 seconds followed by moist heat for 5 minutes, repeating this for about 20 minutes.
- Rhythmically alternating between applying and withdrawing a method may also be very effective, e.g. 30 seconds of heat application and 30 seconds without.

> **KEY POINT:** Although it takes more time and energy, much more pain relief may be achieved by alternating or interrupting cutaneous stimulation techniques every few seconds or minutes.

6. Use more than one method at the same time, e.g. try heat at one site and cold at another site at the same time.
7. Remember to continue to include other appropriate forms of pain relief, e.g. analgesics.

SUPERFICIAL MASSAGE

The *effects* of superficial body massage are usually soothing and relaxing, both physically and mentally. Massage may decrease pain, perhaps mainly by relaxing muscles. It increases capillary circulation and ultimately improves general circulation. Some practitioners feel that massage has such negligible physical effects that its use is a waste of time and energy. However, a massage is enjoyed by almost all who receive it.

Probably the most common *areas of the body* to be massaged are the back and shoulders—the usual back rub. Extremities may be added. When it is inconvenient to do a back rub, massage of both hands or both feet may be equally or more effective.

Superficial massage can be carried out solely as a hands-on technique or in combination with preparations such as essential oils used in aromatherapy.

Appropriate/inappropriate situations for massage

Appropriate uses of massage include:
- A patient restricted to bed or a chair, especially if lying on the back much of the time (massage improves circulation and decreases skin breakdown).
- Assist with sleep disturbance.
- Create an acceptable method of touch for a patient who experiences limited physical contact with others, e.g. a patient isolated from family.
- Pain of any type—the comfort of touch is reassuring and provides a welcome contrast to the feeling of pain.
- Create an opportunity to be with and/or talk with the patient.
- A method of communicating care and concern when verbal communication is limited or impossible, e.g. patient speaks another language or has impaired hearing.

Inappropriate uses or possible contra-indications for massage include:
- A patient who says he/she does not want a massage – attempts to persuade the patient to accept a massage should be avoided. Massage involves a degree of intimacy (physical contact and exposure) that is uncomfortable for some patients. The nurse should not insist that the patient receive a massage.
- Situations in which there is limited time to spend with the patient – other nursing-care activities might be a higher priority.
- Open lesions or skin areas that are tender to touch.
- A patient inclined to make inappropriate sexual advances.
- Whenever it causes pain.

Nursing-Care guidelines and patient/family teaching points for using massage

The patient/family teaching point on massage (see Appendix) contains information and guidelines that are useful to the nurse as well as the patient and family. It is written in the exact words that might be either spoken to the patient or duplicated and given to the patient or a family member who can read.

PRESSURE/MASSAGE

Acupuncture points or trigger points that are related to the patient's pain may be massaged with pressure, or ischaemic pressure may be applied to them. Pain relief may occur at the time pressure is applied because of numbness resulting from ischaemia. Or, if tender acupuncture points or trigger points are stimulated, pain relief may occur after pressure is released. The exact mechanism underlying this type of pain relief is unclear in relation to acupuncture points, but pressure is thought to somehow decrease irritability of trigger points.

Appropriate/inappropriate situations for pressure/massage

Appropriate uses of pressure and/or massage are:

- Patients in whom acupuncture points or trigger points related to pain can be identified. Use Figs. 5.2–5.7 as a guide to finding these sites and apply ischaemic pressure, explained in the next section.
- Muscle spasms or aching, sore muscles, especially muscles not suitable for spray and stretch, i.e. spraying a coolant on the skin over the muscle and stretching the muscle.
- Sharp pain from an acute injury, e.g. a cut. Pressure may relieve pain and reduce bleeding.
- "Back pain during labour," occiput of baby's head pressing on coccyx (apply pressure to lower back, e.g. with fist, especially during contraction).
- IM at deltoid site using the pinch–grasp technique.

Inappropriate uses of pressure and/or massage are:

- Patients with increased bleeding time or who bleed or bruise easily.
- Sites where skin has been injured, e.g. burned or cut.
- Areas of thrombophlebitis.

Patient/family teaching points and nursing-care guidelines for applying pressure/massage

Following are points to consider and possibly discuss with the patient regarding use of pressure/massage:

1. *Acupressure.* When a possible acupuncture point is located (see Figs. 5.6 and 5.7), it can be stimulated with pressure and/or massage, referred to as acupressure. Basically this is acupuncture without needles. Pressure may be applied with the thumb, tip of the index finger, or sometimes the palm of the hand or the fingernail or thumbnail. Pressure is applied as firmly as the patient can tolerate. If massage is done, it is in tiny circles at the rate of about 2–3 circles per second. Pressure is firm enough that contact is maintained with the same area of skin but the tissues beneath are massaged.

For someone untrained in acupressure techniques, it is probably safest to try this for a few seconds to examine the results and then continue it, if desired, for up to 1 minute. Patients can learn to do this for themselves if they can reach the site.

2. *Ischaemic compression of trigger point* (also referred to as myotherapy or pain erasure). The goal is to apply sustained pressure to a trigger point such as those shown in Figs. 5.2–5.5 with sufficient force and for a long enough time to inactivate it. Since acupuncture points and trigger points are often in the same site, this will frequently be almost the same thing as acupressure.

The patient is told to relax the appropriate muscle; he/she must not tense it to resist the pressure. Pressure is then applied over the trigger point with the ball of the thumb or finger and with as much force as the patient can tolerate, up to 20–30lb of pressure. Pressure is continued for up to 1 minute. This may be repeated once after a hot pack has been applied for about 10 minutes or more. Briefer pressure of only 7–10 seconds may be used and repeated several times a day.

Explain to the patient that the force of the compression will be uncomfortable, but pain relief is expected afterward or may begin during the compression. However, excessive pain during compression may lead to failure of the technique, so explain to the patient the importance of letting you know how tolerable the pressure is. Pressure can be increased gradually with feedback from the patient.

Massage may be combined with pressure only if it does not cause a marked increase in pain. This combination is similar to the technique of Rolfing, or skin rolling. Upon release of the compression the skin is white (blanched) at first, then red.

For some trigger points, pressure may need to be applied with a knuckle or elbow, depending on the thickness and depth of the muscle.

For hard to reach trigger points on the patient's back, the patient can be taught to use a *tennis ball.* Instruct the patient to lie on the floor on his/her back with the tennis ball under the back. The patient can move around until the ball presses directly on the sensitive trigger point. Body weight can be used to gradually apply increasing pressure for up to a minute.

TOPICAL ANALGESIC/ANAESTHETIC PREPARATIONS

Appropriate/inappropriate situations for application

Topical analgesics/anaesthetics are usually recommended for the temporary relief of minor aches and pains of muscles and joints, including simple backache, strains, and sprains. The following is a list of more varied uses.

Appropriate uses of topical preparations include:
– Arthritis.
– Various pains of muscles, joints and tendons, e.g. low back pain, tension headache, neck pain and sports injuries.
– Application to appropriately related acupuncture points or trigger points.
– Visceral pain of various origins, e.g. gas pain, menstrual cramps (there may be some reflex dilatation of visceral vessels).
– Sore throat.
– Itch.
– Post-herpetic neuralgia.

Inappropriate uses of topical preparations:
– Open wounds.
– Most mucous membranes.
– Over irritated skin.
– If it increases pain.
– Used in conjunction with heat or tight bandaging.

Possible side effects
– Blistering.
– Skin irritation/allergy.

Caution
– If aspirin is contra-indicated, e.g. due to allergy or bleeding problems, avoid preparations containing salicylate.

Product and Application form	Counter-irritant Ingredients
Algipan Rub (non-greasy cream)	Glycol salicylate 10%, methyl nictinate 1%, capiscum oleoresin (capsicin) 0.1%.
Aspellin liniment	Menthol 1.4%, ammonium salicylate 1%, camphor 0.6%, ethyl and methyl salicylate 0.54%
Difflam cream	Benzydamin hydrochloride 3%
Tranvasin cream	Ethyl nicotinate 2%, hexyl nicotinate 2%, tetrahydrofurfuryl salicylate 14%.

Table 5.1 Examples of non-prescription topical analgesic products.

Topical non-steroidal anti-inflammatory drugs

There are an increasing number of topical preparations containing non-steroidal anti-inflammatory drugs (NSAIDs). In the United Kingdom, these preparations are promoted as an alternative to oral NSAIDs. To date, there have been few clinical trials to confirm the efficacy of these preparations compared to oral NSAIDs. In June 1991, however, the Medicines Resource Centre produced the following summary of their investigation of available topical NSAIDs:*

• There have been few trials comparing topical NSAIDs with conventional therapy. Topical piroxicam has been shown to be as effective as oral ibuprofen, but is many times more expensive. Topical diclofenac has been compared with heparinoid. Most trials have been placebo-controlled.

• Topical NSAIDs are well tolerated. Local reactions can occur, but resolve on withdrawal of therapy. Systemic reactions involving the GI tract and central nervous system, and bronchospasm, have been reported.

* Reprinted with permission from the *MeReC Bulletin*, June 1991, **2**:6, published by the Medicines Resource Centre, Liverpool. This centre is a Department of Health initiative which provides independent information and advice on prescribing for all GPs in England.

- All of these preparations (except benzydamine) are contra-indicated in patients in whom aspirin and other NSAIDs induce symptoms of asthma, rhinitis, angioedema and urticaria.
- Clinically significant drug interactions are unlikely.
- There is a large placebo effect for these preparations. A conventional rubefacient or embrocation, which can be bought without a prescription, may produce as good a response.
- All of the topical NSAIDs are more expensive than the equivalent oral preparations.

SUPERFICIAL HEAT AND COLD APPLICATIONS

For centuries heat and cold have been used for pain relief, but surprisingly, the effects of superficial heating and cooling and the mechanisms that underlie the effects are still largely a matter of speculation. Possible mechanisms by which heat and cold may relieve pain are listed in the box opposite. Some of the effects of heat and cold may be similar, but the mechanisms underlying the effects may be different.

Also, interestingly, the effects of heat and cold are not always limited to the direct local effects; there may be distant effects. The mechanisms underlying this are poorly understood.

Superficial heating methods, with a temperature of approximately 40–45°C (104–113°F)* at point of contact with skin, usually warm only the skin; the muscles and other deeper tissues usually are not affected because they are insulated by the subcutaneous fat. Methods of applying superficial heat that are convenient and commonly available in the home or hospital setting include the following:

1. Packs
   - Rubber hot water bottle (wrap in cover to prevent burns).
   - Electric heating pad, dry or moist (avoid burns by not falling asleep on top of pad since heat output tends to increase; avoid electric shock by proper insulation and following instructions).

*The temperature ranges cited for methods of superficial heating and cooling are merely guidelines in case it becomes necessary to measure the temperature of a heating or cooling method, e.g. in a research project or in a situation where the patient cannot communicate easily regarding the comfort of an application of heat or cold. In daily clinical practice it is rarely necessary to actually use a thermometer since the patient's reported comfort along with close attention to skin reactions are sufficient and maybe better guidelines.

   - Hot moist compresses.
   - Heat packs available through pharmacies or chemists.
2. Immersion in water
   - Bath.
   - Basin.
   - Whirlpool.
3. Radiant heat with 40-watt bulb at a minimum distance of 18 inches (this method of heating avoids touching the area and keeps it dry).
4. Retention of body heat with plastic wrap, e.g. plastic dry cleaner bag taped to itself.

Superficial cooling, around 15°C (59°F) at skin contact, usually cools the skin and, if applied long enough, the muscles. Cold application drops the muscle temperature in slender people after about 10 minutes; in obese people, after about 30 minutes. The effect of cooling on the muscle lasts much longer than the effect of heat on muscle. After heat applications are removed, the muscle rapidly resumes its normal temperature. However, after cold application is discontinued, the fat layer insulates the muscle, and rewarming takes longer depending on the thickness of the fat layer.

Ideally, cold packs should be *sealed* to prevent dripping, *flexible* to conform to body contours, and applied in a manner that produces a *comfortable and safe intensity of cold.* Convenient and readily available, commercially or homemade, *methods of cold application* are:

1. Waterproof bags, e.g. rubber or plastic, filled with ice melting in water.
2. Terry cloth dipped in water with ice shavings, wrung out, and applied repeatedly (frequency of application is an inconvenience).
3. Frozen gel packs. These may be more convenient and may reduce temperature more quickly than the traditional ice bag. (See Fig. 5.8 for uses of flexible cold packs.)
4. Home-made cold packs that are comfortable, quick, and inexpensive:
   - Sealed plastic container (e.g. plastic bag) with one-third alcohol and two-thirds water placed in freezer produces a flexible, unfrozen slush.
   - Sealed plastic container with damp cloth or towel placed in freezer produces flexible cold pack.
   - One-pound bag of frozen green peas or kernels of corn—hit gently to separate peas or corn.

All cold containers, e.g. plastic bags with gel or alcohol and water, should be *wrapped with cloth* to prevent tissue damage and to provide a comfortable intensity of coldness. This slows down the cooling and helps prevent discomfort and tissue damage. A moist cloth allows for faster cooling, if desired.

Appropriate/inappropriate situations for heat and cold

Guidelines for when to use heat or cold are not as clear-cut as originally thought. Conflicting opinions and research results are probably due in part to differences in the methods of applying heat and cold. Although this section is limited to application of heat and cold for superficial, not deep, cooling or warming, there are still considerable differences in the temperatures that may be achieved, the depth of cooling or warming, and the amount of time it takes to achieve this.

For example, water is an excellent conductor of heat. Thus the effects of moist heat are likely to be much greater than the effects of dry heat. Also, since burns are caused by a high rate of heat transmission to the skin, water or moisture must be used cautiously along with heating because of the increased risk of burns. Dry

---

Heat and Cold: Possible Mechanisms of Pain Relief

The following lists of possible effects pertain only to *superficial* heating and cooling:
- Direct effect is limited to the skin and subcutaneous tissues and to the muscle to a limited extent.
- Any deeper effects or effects at a distance are indirect and are probably due to reflex activity.
- In some cases similar effects are obtained from heat and cold.
- In other cases, they achieve opposite effects.

Superficial heating may relieve pain because of the following:

1. Reduces striated muscle spasm, possibly by relieving ischaemia, cooling the muscles by increased blood flow, reducing muscle spindle excitability, or reducing the tension in muscle trigger points. However, if the muscle is inactive, blood flow may remain the same or be reduced.
2. Assists in resolution of superficial, localized infections or inflammations (e.g. thrombophlebitis), partly by increased blood flow.
3. Reduces sensitivity to pain (physiological basis unknown).
4. Reduces joint stiffness.
5. Relaxes smooth muscle, reduces peristalsis, and reduces gastric acidity, possibly by reflex reduction in blood flow to mucous membranes of stomach and intestines (occurs within 5 to 10 minutes when heat is applied to the abdomen).
6. Vasodilatation in skin and increased blood flow to skin.
7. Distant reactions, milder than those at the site of heating. The same reactions that occur at the site of heating may also occur at distant sites, such as contralaterally, but the distant reactions will be milder. For example, if heat is applied to the right leg, vasodilatation there will be greater than the vasodilatation that occurs at distant sites such as the left leg. (These distant reactions are reflexogenic and are referred to as consensual reactions.) Distant reactions are in proportion to the input at the site of heating. Thus distant reactions are greater if the local heat application is more vigorous. That is,
if the intensity of heat is greater, if the area of skin heated is larger, or if the rate of temperature rise is faster, the distant reactions will be greater.
8. Effects of heating do not last as long as effects of cold because the increased blood flow rapidly cools the tissues to normal temperature.

Superficial cooling may relieve pain because of the following:

1. When the cold penetrates deep enough to lower the muscle temperature, it reduces muscle spasm by reducing the muscle spindle response or inactivating trigger points in muscles.
2. Reduces or prevents bleeding and oedema through reflex vasoconstriction. Vasodilatation in response to cold occurs only if the temperature is low enough to be potentially destructive to the tissues.
3. Reduces sensitivity of skin by temperature reduction (cooling) of nerve fibres and receptors.
4. Effects of cold last longer than the effects of heat because the vessels remain constricted after cold application is removed, and rewarming of tissue from inside is delayed accordingly along with delayed warming from the outside. When cold penetrates deep enough to cool the muscle, rewarming of the muscle is further prolonged due to the insulating fat layer.
5. Reduces inflammation, possibly through destruction of enzyme activity.
6. Reduces joint stiffness or perception of stiffness if cooled sufficiently.
7. Increases peristalsis of the stomach, small bowel, and colon if cold is applied to the abdomen.
8. Relieves pain at a distance, possibly because it is placed on a superficial nerve innervating the painful area, an acupuncture point or a trigger point, or because it produces mild but similar effects contralaterally.

---

towelling, a poor conductor of heat, may be used over skin to reduce intensity of heat and risk of burn.

The following lists of indications and contra-indications for using heat or cold are not rigid rules. They are merely suggestions or guidelines. Clearly both heat and cold may be used successfully under the same conditions.

Either heat or cold applied superficially usually relieves the following types of pain, although some exceptions exist and are noted in the separate lists for heat and cold:

- Muscle spasms secondary to underlying pathology.
- Joint stiffness.
- Low back pain.

A. Applied to knee, e.g. for sprain, post knee surgery. Covered with cloth; secured with elastic bandage.

B. Applied over incision to relieve incisional pain.

C. Relief of headache.

D. Applied to neck, e.g. for sore throat, post tonsilectomy, neck pain. Pack is covered with cloth; secured with velcro strips.

E. Applied following rhinoplasty.

Fig. 5.8 Uses of flexible cold gel packs. Some may also be used for heat by warming them in water. Notice that the pack is covered with cloth.

- Myofibrositis (roughly defined as aching muscles of several months duration).

KEY POINT: Use what works best for the individual patient unless it is contra-indicated.

Contrast Bathing: Combined Heat and Cold

Uses: on extremities with severe pain, for pain that responds to both heat and cold, or for joint stiffness (results in increased blood flow).
Supplies: 2 containers of water.
- Cold water at approximately 15°C (59°F).
- Hot water at approximately 40°C (104°F).
Method: Immerse the limb for a total of 30 minutes, alternating as follows:

Time (min) in Hot Water	Time (min) in Cold Water
10	1
4	1
4	1
4	1
4	

(Total of 30 min)

Both heat and cold may be applied whenever heat and cold may be used interchangeably. One technique, contrast bathing, involves alternating immersion of a limb in hot and cold water (see the box above for instructions). Similar results might be obtained by substituting hot and cold packs. Alternating heat and cold or simply intermittent heat has been extremely effective for even severe pain.* Suggestions to patients regarding timing may be similar to those in the box above, or patients may simply develop their own rhythm. Intervals may be very short, e.g. 5–40 seconds.

KEY POINT: Severe pain is likely to be relieved best by intermittent heat applications or by alternating heat and cold. Patients may develop their own rhythm or timing for the intervals.

Obviously, intermittent heat or alternating heat and cold is more time consuming and therefore more inconvenient than constant application of heat or cold. Hence, this is usually reserved for severe pain.

Appropriate uses of superficial heat to relieve pain include the following conditions:
- Muscle spasms secondary to underlying skeletal or neurological pathology, e.g. degenerative joint disease, intervertebral disc disease, nerve root irritation.
- Following trigger point stimulation, e.g. with pressure.
- Painful joint stiffness in arthritis.
- Superficial boils.
- Superficial thrombophlebitis.
- Low back pain, especially acute.
- Gastrointestinal upset with cramping, e.g. viral enteritis.
- Menstrual cramps.
- Reflex sympathetic dystrophy, e.g. shoulder-hand syndrome.
- Tennis elbow during recovery stage, not acute stage.
- During the healing phase of an acute injury after bleeding and oedema have subsided.
- Anorectal pain (especially warm baths).
- Superficial skin breakdown in tissue folds, e.g. perineal or inguinal areas—use radiant heat, e.g. light bulb; avoid higher temperatures that cause cyanosis and pain.
- Myofibrositis.
- Rheumatoid arthritis after the acute state.
- Itching from mosquito bites and poison ivy.
- Haematoma resolution after acute phase to increase rate of absorption—controversial.

Inappropriate uses of or possible contra-indications for superficial heat to relieve pain may include the following conditions:
- Acute trauma (sometimes mild heating is acceptable if injury is minor).
- Bleeding or swelling (almost always contra-indicated for these conditions).
- Impaired sensation or anaesthetic areas.

---

*Intermittent cold does not seem to provide the same contrast of sensations as does intermittent heat, probably because the sensation of cold lasts longer after the removal of a cold pack than does the sensation of heat after the removal of a heating device.

- Unconscious patient—possible tissue damage because patient cannot report when it is too hot.
- Bursitis (unless cold is poorly tolerated).
- Acute state of rheumatoid arthritis (temperatures of about 37°C tend to increase cartilage degeneration).
- Acute and subacute stages of muscle injury when active therapeutic exercise is being used—may increase oedema.
- Tissues with irreversible inadequate vascular supply (heat may increase metabolic demand and cause necrosis).
- Superficial malignancies (may accelerate tumour growth).
- Person prone to orthostatic hypotension should be cautious if heat is applied to large parts of body or if total body is immersed in warm water.
- Person with light sensitivity should avoid radiant heat sources, e.g. light bulb.
- Over topical application of analgesic/anaesthetic preparations.
- Sensitive persons such as those with adrenal suppression, systemic lupus erythematosus, multiple sclerosis, and possibly pregnant women should avoid or be cautious about total body immersion, e.g. hydrotherapy, with temperature maintained at 37.8°C (100°F). For pregnancy, monitor oral temperature and discontinue if it rises above 37.8°C.

Appropriate uses of superficial cold to relieve pain may include the following conditions:

- Muscle spasm secondary to underlying skeletal or neurological pathology, e.g. degenerative joint disease, intervertebral disc disease, nerve root irritation.
- Acute, but not severe, injury, e.g. acute surgical trauma such as episiotomy, minor sports injuries such as sprains (especially combined with compression). Recommended during the first 4–48 hours following injury.
- Following surgical procedures requiring casting, e.g. knee surgery, tendon repair, bone grafts, or fractures, to prevent pain from surgery or potential swelling.
- Joint stiffness in arthritis (if cooled enough; sometimes cold aggravates painful joint stiffness); especially effective for acute stage of rheumatoid arthritis.

- Bursitis.
- Low back pain, especially chronic.
- Back pain during childbirth.
- Therapeutic exercise in subacute stages of muscle injury, especially sports injuries (used with compression prior to and sometimes after therapeutic exercise to reduce oedema).
- Headache, especially migraine, cluster, or mixed headache (migraine plus muscle contraction).
- Myofibrositis.
- Minor burns.
- Itching.

Inappropriate uses of or possible contra-indications for superficial cold for pain relief may include the following conditions:

- Severe acute trauma.
- During the healing phase when bleeding and swelling have subsided following an acute injury (may retard healing).
- Peptic ulcer—application of cold to abdomen may increase gastric acidity.
- Peripheral vascular diseases with arterial insufficiency, e.g. Raynaud's disease.
- Stomach or intestinal cramping—cold packs to abdomen may increase peristalsis.
- Hypersensitivity or cold allergy (rare)—includes wheals, itching, puffiness of eyelids, respiratory distress, and very rarely the severe symptoms of cold anaphylaxis such as shock.
- Occurrence of "hunting reaction" after application of cold. The skin alternately blanches and turns red, signifying vasodilatation. Occurs only if temperature is low enough to be potentially destructive to tissues.

> **KEY POINT:** For some conditions, heat and cold may be used interchangeably. In other conditions, one may be contraindicated or ineffective.

Nursing care guidelines for selecting and using superficial heat and cold applications

The following guidelines along with the patient/family teaching point (see Appendix) summarize important aspects of using heat and cold for pain relief.

1. Be open-minded about the possible uses of heat and cold. Preconceived ideas based on experience or education may unnecessarily limit the possible choices considered. Remember also that research on heat and cold is limited and some results are conflicting.

2. Consider possible contra-indications before using heat or cold. (The remainder of the guidelines assume that this has been done and, if necessary, discussed with and prescribed by the doctor.)

3. Ask the patient if he/she prefers heat or cold. Prior use and results probably heavily influence this choice. Usually the patient's preference is used initially.

4. Help the patient select a method of heating or cooling that is appropriate, practical, and available (see methods listed on this page).

5. If heat has not been effective, encourage the patient to *try cold*. Use the points under Patient/Family Teaching Point: Pain Relief with Heat? Cold? Both? (see Appendix).

6. For severe pain suggest intermittent heat or alternating heat and cold.

7. Most methods of applying heat and cold require wrapping with cloth to prevent tissue damage.

- Moisture or water increases the intensity of the sensation more than dry wrappings (may or may not be desirable).

- For added convenience, especially for the active or ambulatory patient, applications of heat or cold can be secured in place with plastic bandages or cloth pocket-holders with velcro straps.

Patient Example

About 4 hours after labour and delivery, Ms M. reported moderate, very bothersome pain from her episiotomy. Otherwise she felt comfortable, energetic, and wanted to go home, but she was concerned about caring for herself and the baby since the discomfort made walking very difficult. She was breast-feeding and did not want to take medication. To secure a cold pack in place and provide sufficient covering to keep it from being uncomfortably cold, a disposable plastic glove was filled with ice and inserted through an opening torn in a small disposable nappy, placing the absorbent side of the nappy next to the mother. Panties and a sanitary belt held it in place. For increased comfort and convenience, the nurse suggested to the mother that she should purchase two gel packs (about 3 by 10 inches) to keep in the freezer so one would always be ready for use. Ms M. reported significant pain relief and was ready to be discharged early.

Patient/family teaching points for use of heat and cold

When the patient uses heat or cold or both for pain relief, the considerations covered in the patient/family teaching point in the appendix should be discussed with him/her. It is stated in the exact words that may be spoken to the patient, or the list may be duplicated and given to the patient/family who can then read it.

ICE APPLICATION/MASSAGE

Ice application/massage rapidly relieves pain. The mechanisms underlying the effects of ice application are summarized in the box below.

Methods of ice application/massage. The numerous types and sources of ice make it easy to use. Most methods of applying it or massaging with it are inexpensive. Following are common examples of ways to apply ice:

- *Ice cubes/blocks.* Applied directly to skin, not through the barrier of a container. The melting of ice when it is used in direct contact with skin is a safety factor against overchilling. For added safety, use a small surface area of ice, e.g. the corner of a small ice cube rather than the flat surface of the ice cube.

- *Immersion in water* (useful for buttocks, perineal area, hand, foot, elbow). A container with water and melting ice assures a steady temperature of 0°C.

- *Terry cloth* dipped in water with ice shavings, then wrung out and applied rapidly may work for large areas of the body, but must be repeated frequently to maintain freezing temperature.

Caution: the above methods result in an almost instantaneous drop in skin temperature and can cause tissue damage. Muscle temperature drops more slowly, taking longer with thicker layers of fat. In a slender person, muscle temperature may drop after 10 minutes but hardly falls at all in an obese person.

Icing: Possible Mechanisms Underlying Effects

1. *Numbness* or anaesthesia of skin may be caused by decrease in nerve conduction velocity.
2. The discomfort of burning and aching may act as a *counter-irritant,* activating areas in the brainstem which exert inhibitory influences on nerve impulses felt as painful.
3. Pain relief from brief, intense input, such as ice, may *disrupt memory-like processes* caused by prolonged pain, causing pain relief to far outlast the direct effects of ice.
4. *Trigger points* in muscles may be inactivated, resulting in relief of muscle pain or spasm.
5. *Acupuncture points* may be stimulated by ice instead of needling or pressure.
6. Sensation of ice may be felt more strongly than the pain by the patient. Feeling extreme cold may be a distraction or a *"trade-off"* for the pain, perhaps a form of perceptual dominance.

Appropriate/inappropriate situations for ice application/massage

Usually the appropriate and inappropriate uses or contraindications for superficial cold also apply to the use of ice (see p. 141). When the ice is used for only a few seconds, e.g. immediately prior to an injection, there are essentially no contra-indications.

Appropriate uses of ice application/massage:

- Stimulation of trigger points for muscle spasm (see Figs. 5.2–5.5).
- Stimulation of acupuncture points.
- Acute, but not severe, injuries to reduce bleeding and swelling, e.g. in accident and emergency department.
- Myofascial (muscle) pain.
- Stretching muscles that are in spasm. Consult a physiotherapist to determine the correct method for the individual patient.
- Myofibrositis.
- Joint stiffness. (Some studies have shown ice aggravates stiffness; but it may reduce the activity of destructive enzymes such as collagenase, a possible but questionable therapeutic effect for diseases such as rheumatoid arthritis.)

- Tendinitis (ice massage is often considered the treatment of choice).
- Needle punctures, e.g. IM injections, venepuncture (ice at a distance from the needle puncture site or ice pressed into the skin for 15–20 seconds immediately before cleaning area).
- Tennis elbow.
- Sports injuries such as sprains and strains.
- Chronic low back pain.
- Acute bursitis.
- Herpes lesions.
- A substitute for TENS or acupuncture, especially for low back pain.
- Tooth pain, and possibly pain anywhere from the neck up. Ice is applied to the hand by immersing the hand in water with melting ice or using ice massage on the back of the hand at the web between thumb and index finger (Hoku point, see Fig. 5.7) or between the fourth and fifth fingers.
- Headache. The application site can be the area of localized headache, trigger points (see Fig. 5.2), or an ice cube pressed to the roof of the mouth with the tongue.
- Itching.
- Any painful but brief procedure, especially those lasting 10 minutes or less (see the box opposite).

Inappropriate uses of or possible contra-indications for ice are:
- Anterior neck (ice on the vagus nerve can slow the heart).
- Newborns up to about the age of 3 months (ice can coagulate fatty tissue).
- Injuries to the skin, e.g. burn areas.
- Cardiac patients. (Although research on healthy volunteers showed no changes in blood pressure or pulse with use of ice massage, it is wise to check with the doctor.)

Nursing-care guidelines for ice application/massage

1. Many patients are very reluctant to try ice. Express understanding of the patient's view.
2. Explain carefully why ice may be effective. (See reasons listed in the patient/family teaching point: "Ice Application or Massage for Pain Relief," in the Appendix.)
3. Suggest an appropriate method of ice application, e.g. basin of water with melting ice for immersion of hand.

4. Determine if patients can use the ice by themselves. They may need help in preparing it or applying it, especially if they cannot reach the site.

5. Explain that the initial appearance of skin is *erythema* (redness). This is due to a histamine reaction in the skin and should not be mistaken for skin irritation. Interestingly, vasoconstriction does not cause blanching until later.

6. Stress the importance of avoiding tissue damage by discontinuing ice after 10 minutes or when there is numbness, alternating blanching and dilatation of vessels, or shivering.

7. If the patient desires to use ice massage for longer than 10 minutes, e.g. to get longer lasting relief for low back pain, suggest dividing the painful area into several sites, massaging each site for 7 minutes, with a 3-minute waiting period between sites, for a total of 30 minutes.

8. Encourage the patient to try various sites distant to the pain, and explain that the brain's picture of the body is not the same as what we see. For example, a point distant from the pain on the surface of the body may be in the area of pain according to the brain's picture of the body.

Patient Example

In one research study, a patient who had tried ice cube massage to the opposite hip during a bone marrow aspiration surprisingly found that ice massage to the hip successfully relieved rectal pain from fistulas (Collins, 1985). These are unusual findings, but they point out the wisdom of continuing to search for seemingly unrelated sites that might relieve pain when they are stimulated.

Patient/family teaching points for use of ice

When the patient uses ice, discuss with him the patient/family teaching point in the appendix. It is stated in the exact words that may be spoken to the patient, or it may be duplicated and given to the patient or family member who can read.

VIBRATION

Vibration is a form of electric or vigorous massage. It is not widely used for pain relief, but research suggests it may be very effective, possibly as a substitute for TENS for some patients.

Ice Massage for Painful Procedures

Any brief but painful procedure, especially one that lasts 10 minutes or less, may be felt as less painful or be better tolerated if ice massage is used.
Examples of procedures are:
Biopsy under local anaesthesia.
Bone marrow aspiration.
Catheterization.
Chest tube removal.
Injection into joints.
Lumbar puncture.
Suture removal.
Technique of ice massage for procedures:

1. Begin 1–5 minutes prior to the procedure.
2. Apply the ice directly to the skin or through a porous covering.
3. Keep a cloth available to wipe up melting ice.
4. Immediately prior to the procedure, if it can be timed appropriately, numb the site of the procedure with ice. Then move to a distant point.
5. Massage with ice at a distance from the site of the procedure, e.g. contralaterally.
6. If the procedure unexpectedly lasts longer than 10 minutes or if ice must be discontinued to prevent tissue damage, try a completely different distant site.
7. If the procedure can be predicted to last longer than 10 minutes, try intermittent ice massage, e.g. 2 minutes of massage followed by a rest period that allows skin to begin to return to normal colour. Or, divide the area into several sites and change massage sites every few minutes.

One mechanism underlying pain relief from vibration is that some types, especially from a hand-held vibrator applied with moderate pressure, cause numbness, paraesthesia, and/or anaesthesia of the area stimulated. Thus pain relief may occur during vibration. If this type of vibration is continued for 25 minutes or longer, pain relief may last for several hours after stimulation. If vibration is effective at trigger points or acupuncture points, it may also relieve pain following stimulation. Vibration may also change the character of the sensation, e.g. from sharp to dull.

A number of different *types of vibrating devices* are available commercially, and many have adjustable speeds. Common types are:

Hand-held vibrators, using batteries or mains current. Pressure and movement are provided by the operator. Frequencies and amplitudes vary widely, coarser movement oscillating at 10–50 Hz and finer movements at 100–200 Hz, the latter probably being more common and comfortable. Many have interchangeable applicators of different shapes and sizes made of plastic or rubber. Those with the rounded tips, e.g, shaped like a phallus, are particularly good for getting at certain acupuncture or trigger points. Battery-operated ones are also convenient to use. However, they may be embarrassing to the patient. Some small vibrators are strapped to the dorsum of the hand, allowing the human hand to be in contact with the patient's skin. This type allows better adaptation to the contours of the body.

Stationary vibrators. Vibrating pads may resemble a seat cushion or be incorporated in an armchair or bed mattress. These are probably best suited to provide superficial massage. The body part, such as the back, is placed against the surface. Some are constructed especially for massaging the feet. Some have heating elements incorporated.

Appropriate/inappropriate situations for using vibration

Appropriate situations for use of vibration may include:
- Muscle pain or spasm, acute or chronic, e.g., back pain or neck pain.
- Tension headache.
- Itch (either to site or contralateral).
- Near injection site, e.g. during IM injection.
- Neuropathic pain, e.g. post-herpetic neuralgia (surround the area if site of pain is too sensitive) or other pain of a neuralgic nature in the thoracic regions radiating along the course of an intercostal nerve.
- Phantom limb pain.
- Rheumatoid arthritis.
- Orofacial pain, acute or chronic (use at the Hoku point (Fig. 5.7) or at the site of pain), e.g. dental pain.
- Acute tendinitis.
- As a substitute for TENS.

- Many types of chronic non-malignant pain not listed above, as long as they are well-localized and can be covered with the vibrator.

Inappropriate uses of vibration usually include:
- Patients who bruise easily.
- Areas of thrombophlebitis.
- Sites where skin has been injured, e.g. burned or cut.
- Causalgia or other conditions that cause hypersensitivity to mechanical stimulation.
- Migraine headache or any headache that worsens with movement or sound.
- Marked increase in pain.

Nursing-care guidelines and patient/family teaching points for using vibration

The following points may be discussed with the patient who is willing to try vibration for pain relief:

1. Be open-minded about the uses and possible effectiveness of vibration for pain relief. It tends to be under-used.
2. Experiment with vibration applied for 1 minute to various sites to determine which site results in the best pain relief. Since one of the main immediate effects of vibration is partial loss of sensation, the best site for stimulation with vibration is often in the area of pain. However, some success has been achieved with application to areas surrounding the pain, especially distal to the pain, and stimulation of acupuncture points or trigger points.
4. A hand-held vibrator applied with moderate pressure may provide the best relief.
5. The length of time for using a vibrator commonly varies from 20 seconds to 15 minutes, but there tends to be very little post-stimulation pain relief. However, vibration for 25–45 minutes may provide up to several hours of pain relief. Intermittent use may be the most effective approach, applying and withdrawing every few seconds.
6. After 45 minutes of vibration, a common skin reaction is redness and a feeling of warmth along with some loss of sensation. Itching may also occur.
7. High-frequency vibration, as opposed to slow, coarse vibration, tends to be the most effective.
8. Vibration should be non-painful.
9. For chronic pain, use of vibration for as long as 30–45 minutes may best be limited to twice a day.

Over a period of months, using it four times a day or more may lead to shorter periods of pain relief after vibration.

10. When pain relief extends beyond the period of vibration, warn the patient to be careful of injury afterward. Care should be taken not to perform physical activities that would injure the muscles, but supervised therapeutic exercises may be appropriate.

11. Vibration is easily self-administered and very suitable for home use.

TRANSCUTANEOUS ELECTRICAL NERVE STIMULATION (TENS)

Transcutaneous electrical nerve stimulation is commonly referred to as TENS (pronounced like the plural of the number ten). TENS is a method of applying controlled, low-voltage electricity to the body via electrodes placed on the skin. Most TENS units are small, portable, and battery operated, consisting of three major parts: (1) box with energy source, (2) lead wires, and (3) electrodes (two or more electrodes may be used). These three components with two electrodes placed on an adult body are illustrated in Fig. 5.9.

The sensation felt by the patient from TENS is usually described as tingling, vibrating or pulsating; however, some settings produce discomfort. TENS stimulation may be constant or intermittent.

The primary purpose of TENS is to relieve pain, either while natural healing takes place, e.g. postoperatively, or to enable appropriate therapy to be used, e.g. stretching and strengthening muscles to alleviate the source of chronic low back pain. It is a safe, non-invasive method of pain relief that is easy to use under the guidance of appropriately trained health professionals. The success rate of TENS varies. For relief of chronic non-malignant pain, estimates of good results range from 20% to 40%; for relief of postoperative incisional pain, 70% to 90%.

TENS is usually approved by a doctor, but treatment with TENS is usually administered by physiotherapists or trained nurses who have had teaching education in the use of TENS. The success of TENS is strongly dependent upon the skill of the person administering it. It is highly recommended that the person administering TENS has been trained and has experience in the complexities of this treatment, such as electrode placement, stimulation modes, and

Fig. 5.9 Three major components of a TENS unit with two electrodes placed on the upper back of the patient to relieve shoulder pain. This shows the size of the TENS unit in relation to an adult body, illustrating that it is small and portable.

appropriate adjunctive therapies. It is beyond the scope of this book to provide such instruction. For a comprehensive guide to the use of TENS, refer to Mannheimer and Lampe, 1984, or to individual companies' instruction manuals.

The purpose of this section on TENS is limited to assisting the nurse to obtain sufficient knowledge to do the following:

- Know when it is appropriate to recommend TENS for pain relief.
- *Discuss its use, limits, and potential problems* with health-care team members and patients/families.
- Suggest *resources for assisting* the health-care team and patient/family with TENS.

The *mechanisms* underlying the effectiveness of TENS in relieving pain are unclear. Since there are several distinctly different electrical stimulation modes and many different methods of electrode placement, it is likely that different methods of TENS provide pain relief by different mechanisms. Some types of TENS, but not all, appear to relieve pain at least in part by increasing the patient's endorphin, or natural morphine. Another explanation is that TENS acts as a counter-irritant, masking the pain or activating a complex neural inhibitory system that alleviates more intense or prolonged pain at near or distant sites.

Appropriate/inappropriate uses of TENS

Although TENS is no panacea, the indications for TENS are almost limitless as long as the pain is reasonably well localized. This makes it virtually impossible to list all the painful conditions that might be relieved by TENS. However, TENS is not an alternative to the diagnosis and appropriate treatment of the underlying cause of pain, nor does it usually replace all other methods of pain relief. *Common appropriate uses of* TENS may be divided into the two following, somewhat overlapping, categories, accompanied by examples that are also somewhat overlapping:

1. TENS *along with physiotherapy;* i.e. TENS as one part of a comprehensive programme of pain management aimed at rehabilitation of the patient with musculoskeletal problems. TENS is usually used to prevent or break the three-part pain cycle, consisting of pain (1) leading to muscle spasm and guarding (2), leading to dysfunction (3), leading to more pain (1), as shown in Fig. 5.10. TENS relieves pain so that muscles can receive appropriate therapy, e.g. stretching and strengthening exercises, and so that function can be restored automatically or with assistance, e.g. proper body mechanics. Examples of conditions in which TENS is used for pain relief along with appropriate physiotherapy are:

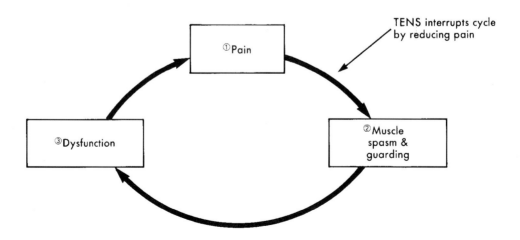

Fig. 5.10 The three-part pain cycle. TENS interrupts this cycle by relieving pain.

- Stimulation of trigger points or acupuncture points related to musculoskeletal problems.
- Back pain, chronic or acute.
- Sciatic pain.
- Arthritis, e.g. wrist pain of rheumatoid arthritis.
- Temporomandibular joint (TMJ) syndrome.
- Cervical spine pain post-laminectomy.
- Neck pain, e.g. chronic cervical strain, whiplash.

2. *Analgesia for acute pain in which the underlying disorder will more or less spontaneously resolve*, e.g. healing of postoperative incisional pain or periodic migraine. These are often conditions that ordinarily require analgesics such as aspirin or a narcotic. TENS may be used to provide part or all of the pain relief. Examples include:

- Postoperative pain.
- Trauma typically seen in accident and emergency departments, especially when medications are withheld pending medical evaluation.
- Fractured ribs.
- Under the cast covering a fractured bone.
- Prior to painful dressing changes.
- Thrombophlebitis.
- Pancreatitis.
- Phantom limb pain.
- Cancer pain (research is very limited in this area, but if pain is localized, even if the patient is on narcotics, TENS may be helpful).
- Headache due to tension, fever, hangover, or sinus conditions; possibly migraine and cluster headaches.
- Dysmenorrhoea (menstrual pain).
- When narcotics are contra-indicated, e.g. allergy to narcotics, desire of recovering substance abuser to abstain, during pregnancy or childbirth, a nursing mother following caesarean section.
- Itch.

Possibly inappropriate uses of TENS, or situations in which precautions are warranted, include:

- In the presence of a cardiac pacemaker, especially a demand pacemaker.
- Over the carotid sinuses (front and sides of the throat) because of a possible hypotensive effect secondary to a vasovagal reflex.
- Over the eyes. However, electrodes may be placed on the boney orbit of the eye.

- Head and neck regions in patients with vascular or seizure disorders. These patients should be monitored carefully.
- Over burns or open wounds (electrodes can, of course, be placed nearby).
- Over skin that is already irritated, e.g. dryness or rash.
- Internal use, e.g. mouth or vagina. Mucosal linings probably would not tolerate the electrical stimulation.
- Anterior chest wall in cardiac problems (until more is known about the effects of this).
- Pregnancy, possibly. However, TENS has been used successfully without complications for pain during labour and delivery and in pregnant women with back pain with no adverse side effects.
- As a substitute for appropriate medication or other therapy.
- Incompetent patients, for example those with mental impairment, the very old and very young. The patient should be carefully monitored and safety precautions taken, e.g. securing the settings for electrical output.

Special attention needs to be directed toward the appropriateness of TENS for a *patient who is already taking narcotics*. Some studies have revealed that postoperative use of TENS significantly reduces the narcotic intake of patients who have not used narcotics preoperatively but does not reduce postoperative narcotic intake of those who used narcotics preoperatively (Solomon, Viernstein, and Long, 1980). However, not only are there few studies on this subject, but the studies of postoperative TENS are not sufficiently well controlled to be considered conclusive.

One major flaw in some studies of postoperative TENS is that the measure of effectiveness of TENS is not based on patients' ratings of pain but on the amount of narcotic required or given. This does not accurately reflect the amount of pain the patient may have had. Patients with significant pain may not request narcotics, and those who request them may not receive them. Thus it is possible that patients who used narcotics prior to surgery are more comfortable or assertive about requesting narcotics, while those who have not taken narcotics may fail to request them due to exaggerated and unrealistic fears about the dangers of narcotics.

Further, several studies have been done using postoperative TENS on patients who more than likely took narcotics preoperatively, e.g. patients who had had low back surgery, knee surgery, and hip replacement (a procedure almost always done solely for pain relief). These studies have shown that TENS reduced postoperative narcotic intake compared to control groups that did not have TENS (Pike, 1978; Schuster and Infante, 1980; Stabile and Mallory, 1978). Further, several clinical reports state that TENS is helpful for cancer pain (Mannheimer and Lampe, 1984), and these patients also are likely to have received narcotics prior to TENS use.

> **KEY POINT:** There is insufficient evidence to automatically conclude that TENS will be ineffective for a patient who is or has been taking narcotics. A trial of TENS is warranted.

One final point in rebuttal to avoiding TENS if the patient is taking narcotics is that not all TENS relieves pain by increasing endorphins. Patients taking narcotics may develop tolerance to narcotic analgesia. Some have argued that if TENS relieves pain by increasing endorphins, the patient on narcotics may be tolerant to this analgesia as well. However, in some studies pain relief from TENS is not reversible by naloxone, a narcotic antagonist (Hansson, Ekblom, Thomsson, and Fjellner, 1986). Some types of TENS apparently relieve pain by mechanisms other than increasing endorphins, and therefore it is at least theoretically possible for TENS to provide effective pain relief for patients who are tolerant to narcotics.

Nursing-care guidelines for general use of TENS

1. Recommend TENS as early as possible, e.g. pre-operatively for postoperative pain, or immediately following a musculoskeletal injury before pain becomes chronic.
2. A doctor's agreement is usually necessary for the use of TENS.
3. Identify an "expert" resource person who can assist the health care team and patient/family. One or more of the following may be appropriate:

- Within the hospital, one person or one department, e.g. Physiotherapy or Pain Relief Unit, or Acute Pain Service, is usually responsible for TENS units and treatment.
- It is useful to be aware of TENS manufacturers for either advice on individual machines or for purchasing/maintenance details. Some UK firms are listed at the end of this section.

4. Thorough patient/family teaching is essential to the success of TENS. When the patient receives a TENS unit, ensure that the patient is given written instructions, whether the patient is either in or out of the hospital.
5. The most common, although not frequent, complication of TENS is an adverse skin reaction. This may be caused by a variety of factors such as electrical reactions or irritation from electrode gels or adhesive tape. Simple measures, such as altering electrode sites and/or gel or using cortisone cream or self-adhesive electrodes, usually alleviate the problem.
6. If the patient has problems using the TENS unit, all of the following are logical options:

- Contact the resource person from the hospital or manufacturer.
- Consult the written instructions. Most patients who are using TENS units have received written instructions developed by the resource person or the manufacturer. Ask the patient for these instructions, suggest that they are reviewed, and offer to go over them with the patient/family, if time permits.
- If all efforts to resolve the problem fail, suggest that TENS be discontinued until assistance is found.

7. If the patient asks about the cost of purchasing/renting TENS, investigate the specific situation, keeping in mind the following:

- When TENS is used on an out-patient basis for chronic pain, the usual recommendation is that a unit should not be purchased until treatment has been successful over a recognized trial period, e.g. an agreed number of treatments or time scale. (This often depends on the clinical situation and resources available.)
- Some third-party providers may fully or partially reimburse the rental and purchase cost.

- Some patients on low incomes or with particular disease processes requiring TENS as part of their rehabilitation programme may be able to obtain NHS/social service assistance in the purchase of the machine.
- It is worthwhile contacting different companies for specifications, quotes and details of follow-up service.

NURSING-CARE GUIDELINES FOR USE OF TENS POSTOPERATIVELY

The use of TENS has now become far more extensive, and is used in post-operation pain management. This can involve a pain nurse specialist, doctor or physiotherapist in the placement of electrodes and connection of the machine. In the clinical area the nurse is the only health-care team member immediately available to the patient 24 hours a day as the latter uses the TENS unit during his recovery.

Instructions about the particular TENS unit and guidelines for its use from the preoperative through to the postoperative period usually can be obtained either from the in-house person/department resource or the manufacturer. The nurse may not be responsible for preoperative teaching, but should be knowledgeable enough to answer the patient's questions about TENS, be supportive of its use, and check to see that appropriate preoperative teaching has been done. Postoperatively, the nurse may need to remind the patient to use TENS or increase stimulation for painful events and be able to troubleshoot common problems.

Following is an overview of how TENS is initiated and used for postoperative pain, including nursing responsibilities.*

Contra-indications

1. Cardiac pacemakers.
2. Application over a uterus in pregnancy.
3. Senility.
4. Application over the carotid sinus.

*The material about postoperative use of TENS is copyrighted as Lampe, J, and Meyer, D: *Postoperative T.E.N.S. Analgesia: Protocol, Methods, Results, and Benefit*, Pain Control Services, Inc., Kansas City, 1978. Recently the material, along with additional information, was published in Mannheimer, JS, and Lampe, GN: *Clinical Transcutaneous Electrical Nerve Stimulation*, pp. 514–515, FA Davis Company, Philadelphia, 1984. It is reprinted here with permission from Gerald N. Lampe.

Postoperative ward procedure

1. The doctor should leave a standing order for TENS to be discontinued immediately if any complications develop.
2. Normal length of usage is 3–5 days.
3. The skin should be checked every 12 hours for rash or irritation. This is done by lifting a corner of the electrode and looking under the pad.
4. Depending on the sterile electrode materials employed and the condition of the patient's skin or incision, electrodes may require replacement during recovery. If the conducting medium should dry out or the electrodes come loose, stimulation will be uncomfortable, indicating a need to secure or change the electrodes.
5. If replacing the electrodes is necessary, place each one parallel to the incision, approximately 2–3 inches from the sutures. If any skin irritation is present and stimulation is to be continued, place the electrodes at alternate sites parallel to the suture line to avoid the irritation.
6. The patient should reset the amplitude knob to a comfortable effective setting.
7. Increase generator output prior to coughing and increased physical activity, which may increase noxious input.
8. Chart on the postoperative analgesia record all pertinent information relative to the use of TENS throughout the recovery period.

The continuous-assessment sheet on p. 38 may be used to record hourly pain ratings given by the patient, along with analgesic requirements and any problems. This can serve as the postoperative analgesia record referred to above.

Placement of electrodes for postoperative pain varies somewhat, but electrodes are often placed parallel to the incision, about 1 inch or more from the incision (Fig. 5.11).

Nursing-care guidelines and patient/family teaching points for use of TENS in the home

TENS is most often used on an out-patient basis for chronic pain problems, especially chronic non-malignant pain such as back or neck pain. Sometimes TENS is used for chronic cancer pain.

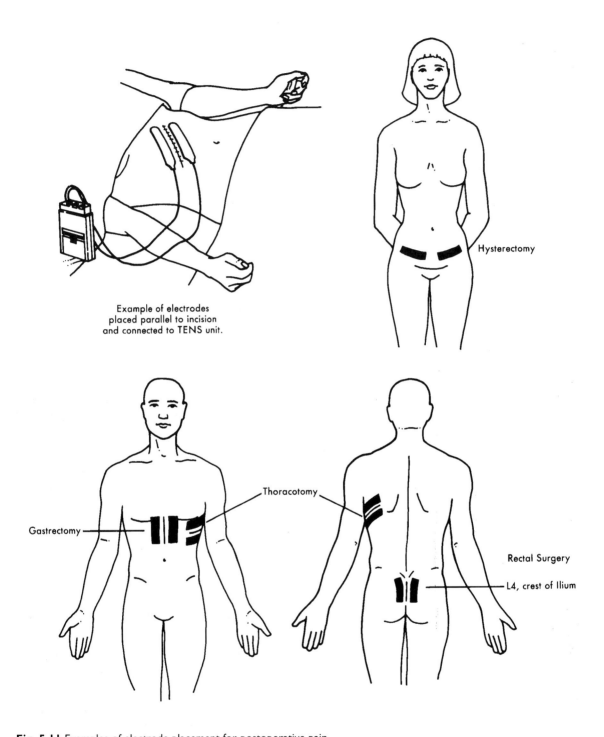

Example of electrodes
placed parallel to incision
and connected to TENS unit.

Hysterectomy

Gastrectomy

Thoracotomy

Rectal Surgery

L4, crest of Ilium

Fig. 5.11 Examples of electrode placement for postoperative pain.

Redrawn with permission from Mannheimer, JS, and Lampe, GN: *Clinical Transcutaneous Electrical Nerve Stimulation*, pp.. 518–522, F.A. Davis Co., Philadelphia, 1984.

Once again, unless the nurse has had training in the use of TENS, the nurse is not expected to instruct the patient or provide follow-up in the home for the use of TENS. However, if the nurse is caring for a patient in or out of the hospital who is using TENS on an out-patient basis or is a candidate for this, the nurse will need to know enough about TENS to identify the patient's needs and obtain appropriate assistance.

If TENS is not relieving the patient's pain, probably the most important nursing actions are:

- Help the patient obtain assistance from a physio-therapist/resource person associated with the hospital or the manufacturer.
- Offer to review with the patient the written home instructions. These instructions usually provide the following information:

Basic operation and care of the unit

Sites for electrode placement. Figure drawings usually show electrode placement, and often alternative sites for electrode placement (alternative sites might be used when other sites do not provide relief).

Stimulation modes. TENS units usually have three dials that can be adjusted: (1) pulse rate, (2) pulse width, and (3) amplitude.

- Encourage the patient to continue to try, under supervision, various stimulation modes and electrode placements. For some patients, numerous attempts may be necessary before an effective approach is found.

Stimulation modes and electrode placement for chronic pain can be complicated and should be carefully determined by a health professional with training in this. To illustrate the complexity of electrode placement, chronic low back pain may be treated with four or more electrodes connected to two different channels originating from the same battery-operated power source, placed on the site of pain as well as distant sites.

List of TENS manufacturers in the UK

Medaid Ltd
Medaid Health Products
Church View, Grange Road, Felmersham
Beds MK43 7EU
0234-781480

Mini-Tens
N.H. Eastwood & Son Ltd
118 East Barnet Road, Barnet, Herts EN4 8RE
081-441 9641

Neen Ltd
Old Pharmacy Yard, Church Street, East Dereham
Norfolk NR19 1DY
0362-698967

Promedics. Dynatens.
Clarendon Road, Blackburn, Lancs BB1 9TA

RDG Medical
429 Brighton Road, Croydon, Surrey CR2 6UD
081-660 4374

Spembley Ltd.
Newbury Road, Andover, Hants SP10 4DR
0264-65741

Voltastar Ltd
20 Bailiff Street, Northampton, NN1 3DY
0604-22341

3M Healthcare
Morley Street, Loughborough, Leicestershire
0509-611811

SELECTED ANNOTATED REFERENCES THAT CITE RESEARCH OR GIVE CLINICAL SUPPORT

Many of the non-invasive pain relief measures, such as cutaneous stimulation, have not yet been adequately researched. This sometimes makes it difficult to document or justify the use of these techniques. The following brief, annotated list provides some clinical or research support for use of cutaneous stimulation techniques as discussed in this chapter.

Bini, G, Cruccu, K-EH, Schady, W, and Torebjork, E: Analgesic effect of vibration and cooling on pain induced by intraneural electrical stimulation, *Pain* 18:239–248, 1984. Moderate or intense pain was experimentally produced by electrical stimulation in volunteers to examine the pain relieving effects of 20–60 seconds of vibration, pressure, cooling, or warming within or near the painful area of skin. The most effective results were obtained for moderate pain when vibration was applied within the area of pain. Pressure and cooling provided some pain relief, but mild warming produced inconsistent results. Vibration was applied contralaterally in only four subjects and was not effective. Sometimes vibration used for intense pain merely changed the sensation from sharp to dull.

Collins, PM: Contralateral ice massage during bone marrow aspiration, Masters thesis, University of Miami, June 1985. Ten patients received contralateral ice massage during one bone marrow aspiration (BMA) and a control treatment of an EKG patch during another BMA. Ice wrapped in a piece of gauze was gently massaged on the contralateral iliac crest beginning 5 minutes prior to the injection of the local anaesthetic and continued until the completion of the procedure. Six of the ten patients had less pain with ice massage than with the EKG patch; one said both the ice and the patch helped; two said neither helped; one replied that the patch helped. An incidental finding was that one patient with a very painful rectal fistula said the ice massage decreased this pain, and he continued ice massage to the hip periodically on his own for his rectal pain.

Cooling more effective, *Aches & Pains*, **3**:37, 1982. In 100 patients with rheumatoid arthritis and knee pain, a heating or cooling device was placed around one knee for 20 minutes twice a day. Patients preferred heat, probably because of the initial discomfort of cold, but cooling produced more pain relief.

Ekblom, A, and Hansson, P: Extrasegmental transcutaneous electrical nerve stimulation and mechanical vibratory stimulation as compared to placebo for the relief of acute oro-facial pain, *Pain*, **23**:223–229, 1985. Only 10 of the 30 patients receiving actual stimulation (low frequency TENS of 2Hz, high frequency TENS of 100Hz, or 100Hz vibration) to the Hoku point reported pain relief. However, several patients spontaneously reported paresthesia and/or anaesthesia from the stimulated hand area. Vibration showed a slight tendency toward relieving orofacial pain in a larger number of patients than did either form of TENS.

Gammon, BD, and Starr, I: Studies on the relief of pain by counterirritation, *J Clin Invest*, **20**:13–20, Jan 1941. This report on several experiments continues to be cited as a basic reference in the literature on cutaneous stimulation. Selected findings are as follows. The *most effective intensity* of counter-irritation was slightly less than that which produced discomfort. After the application of a counter-irritant and after it was removed, there was often a period of sharp, but transient, increase in pain followed by pain relief. Relative *effectiveness of counter-irritants* in descending order: cold (4–10°C), electrical stimulation (single shocks sufficient to cause muscle twitching), heat (40°C), tactile stimulation (rubbing with cotton or scratching with wooden edge), vibration, and air jet. However, sometimes heat or cold would relieve one pain and exaggerate another. In other cases both heat and cold were equally effective. By far the *greatest relief*, even for severe discomfort, was attained by interrupted counter-irritation, consisting of a rhythm of approximately 5 seconds of application and 10 seconds without. When patients chose their own rhythms with heat and cold, the majority preferred alternating heat and cold or intermittent heat without cold. Intervals selected were generally about 40 seconds of heat and 30 seconds without it. The patients always preferred heat or cold to electrical or tactile counter-irritation. The most effective *site of stimulation* for pain in the arm was over the pain, followed by a site 6 inches proximal to the painful area along the course of the nerve supplying it. Less, but clearly detectable, relief occurred with counter-irritation distal to the pain, the back, or the contralateral arm.

Hansson, P, Ekblom, A, Thomsson, M, and Fjellner, B: Influence of naloxone on relief of acute oro-facial pain by transcutaneous electrical nerve stimulation (TENS) or vibration, *Pain*, **24**:323–329, 1986. Out of 28 patients with orofacial pain, 20 reported pain reduction during 100Hz vibratory stimulation, low-frequency (2Hz) TENS, or high-frequency (100Hz) TENS. Application site was the skin overlying the painful area. This pain relief was *not* influenced by naloxone in 19 of the 20 patients. A review of research shows somewhat contradictory results regarding the naloxone reversibility of pain relief obtained with afferent stimulation, such as acupuncture and high frequency TENS. Relief of chronic pain from low-frequency TENS appears more likely to be reversed by naloxone, but not always. Thus pain relief from vibration or TENS is not necessarily mediated by opioid mechanisms.

Heng, MCY: Local necrosis and interstitial nephritis due to topical methyl salicylate and menthol, *Cutis*, **39**:442–444, May 1987. A case report of a 62-year-old man illustrates the danger of using heat over the topical application of methyl salicylate and menthol. Used alone, these topical applications seldom cause significant problems; but combined with heat, skin necrosis and other complications may result. This particular patient suffered full-thickness skin and muscle necrosis as well as persistent interstitial nephritis following 15–20 minutes of heat over topical applications of Ben-Gay on several areas of his body, including both legs and arms.

Hillman, H, and Jarman, D: Freezing skin, *Nurs Times*, **82**:40–41, May 1986. Immediately after a cube of ordinary ice was applied with slight pressure for 15–20 seconds to the upper arm of 10 subjects, sensations of touch and sharpness in the skin in that area were reduced. This use of ice was suggested as an inexpensive and safe way to decrease the discomfort of needle injections, e.g. IV or IM.

Hillman, SK, and Delforge, G: The use of physical agents in rehabilitation of athletic injuries. In Harvey, JS, ed: Rehabilitation of the injured athlete, *Clin Sports Med*, **4**:431–438, July 1985. It is a common misconception that heat is invariably appropriate after 24 or 48 hours following an acute soft tissue injury. Application of cold, especially prior to therapeutic exercise, is recommended to reduce edema that commonly occurs when active exercise is used early in the recovery period, as is often done with athletes to avoid delay in return to competition.

Kunesch, E, Schmidt, R, Nordin, M, Wallin, U, and Hagbarth, K-E: Peripheral neural correlates of cutaneous anaesthesia induced by skin cooling in man, *Acta Physiol Scand*, **129**:247–257, Feb 1987. Cooling of the skin by ice application for 3–5 minutes or by ethyl chloride spray for about 10 seconds resulted in "needle" or "sharpness" sensations being felt as blunt. Sensations for sharpness and pain did not fully return for 2–5 minutes.

Lehmann, JF, and de Lateur, BJ: Cryotherapy. In Lehmann, JF, ed: *Therapeutic Heat and Cold*, ed 3, pp. 563–602, Baltimore, 1982, Williams & Wilkins. This is an extensive review of the therapeutic uses of local applications of cold – cryotherapy. Cold applications reduce *muscle spasm* secondary to underlying skeletal and joint pathology or nerve root irritation by breaking the cycle of secondary muscle spasm, ischaemia, pain, and more muscle spasm. Arthritic joints are also treated with cold to reduce inflammation and pain. Cold produces an almost instantaneous drop in skin temperature with a slow reduction of muscle temperature, depending on thickness of subcutaneous fat. To reduce muscle temperature, cooling for a slender person should last longer than 10 minutes; for an obese person, longer than 30 minutes. When the muscle temperature does drop, it takes a long time to rewarm because the fat layer acts as an insulator. By contrast, a warmed muscle resumes normal temperature within a few minutes. Cold packs applied to the abdomen produce an increase in *peristalsis* in the stomach, small bowel, and colon.

Lehmann, JF, and de Lateur, BJ: Therapeutic heat. In Lehmann, JF, ed: *Therapeutic Heat and Cold*, ed 3, pp. 404–562, Baltimore, 1982, Williams & Wilkins. This extensive review of the uses of heat includes the following information. The effect of heat on the contralateral extremity is referred to as *consensual reaction*. Heating the skin of one extremity increases the blood flow to that extremity and also to the contralateral extremity but to a lesser degree. The degree of this reflex response is in proportion to the intensity of heat and the area of skin affected. When the skin of the abdominal wall is heated, e.g. with hot water bottles, within 5 to 10 minutes there is a reflex *reduction in blood flow to the mucous membranes of the stomach and intestines* along with relaxation of smooth muscle and a reduction in peristalsis and gastric acidity. *Contrast bathing*, a method of alternating heat and cold, results in increased blood flow and decreased joint stiffness. Initially the limb

is immersed for 10 minutes in hot water (approximately 40°C, 104°F), followed by 1 minute in cold water (approximately 15°C, 59°F). Then 4 minutes in hot water and 1 minute in cold water is repeated for a total treatment time of 30 minutes.

Lundeberg, T, Nordemar, R, and Ottoson, D: Pain alleviation by vibratory stimulation, *Pain*, **20**:25–44, 1984. In this study of 366 patients with acute or chronic musculoskeletal pain of various origins, 69% reported pain relief during vibratory stimulation at 100Hz, most eventually reporting pain reduction of 50% or greater. The best site was the area of pain, the affected muscle or tendon, the antagonistic muscle, or a trigger point outside the painful area. Vibration applied with moderate pressure over a large area (i.e. a 200cm cushioned applicator as opposed to 6cm probe) produced the best pain relief. Maximal pain relief was experienced within about 10 to 20 minutes for most patients. After 45 minutes of vibration, many experienced pain relief for 3–12 hours.

Mannheimer, JS, and Lampe, GN: *Clinical Transcutaneous Electrical Nerve Stimulation*, Philadelphia, 1984, FA Davis Co. This is a comprehensive text on the use of TENS for pain relief, both as adjunctive treatment while appropriate rehabilitation treatment occurs and as an analgesic while the body spontaneously heals, e.g. postoperatively. The book is heavily referenced and gives very specific guidelines regarding evaluation of numerous pain syndromes, electrode placement, stimulation modes, patient teaching, limitations of TENS, and available TENS units. This book is an invaluable guide to the appropriate use of TENS.

Melzack, R: Hyperstimulation analgesia. In Brena, SF, and Chapman, SL, eds: *Clin Anaesthesiol*, **3**:81–92, Jan 1985. Hyperstimulation analgesia is identified as moderate to intense sensory input for a few seconds to 20–30 minutes, sometimes applied to a site distant to the site of pain, that may relieve pain for days. Pain relief may be due to neural inhibitory mechanisms followed by increased physical activity in the absence of pain that prevents the recurrence of memory traces of pain.

A review of research shows that stimulation of acupuncture points or trigger points may effectively relieve pain. However, not only are the locations of trigger points very similar to those of acupuncture points, but at these locations are not always discrete points—they may be a large area. That is, stimulation of exactly the precise point is sometimes the most effective, but other times stimulation over a large area is equally effective. As an example, ice massage of the back of the hand between the thumb and index finger (where the Hoku point is located) on the same side as the pain decreases dental pain by 50% or more in most patients, but it may be equally effective to stimulate between the fourth and fifth fingers where no acupuncture point for the face is located. The entire hand or any point on it may be effective. As another example, research has shown that spinal cells excited by stimulation of the leg are inhibited by intense stimulation of the other leg or either hand.

The brainstem areas with mechanisms that exhibit a powerful descending inhibitory control appear to have a gross, complex somatotopic organization characterized by large receptive fields, making it possible for pain to be affected by stimulation at a distant site.

Melzack, R, and Bentley, KD: Relief of dental pain by ice massage of either hand or the contralateral arm, *Can Dent Assoc J,* **49**:257–260, Apr 1983. An ice cube held in a gauze pad was used on 22 patients with dental pain to massage four sites for 7 minutes or until patient reported it was too painful to endure any longer. This was compared with a control procedure of tactile massage. Pain intensity was decreased by 40–50% after ice massage of the Hoku points (back of hand between thumb and index finger) ipsilateral and contralateral to the dental pain and ice massage of the contralateral arm (near the elbow) but not the ipsilateral arm. Pain relief was comparable to that obtained from TENS and acupuncture. This study and others suggest that intensity of stimulation is the significant factor rather than the precise site or mode of stimulation.

Melzack, R, Jeans, ME, Stratford, JG, and Monks, RC: Ice massage and transcutaneous electrical stimulation: comparison of treatment for low-back pain, *Pain,* **9**:209–217, 1980. The results indicate that brief, intense cold from gentle massage with ice for lower back pain has analgesic effects comparable to those produced by transcutaneous electrical stimulation (TES). After being treated with TES and ice, 13 patients chose TES, 9 chose ice (even though some reported it was more painful than TES), and 5 asked for other therapy. Ice massage was performed for 7 minutes or less at each site with a 3-minute rest interval between stimulation until a total time of 30 minutes had elapsed. Treatment was stopped if the patient reported pain. Typically the sequence of sensations reported was cooling, burning, aching, and numbness. It was suggested that the analgesic effects of ice massage were a result of intense cold activating brainstem mechanisms that are known to exert descending inhibitory influences on pain signals.

Melzack, R, Stillwell, DM, and Fox, EJ: Trigger points and acupuncture points for pain: correlations and implications, *Pain,* **3**:3–23, 1977. This study of trigger points and acupuncture points revealed a high degree of correspondence between them. Figures and tables clearly identify locations of numerous trigger points and acupuncture points.

Ramler, D, and Roberts, J: A comparison of cold and warm sitz baths for relief of postpartum perineal pain, *J Obstet Gynecol Neonatal Nurs,* **15**:471–474, Nov-Dec 1986. In a study of 40 postpartum patients with episiotomies who took both cold (15.6–18.3°C) and warm (36.7–44.4°C) sitz baths, cold sitz baths were significantly more effective in relieving perineal pain. However, pain relief following the cold bath was of no longer duration than with the warm bath. The latter differs from Droegemueller's (1980) findings of longer duration of pain relief following cold sitz baths, but he probably used colder water. Although 20 (50%) of the women in the study stated they preferred the cold to the warm bath, it is noteworthy that 119 women refused to participate in the study because they did not want to take a cold sitz bath. Of those 119, 58 stated they would not take a cold sitz bath no matter how severe their pain. This suggests that willingness to try a pain-relief measure may be strongly influenced by beliefs or prior use.

Shere, CL, Clelland, JA, O'Sullivan, P, Doleys, DM, and Canan, B: The effect of two sites of high frequency vibration on cutaneous pain threshold, *Pain,* **25**:133–138, 1986. Cutaneous pain threshold was measured prior to, during, and following 5 minutes of vibration applied either proximal or distal to the site of pain. Significantly more temporary analgesia occurred when vibration was placed distally than when it was placed proximally, especially during vibration rather than before or after.

Talbot, JD, Duncan, GH, Bushnell, MC, and Boyer, M: Diffuse noxious inhibitory controls (DNICs): psychophysical evidence in man for intersegmental suppression of noxious heat perception by cold pressor pain, *Pain,* **30**:221–232, 1987. Submerging the hand in painfully cold water (cold pressor pain) significantly, although not completely, reduced perception of painful heat stimuli applied to the face, and this effect continued briefly after the hand was removed from the cold water.

Travell, JG, and Simons, DG: *Myofascial Pain and Dysfunction: The Trigger Point Manual,* Baltimore, 1983, Williams & Wilkins. This is the first of two planned volumes. It contains trigger points and related information for the upper half of the body. Numerous drawings clearly identify trigger points and pain patterns along with other details of the problem and its treatment.

Waylonis, GW: The physiologic effects of ice massage, *Arch Phys Med Rehabil,* **48**:37–42, 1967. Ice massage to the thigh or calf for 5–10 minutes decreased skin temperature by as much as 19.2°C, but not enough to present a danger of frostbite. Surface anaesthesia occurred after 4.5 minutes and persisted for 30 minutes to 3 hours. Temperature reductions were smaller than those obtained with ice packs or ethyl chloride. No changes in blood pressure or pulse were observed. It was concluded that ice massage was safe even in inexperienced hands.

White, JR: Effects of a counterirritant on perceived pain and hand movement in patients with arthritis, *Phys Ther*, **53**:956–960, Sept 1973. In 30 patients with either rheumatoid arthritis or osteoarthritis, a placebo cream was applied to one hand and a counter-irritant (10% menthol and 15% methyl salicylate, similar to Ben-Gay Greaseless/Stainless) to the other hand. Both significantly increased range of motion, but the counter-irritant resulted in a significantly greater increase. Only the counter-irritant reduced pain.

REFERENCES AND SELECTED READINGS

Aronoff, GM: Ice massage for pain, *Aches & Pains* **3**:33–36, Feb 1982.

Aronoff, GM: Massaging with ice, *RN* **48**:84, June 1985.

Arvidsson, I, and Eriksson, E: Postoperative TENS for pain relief after knee surgery: objective evaluation, *Orthopedics* **9**:13461351, Oct 1986.

Cailliet, R: Physical modalities and low back pain management. In Stanton-Hicks, M, and Boas, R, eds: *Chronic Low Back Pain*, pp 171–176, New York, 1982, Raven Press.

Cold may ease arthritis pain, *J Gerontol Nurs* **8**:471, Aug 1982.

Cooling more effective, *Aches & Pains* **3**:37, Sept 1982.

Crue, BL, Jr, and Hubrecht, G: Cutaneous vibrator—two models. In Crue, BL, Jr, ed: *Pain: Research and Treatment*, pp. 293–296, New York, 1975, Academic Press.

Crue, BL, Jr, Todd, EM, and Maline, DB: Postherpetic neuralgia—conservative treatment regimen. In Crue, BL, Jr, ed: *Pain: Research and Treatment*, pp. 289–292, New York, 1975, Academic Press.

Cyriax, JH: Clinical applications of massage. In Basmajian, JB, ed: *Manipulation, Traction and Massage*, ed 3, pp. 270–288, Baltimore, 1985, Williams & Wilkins.

Dalton, JA: Education for pain management: a pilot study, *Pat Educ Counsel*, **9**:155–165, 1987.

Day, JA, Mason, RR, and Chesrown, SE: Effect of massage on serum level of b-endorphin and b-lipotropin in healthy adults, *Phys Ther*, **67**:926–930, June 1987.

Diamond, S, and Freitag, FG: Cold as an adjunctive therapy for headache, *Postgrad Med*, **79**:305–309, Jan 1986.

Dodi, G, Bogoni, F, Infantino, A, Pianon, P, et al: Hot or cold in anal pain? *Dis Colon Rectum*, **29**:248–251, Apr 1986.

Droegemueller, W: Cold sitz baths for relief of postpartum perineal pain, *Clin Obstet Gynecol*, **23**:1039–1043, 1980.

Fine, PG, Milano, R, and Hare, BD: The effects of myofascial trigger point injections are naloxone reversible, *Pain*, **32**: 15–20, 1988.

Green, BG: Menthol inhibits the perception of warmth, *Physiol Behav*, **38**:834–838, 1986.

Halverson, GA: Sports-related injuries. In Kaplan, PE, ed: *The Practice of Physical Medicine*, pp. 490–525, Springfield, Ill, 1984, Charles C Thomas.

Harvie, KW: A major advance in the control of postoperative knee pain, *Orthopedics*, **2**:26–27, 1979.

Hendrixson, K: Alcohol on ice, *Nursing*, **12**:127, Nov 1982.

Hofkosh, JM: Classical massage. In Basmajian, JB, ed: *Manipulation, Traction and Massage*, ed 3, pp. 263–269, Baltimore, 1985, Williams & Wilkins.

Howard-Ruben, J: Controlling pain from stomatitis, *Oncol Nurs Forum*, **11**:92, Jan-Feb 1984.

Hymes, AC, Raab, ED, Yonehiro, EG, Nelson, GD, and Printy, AL: Electrical surface stimulation for control of acute postoperative pain and prevention of ileus, *Surg Forum*, **24**:447–448, 1973.

Hymes, AC, Raab, ED, Yonehiro, EG, Nelson, GD, and Printy, AL: Acute pain control by electrostimulation: a preliminary report. In Bonica, JJ, ed: *Advances in Neurology*, vol 4, pp. 761–767, New York, 1974, Raven Press.

Hymes, AC, Yonehiro, EG, Raab, DE, Nelson, GD, and Printy, AL: Electrical stimulation for the treatment and prevention of ileus and atelectasis, *Surg Forum*, **25**:222–224, 1974.

Ice massage, *Nursing*, **17**:94, Aug 1987.

Kamenetz, HL: Mechanical devices of massage. In Basmajian, JB, ed: *Manipulation, Traction and Massage*, ed 3, pp. 289–308, Baltimore, 1985, Williams & Wilkins.

Kirk, JA, and Kersley, GD: Heat and cold in the physical treatment of rheumatoid arthritis of the knee. A controlled clinical trial, *Ann Phys Med*, **9**:270–274, Aug 1968.

Lehmann, JF, and de Lateur, BJ: Diathermy and superficial heat and cold therapy. In Kottke, FJ, Stillwell, CK, and Lehmann, JF, eds: *Krusen's Handbook of Physical Medicine and Rehabilitation*, pp. 275–350, Philadelphia, 1982, WB Saunders Co.

Lehmann, JF, and de Lateur, BJ: Ultrasound, shortwave, microwave, superficial heat and cold in the treatment of pain. In Wall, PD, and Melzack, R, eds: *Textbook of Pain*, pp. 717–724, New York, 1984, Churchill Livingstone.

Levin, J: Fearless venipuncture, *Consultant*, **27**:122, Mar 1987.

Licht, S: History of therapeutic heat and cold. In Lehmann, JF, ed: *Therapeutic Heat and Cold*, ed 3, Baltimore, 1982, Williams & Wilkins.

Locsin, RG: Pinch-grasp technique, *Pain Res News Forum*, **4**:4–5, Mar-Apr 1985.

Lublanezki, NC, and Cleary, RW: External analgesic products. In *Handbook of Nonprescription Drugs*, ed 8, pp. 547–556, Washington, DC, 1986, American Pharmaceutical Association.

Lundeberg, T: Long-term results of vibratory stimulation as a pain relieving measure for chronic pain, *Pain*, **20**:13–23, 1984.

Lundeberg, T, Ottoson, D, Hakansson, S, and Meyerson, BA: Vibratory stimulation for the control of intractable chronic orofacial pain, *Adv Pain Res Ther*, **5**:555–561, 1983.

Lundstrom, R, and Johansson, RS: Acute impairment of the sensitivity of skin mechanoreceptive units caused by vibration exposure of the hand, *Ergonomics*, **29**:687–698, 1986.

Marshall, CM: The use of ice-cube massage for the relief of chronic pain following herpes ophthalmicus, *Physiotherapy*, **57**:374, Aug 1971.

Mehus, AF: Cold comfort, *Nursing*, **11**:96, Oct 1981.

Melzack, R, Guite, S, and Gonshor, A: Relief of dental pain by ice massage of the hand, *Can Med Assoc J*, **122**:189–191, 1980.

Melzack, R, and Schechter, B: Itch and vibration, *Science*, **147**: 1047–1048, Feb 26, 1965.

Melzack, R, Stillwell, DM, and Fox, EF: Trigger points and acupuncture points for pain: correlations and implications, *Pain*, **3**:3–23, 1977.

Mennell, JM: The therapeutic use of cold, *Am Osteopath J*, **74**: 1146–1157, Aug 1975.

Ordog, GJ: Transcutaneous electrical nerve stimulation versus oral analgesic: a randomized double-blind controlled study in acute traumatic pain, *Am J Emerg Med*, **5**:6–10, Jan 1987.

Parsons, CM, and Goetzl, FR: Effect of induced pain on pain threshold, *Proc Soc Exp Biol Med*, **60**:327–328, 1945.

Perdikis, P: Transcutaneous nerve stimulation in the treatment of protracted ileus, *South Afr J Surg*, **15**:81–86, 1977.

Pike, PMH: Transcutaneous electrical stimulation, *Anesthesia*, **33**:165–171, 1978.

Price, DD: Modulation of first and second pain by peripheral stimulation and by psychological set. In Bonica, JJ, and Albe-Fessard, D, eds: *Advances in Pain Research and Therapy*, vol 1, pp. 427–431, New York, 1976, Raven Press.

Prudden, B: *Pain Erasure: The Bonnie Prudden Way*, New York, 1980, M Evans & Co.

Roberts, DJ, Walls, CM, Carlile, JA, Wheaton, CG, and Aronoff, GM: Relief of chronic low back pain: heat versus cold. In Aronoff, GM, ed: *Evaluation and Treatment of Chronic Pain*, pp. 263–266, Baltimore, 1985, Urban & Schwarzenberg.

Russell, WR: Discussion on the treatment of intractable pain, *Proc R Soc Med*, **52**:983–991, Nov 1959.

Russell, WR, Espir, MLE, and Morganstern, FS: Treatment of post-herpetic neuralgia, *Lancet*, **1**:242–245, 1957.

Schuster, GD, and Infante, MC: Pain relief after low back surgery: the efficacy of transcutaneous electrical nerve stimulation, *Pain*, **8**:299–302, 1980.

Snyder, M: *Independent Nursing Interventions*, New York, 1985, John Wiley & Sons.

Solomon, RA, Viernstein, MC, and Long, DM: Reduction of postoperative pain and narcotic use by transcutaneous electrical stimulation, *Surgery*, **87**:142–146, 1980.

Stabile, ML, and Mallory, TH: The management of postoperative pain in total joint replacement, *Orthop Rev*, **7**:121–123, 1978.

Strodhoff, CC: Pathophysiology of rheumatoid arthritis, *Nurs Pract*, **7**:32, June 1982.

Swezey, RL: Low back pain in the elderly: practical management concerns, *Geriatrics*, **43**:39–44, Feb 1988.

Taub, HA, Beard, MC, Eisenberg, L, and McCormack, RK: Studies of acupuncture for operative dentistry, *J Am Dent Assoc*, **95**: 555–561, 1977.

Veehoff, D: Put herpes pain on ice, *RN NV*,:79, Oct 1985.

Wachter-Shikora, HL: Does mechanostimulation control pain? *Am J Nurs*, **82**:81, Jan 1982.

Wagman, IH, and Price, DD: Responses of dorsal horn cells of M. *mulatta* to cutaneous and sural nerve A and C fiber stimuli, *J Neurophysiol*, **32**:803–817, 1969.

Wakim, KG: Physiologic effects of massage. In Basmajian, JB, ed: *Manipulation, Traction and Massage*, ed 3, pp. 256–262, Baltimore, 1985, Williams & Wilkins.

Wing, DM: A different approach to IM injections, *Am J Nurs*, **76**:1239–1240, Aug 1976.

Yeatman, GW, and Dang, VV: Cao gio (coin rubbing): Vietnamese attitudes toward health care, *JAMA*, **244**:2748–2749, Dec 19, 1980.

6

Non-Invasive Pain-Relief Measures

Relevant Patient/Family Teaching Points (see appendix):
- Ball of Healing Energy
- Breathing Out Pain
- Deep Breath/Tense, Exhale/Relax, Yawn for Quick Relaxation
- Distraction for Brief Pain by Describing a Series of Pictures
- Distraction for Brief Pain with Slow Rhythmic Breathing
- Emptying the Sandbag
- Handling Boring or Strange Days
- Heartbeat Breathing for Relaxation
- Humour for Relaxation
- Learning and Using Relaxation Techniques
- Using Imagery for Pain Relief

Distraction

DEFINITION OF DISTRACTION

Distraction from pain may be defined as *focusing attention on stimuli other than the pain sensation.* At times, however, the focus may be on less bothersome qualities of the pain sensation such as pressure or warmth. Distraction is a kind of sensory shielding, i.e. patients shield themselves from the sensation of pain by increasing other sensory input, especially auditory, visual, and tactile-kinesthetic (hearing, seeing, touching, and moving). Attention to pain is sacrificed in favour of attention to other stimuli. The stimuli may be internal or external, e.g. patients may hear music from a headset (external auditory stimuli) or may hear themselves singing mentally but silently (internal auditory stimuli).

In summary, the characteristics of distraction are:
- Attention is focused on stimuli other than the unpleasantness of pain.
- Pain is on the edge or periphery of awareness.
- When distracting stimuli cease, attention is again focused on pain.

This section focuses on two types of distraction:
1. Strategies for brief episodes of pain, and

> **KEY POINT:** Usually distraction only makes pain more bearable and does not make the pain go away.

2. Maintaining a "normal" level of sensory input on a daily basis for ongoing or chronic pain.

BENEFITS AND LIMITS OF DISTRACTION

Table 6.1 summarizes the assets and liabilities of using distraction, and it also corrects a common misconception.

DISTRACTION STRATEGIES FOR BRIEF EPISODES OF PAIN

Appropriate/inappropriate situations/patients

The distraction strategies described in the patient/family teaching points (see appendix) are appropriate for episodes of pain lasting a matter of minutes up to 1 hour. They are not appropriate for managing pain that lasts for hours, except under extreme circumstances where other methods of pain relief are not available. *Examples of brief episodes of pain* that might be made more bearable with a structured distraction strategy are:

Misconception: The patient who can be distracted from pain does not have very severe pain, or the pain is not as severe as the patient would have us believe.

Correction: Research and clinical observations show that distraction strategies are powerful techniques for making even severe pain more bearable for the patient.

Assets of Using Distraction:
↑ Pain tolerance
↑ Self-control
↓ Pain intensity
Renders quality of pain more acceptable, e.g. changes from sharp to dull.

Liabilities of Using Distraction: Others doubt the existence or severity of pain because the patient does not look like he/she is in pain.
After the distraction is over:
↑ Awareness of pain
↑ Fatigue
↑ Irritability
Patient needs a pain-relief measure that allows rest—usually asks for analgesic; health-care team reluctant to administer it since the patient did not look like he/she was in pain a short time earlier.

TABLE 6.1 Assets and Liabilities of Distraction

- Lumbar puncture.
- Bone marrow aspiration.
- Tanking/debridement of burn or other wound.
- Suture removal.
- Dressing change.
- Removal of drainage tubes.
- Period of time between onset of pain and the onset of relief from an analgesic.
- Biopsy under local anaesthetic.
- Unusually painful injections.
- Difficult venepucture.
- Pain on movement, e.g. transfer from bed to chair.
- Uterine contractions during childbirth.

The *types of patients* who might be able to use and benefit from the distraction strategies are children or adults who:

- Understand the instructions.
- Possess the physical ability and energy to perform the activities.
- Are able to attend to, and preferably concentrate on, the stimuli being offered.
- Are willing to try the technique, i.e. open-minded (initially the patient need not be convinced the technique will work).
- Desire some self-control over the painful experience.

Inappropriate patients/situations for structured distraction techniques may include:

- Patients who are hypersensitive to stimuli, e.g. patients with migraine or meningitis. Distraction may make them more uncomfortable.
- Long periods of moderate to severe pain. Structured distraction techniques require too much time and energy to be used repeatedly for long periods. The patient is also unable to engage in something else that may be a better contribution to quality of life.

Patient/family teaching points and nursing guidelines for developing and using distraction for brief episodes of pain

Both patients and nurses spontaneously devise effective distraction techniques for many unpleasant situations, including pain. Most people are accustomed to using distraction to some extent, e.g. watching TV to avoid thinking about or doing something unpleasant. To make distraction for brief episodes of pain more deliberate and structured, and hopefully more effective, both the nurse and the patient need to consider the following guidelines:

1. Individualize the content of the distraction technique. Assess whether or not the patient has used distraction successfully for pain relief. If so, try to utilize what has been done, perhaps improving upon it with the ideas that follow. Ask specifically if the patient (man or woman) has attended childbirth education classes. If so, the patient may already know distraction techniques such as rhythmic breathing patterns but may not realize that these may work for any brief episode of pain. If the patient does not have a useful technique to suggest, assess his/her interests and use them to give choices of distraction techniques.

2. Suggest distraction techniques consistent with the patient's energy level and ability to concentrate.

3. In developing the actual distraction strategy, use as many of the following as possible:
   - As pain increases in intensity, increase the complexity of the distraction, i.e. increase stimuli when pain increases. However, with very high intensities of pain, consider simple distractions since the patient may have limited energy and may not be able to concentrate well.
   - Try to provide stimuli through all the major sensory modalities, such as:

Auditory: something to listen to, e.g. music.

Visual: something to look at, e.g. picture, spot. (If the patient wishes to close the eyes, suggest a mental image or picture so that the patient will not begin to picture the pain or its cause.)

Tactile: something to touch, rub, or hold.

Olfactory: something to smell, e.g. essential oils.

Kinesthetic: movement such as nodding or tapping.

- Avoid external or internal stimuli related to pain, e.g. looking at or mentally picturing the pain. Focus is away from pain.

- Include and emphasize rhythm, e.g. use music and ask the patient to keep time to music by tapping finger or foot. Keeping time to the music makes it necessary to pay attention to the music so less attention is paid to the pain; or alternatively, teach some type of rhythmic breathing and ask the patient to maintain the rhythm with silent counting or words or by nodding the head. (Characteristics of effective distraction strategies for brief episodes of pain are summarized in the box below.)

4. Perfect performance of the distraction is not necessary for success nor does it guarantee success. The patient can actually be distracted from pain by trying to learn a technique of distraction.

5. Identify the need for additional pain relief, i.e. an analgesic, during or after the distraction.

Characteristics of Effective Distraction Strategies for Brief Episodes of Pain

1. Interesting to the patient.
2. Consistent with patient's energy level and ability to concentrate.
3. Rhythm is included and emphasized, e.g. keeping time to music.
4. Stimulates the major sensory modalities:
   - Hearing
   - Vision
   - Touch
   - Smell
   - Movement.
5. Capable of providing a change in stimuli when the pain changes, e.g. ↑ stimuli for ↑ pain.

---

6. Plan to use distraction for a limited period of time, i.e. not for hours. Remember that most patients cannot use distraction for hours at a time as the only form of pain relief.

7. Whenever possible, practise the distraction technique with the patient prior to the time it is needed.

8. Use a preventive approach. Begin the distraction strategy before the pain begins or increases, or as soon as possible after the pain begins.

9. Inform others (health-care team, family) of what the patient will be doing, when, and why. This may help decrease the patient's self-consciousness about doing something different and avoid ridicule from those who do not understand the value of distraction. Explaining when the patient plans to begin the distraction, i.e. the importance of the preventive approach, may assure that the patient is warned prior to a painful procedure.

10. Consider giving the patient written instructions about how and when to use the distraction strategy.

Specific distraction strategies

Criteria for selection. The distraction strategies described in the patient/family teaching points in the appendix were selected with both the nurse's and patient's needs in mind. Most require little, if any, equipment; can be taught quickly and easily by the nurse; and have been shown to be effective on the basis of clinical experience or research. The directions for each strategy are stated in exactly the way the nurse might say them to the patient, or the directions may be duplicated and a copy given to the patient. For the patient's benefit, most of the distraction strategies require very little physical exertion or intellectual ability and are low risk.

Problems and possible solutions

Getting the patient's attention. When the patient is very frightened about impending pain or is already experiencing severe pain, it may be difficult to distract him/her. All of the patient's attention may be narrowly focused on the pain or fears. To get the patient's attention, try the following:

- Whisper in the person's ear.
- Use the person's first name.

- Ask a very simple question that focuses on you, e.g. How many fingers am I holding up? Or, what colour is my hair?
- Begin with a very simple distraction such as "visual concentration and rhythmic massage," previously described.
- Perform the distraction with the person and maintain eye contact.

Patient monitoring painful event. Some patients may feel a need to watch a painful procedure. This may give them a sense of control or reassurance that they are safe from or can prevent unnecessary harm to themselves. Naturally, while patients are watching the painful event, they cannot be distracted from it. Try the following:

IMMEDIATE HELP FOR DISTRACTION

Time involved: Reading time, 5 minutes; implementation time, 5 minutes.

Sample situation: A brief episode of pain, hopefully only a matter of a few minutes. The patient, Mr T. talks to you about this, saying he is afraid and he anticipates or is experiencing a lot of pain. The pain is sudden or unexpected and you have no special equipment, just yourself and a patient who wants help.

Possible solution: A structured distraction strategy.

Expected outcome: The patient says that the pain is more tolerable while he is using the distraction.

Do's

Assure the patient you believe he hurts as much as he says he does.

If the patient is very frightened and if it is difficult to get his attention, start by asking the patient to look you in the eye. Then tell him your name and ask him to take a deep breath, hold it a moment, and then breathe out.

Tell him you will suggest, and help him do, a distraction method.

Tell him that you know distraction will not take away the pain but that you do know distraction can make pain a little more bearable.

Tell him you know that what you are about to suggest may sound silly or even disrespectful of his pain but that it may help.

Tell him you will do it with him so he will know you're serious and so he won't feel as self-conscious.

Explain that the two of you do not have much time to develop a plan so you will give him two ideas to choose from and make suggestions about.

Tell the patient you can help him do *either* of the following:

• Describe out loud each object he can see or use a magazine with pictures if one is available (see appendix,

patient/family teaching point regarding describing a series of pictures).

or

• Sing silently, whispering or mouthing out the words, a song such as "Jingle Bells" or "Happy Birthday". The latter can be sung over and over again to everyone he can think of including you and himself. Any song he knows is acceptable.

Ask the patient which he prefers.

If he chooses to describe objects in the room or a magazine, ask him to look at one picture or object at a time and ask him questions as often as necessary to help him keep talking.

If he chooses a song, ask him to look you in the eye and you will whisper or mouth out the words with him. Suggest he taps out the rhythm.

With either method, explain that when he hurts more he can talk or sing faster, slowing down when he hurts less.

Start the distraction *before the pain starts* if possible.

Explain to others present what you and the patient will be doing and why.

After the distraction and pain are over, or during the event, ask the patient if this helps him.

Regardless of the results, praise the patient for making the effort or being willing to listen to your ideas.

Don'ts

Do not expect or suggest that distraction will take away the pain.

Do not tell the patient he is just anxious or his pain is not as bad as he thinks.

Do not tell the patient everything will be all right.

Do not be afraid to laugh with the patient, *if* the patient begins to laugh as he tries to perform the distraction strategy. Laughter can be extremely effective.

Non-Invasive Pain-Relief Measures

- Discuss the painful event with a patient prior to its occurrence. Ask if he/she wants more information or wants to be sure that the procedure is done in a particular manner.
- If the patient continues to monitor the procedure, respect the desire to do this, and suggest that he/she consider using the distraction before and/or after the painful procedure.
- Use another type of pain relief during the painful procedure, e.g. analgesic or application of cold near the site of pain.

Bedtime. Active involvement with distraction may very well prevent the patient from going to sleep. For distraction at bedtime, when sensory input needs to be reduced to allow the patient to go to sleep, try the following:

- Passive involvement with a distraction, e.g. simply listen to calming music or watch a calming TV programme and perform no other activities along with this.
- Use another pain-relief measure with or instead of distraction, e.g. analgesic or back rub.

INDIVIDUALIZED NURSING-CARE PLAN

Patient with Brief Pain Who May Benefit from Distraction
Patient Description: An adult undergoing bone marrow aspiration (BMA).

Assessment	Potential Nursing Problems	Planning/Intervention	Evaluation/Expected Outcomes
Identify the following: • Knowledge of the type of pain usually felt during a BMA. • Types of distraction, if any, used previously and their effectiveness. • Mental ability to understand instructions and concentrate. • Level of physical energy. • Desire for some personal control over pain and behaviour during BMA. • Special interests, e.g. music, family, shopping.	Pain related to BMA. Fear related to how pain will be managed. Knowledge deficit related to structured distraction techniques to use during BMA.	Describe benefits, limits, and types of distraction (see Table 6.1 and the appendix). Allow patient to choose the distraction he/she wishes to use and modify it to match interests and abilities. Provide written instructions if needed. Practise technique with patient prior to BMA, if possible. Explain the importance of using the distraction before pain begins or increases. Inform person performing BMA and any assistants, of the specific distraction the patient will use, stressing need to forewarn patient of pain so technique can be used preventively.	Patient reports pain during BMA is more bearable when distraction is used. Patient may report that distraction makes the pain sensation more acceptable, e.g. more dull than sharp, and perhaps less intense. Patient may feel a sense of pride in being able to handle part of the discomfort on his/her own. If future BMAs are anticipated, patient says he/she wishes to use distraction again and reports feeling less fearful of subsequent BMAs.

Emotional reactions. The specific content of the distraction may be unexpectedly upsetting to the patient. Fast music may make the patient feel more anxious. Certain pictures may remind the patient of a sad or irritating event. Obviously, these stimuli can simply be changed. However, not all emotional reactions, even sadness, are necessarily undesirable. For example, if a patient with pain knows he is terminally ill, using family photographs may precipitate part of the grieving process. The patient may actually benefit from this.

Ineffective technique. With each distraction strategy described, suggestions are given for making it more effective. If the patient is able to perform the technique reasonably well and if the suggested variations have failed to make the technique effective, try the following:

- If the patient says it is too simple, find a more complex technique.
- If the patient says it is too difficult to perform for very long, try a less complex technique.
- If the distraction involves an activity the patient does not usually like anyway, such as the amount of talking that is involved with describing a series of pictures, switch to an entirely different distraction, such as listening to music.
- Use another method of pain relief, e.g. analgesia or relaxation.

MAINTAINING NORMAL SENSORY INPUT FOR ON-GOING PAIN

A common problem for the patient with on-going or chronic pain is frequent or almost constant exposure to a boring or monotonous environment. The level of sensory input may be less than usual simply because he/she is not engaged in normal activities of daily living. Other patients may be exposed to excessive input that is largely meaningless to them, such as monitoring equipment in intensive-care units.

In either case, the patient is deprived of sensory input that usually occupies time and attention. This may result in the patient focusing more attention on the pain, making it seem more intense or less tolerable. Such environments may also contribute to anxiety or depression.

Appropriate/inappropriate situations/patients

Examples of situations where there tends to be a lack of normal sensory input are:

- Isolation, protective or for infections.
- Decreased ability to be physically active, e.g. body traction, debilitating illness, arthritis, or artificial ventilation.
- Living alone with limited access to outside activities.
- Sedating medications (these decrease activity and interaction with others).
- Intensive-care units.
- Hospitalized patient from a different culture and/or with language barrier.

Types of patients with pain who may benefit from plans to provide a more normal level of daily sensory input are adults and children who:

- Possess the physical energy and ability to engage in some activities similar to those in their previous daily lives.
- Are willing or motivated to make an effort to engage in more activities.
- Desire to regain some of their previous function or quality of life.
- Are aware of being adversely affected by the present environment, e.g. express feelings of loss, depression, frustration, or apprehension.
- Occasionally over-extend themselves, i.e. "do too much," and precipitate more pain or retard their recovery.

Patients who may not be appropriate are:

- Those whose pain has produced an almost complete disability. The simple approaches recommended here may be insufficient. The patient may require a multidisciplinary approach in a structured prog-ramme for several weeks along with systematic follow-up. This is discussed in greater detail in Chapter 7.
- Very withdrawn. Some patients feel very threatened by illness and the treatment inflicted upon them. They feel they have no control over the external environment, so they retreat into their internal environment. Such patients may first need to be given many choices about their care. Then they may be ready to participate more actively in creating a more normal day for themselves.

Nursing-care guidelines and patient/family teaching points for maintaining normal sensory input

Here the focus is on simple and practical approaches to normalizing daily sensory input so that pain is more tolerable. This is done by avoiding an undue focus on pain and minimizing anxiety and depression. *Nursing-care guidelines*, in addition to the patient/family teaching point "Handling boring or strange days" in the appendix, are:

1. Include some normal sensory input at regular intervals throughout the patient's waking day.

2. Identify the need for any pain-relief methods that would allow the patient to engage in normal activities, e.g. aspirin and a cold pack prior to walking.

3. Identify the need for any special assistance needed for the activity, e.g. asking the patient's friend to bring in a videotape or referring to physiotherapy to provide range of motion and stretching of muscles for the inactive patient.

4. Realize the importance of providing input through all the major sensory modalities, e.g. music for auditory stimuli, essential oils for olfactory stimuli,

INDIVIDUALIZED NURSING-CARE PLAN

Patient Who May Benefit from Maintaining Normal Sensory Input

Patient Description: An adult male in isolation with antibiotic resistant infected lesions on both legs.

Assessment	Potential Nursing Problems	Planning/Intervention	Evaluation/ Expected Outcomes
Identify the following: • Feelings of boredom, confusion, pain seems endless and tiring. • Amount of time focused on pain vs. amount focused on activity not related to illness. • Differences between activities now and those prior to illness. • Physical and mental ability to perform more activities. • Willingness to try some activities similar to normal day listening to music visiting with family and friends physical exercise • Special treats not now used. • Need for pain-relief measures to facilitate more activity.	Pain related to infected, open lesions on legs. Diversional activity deficit related to isolation to prevent spread of infection and to inability to walk.	Patient and nurse write a daily diary with an hourly schedule of activities these may include daily: music (×2) physical activity (×1) involvement with friends and family, visits or telephone (×2–3) different special treats at end of each day rest periods. Nurse acknowledges/compliments patient at conclusion of each scheduled activity. Inform others that patient will be more active but that this does not mean pain has subsided. Provide analgesics or other pain relief as needed to facilitate patient's schedule of activity. Patient states pain is less bothersome more of the time. Patient expresses positive feelings about the effects of activities, e.g. less bored, feels happier. Patient begins to initiate additional activities.	Patient states pain is less bothersome more of the time. Patient expresses positive feelings about the effects of activities, e.g. less bored, feels happier. Patient begins to initiate additional activities.

physical exercise for tactile–kinesthetic stimuli, and selected TV viewing or magazines for visual stimuli.

5. Consider using the Daily Diary format (see appendix) for you and the patient to formulate a written daily plan. The first and last columns may be helpful—each hour already written in with a space to enter the major activity.

6. Expect resistance from some patients. Some are self-motivated and will require little assistance. But many people need to have structure and well-stated expectations in order to perform. In a way, this is similar to the difference between a person who is self-directed and one who is not. To complicate the problem further, remember that for reasons not well understood, *boredom tends to lead to more boredom.* While bored patients suffer the consequences of boredom such as disinterest, difficulty in thinking, and less tolerance for pain, many are also surprisingly lacking in frustration. They become passive victims, even those who want to resume a more normal life-style. This circular process is illustrated below.

7. For patients who are able to read, consider duplicating the patient/family teaching point "Handling Boring or Strange Days" and giving it to the patient and family. The teaching points are stated in a manner suitable for the patient to receive.

8. Inform other members of the health-care team of efforts to normalize the patient's day, explaining that this may increase pain tolerance and possibly decrease the need for analgesics. However, warn the health-care team not to mistake more-normal behaviour for an absence of pain. When the patient engages in more activities, he/she may not look or act like he/she is in pain, but the pain is still there.

Relaxation

DEFINITION OF RELAXATION

Relaxation may be defined as *a state of relative freedom from both anxiety and skeletal muscle tension,* a quieting or calming of the mind and muscles. Subjectively, the person usually feels minimal or no anxiety or apprehension. Actually, the complete absence of anxiety is rare and not necessarily beneficial, since some level of arousal or anxiety is useful in alerting or motivating a person to take appropriate action.

In the strictest sense, relaxation should produce the relaxation response. Physiologically, the relaxation response is the opposite of the fight-or-flight response. It is characterized by a normal level of physiological functioning or a decrease in autonomic nervous system activity. However, many people use a relaxation technique and report feeling more relaxed and less distressed without necessarily demonstrating the traditional relaxation response, as summarized in the box below.

Relaxation Response

Physiological characteristics of the relaxation response are:
1. ↓ Oxygen consumption
2. ↓ Respiratory rate
3. ↓ Heart rate
4. ↓ Muscle tension
5. Normal blood pressure (↓ in patients with high blood pressure)
6. ↑ Alpha waves

Reference: Benson, H, Beary, JF, and Carol, MP: The relaxation response, *Psychiatry* **37**:37–46, Feb 1974

Pain + Boring or meaningless environment
↓ Stimulation to think or act
↓ Attention to external events
↑ Focus on pain (internal event, available stimuli)
↓ Pain tolerance
↓ Motivation or energy to change situation

Knowing *what relaxation is not,* is important since many health-care team members, as well as patients, have naive attitudes about relaxation. Relaxation is *not* plopping down in front of the television set, sleeping, resting, sitting quietly, reading a book, working in the garden, or playing tennis. These activities may *promote* relaxation but should not be equated with it. During sleep, for example, dreams or subconscious thoughts can maintain or increase muscle tension. Further, even when the muscles are not being used, high levels of muscle tension may exist. In essence, people often think they are relaxed when in fact they are not. Most people must make a conscious attempt to relax, and many must learn the skill—it does not necessarily come naturally.

> **KEY POINT:** It is common for people to think they are relaxed when they are not.

Techniques for accomplishing or learning relaxation comprise a wide variety of methods, including meditation, autogenic training, yoga, religion, and music. Some techniques are simple or utilize what the patient has already learned, while others constitute a training programme of building skill in relaxation and incorporating this into daily life. Sometimes biofeedback in the form of skin temperature or muscle tension is used to help a person learn when he/she is relaxing, although there is little evidence that biofeedback is necessary or even helpful for learning relaxation (Roberts, 1987; Turner and Chapman, 1982).

The benefits of nurses being able to teach some relaxation techniques are now becoming recognized. Relaxation techniques are incorporated in programmes that have a multitude of purposes, such as stress reduction for those who have stressful life-styles, aiding weight reduction or abstinence from abused substances, reduction of nausea and vomiting during chemotherapy, and treatment for hypertension. Here the focus is on using relaxation techniques to help people with pain.

> **KEY POINT:** Relaxation may not relieve pain, but it has many other potential benefits for people with pain.

BENEFITS AND LIMITS OF RELAXATION

The widely held belief that relaxation may be beneficial to patients with pain is illustrated by its use in almost every programme for prepared childbirth, and for management of pain for patients with chronic non-malignant pain. On the other hand, there is very little research to justify this widespread use. In fact, the exact benefits of relaxation for people with pain remain largely unknown. Thus relaxation should be used judiciously, not automatically.

> **KEY POINT:** Muscle tension, anxiety, and pain may perpetuate each other and become a spiralling process.

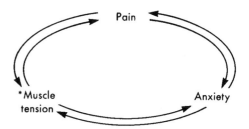

*Interrupting the cycle here with skeletal muscle relaxation may have many benefits, such as preventing the situation from worsening.

For the person with pain, the *potential benefits* of using relaxation are related to the interaction between pain, muscle tension, and anxiety. The usual responses to pain, especially initially and when it cannot be avoided, are some anxiety-like feelings such as apprehension, fear, or panic, and some muscle tension such as restriction of movement, jaw-clenching, or splinting. The anxiety, pain, and muscle tension tend to intensify each other, and the situation proceeds from bad to worse. To help the patient with pain, relaxation attempts to interrupt this spiralling process with skeletal muscle relaxation. Quieting the body often quiets the mind.

Relaxation, especially when it is used preventively, may produce one or more of the following *specific benefits* for the person with pain (this list has been developed from research findings and clinical observations):

1. Aids sleep by helping the patient get to sleep faster, improving the quality of sleep by decreasing physical and mental tension, and helping the patient with frequent awakenings get back to sleep more quickly.

2. Strengthens the nurse–patient relationship through individualized attention. The manner in which the nurse offers to help the patient with relaxation can reassure the patient that the nurse is aware of distress felt and wants to be of help.

3. Improves problem-solving and increases the likelihood that positive, adaptive ideas will reach consciousness.

4. Minimizes the detrimental effects of continued or repeated stress from pain or other sources. The patient may be able to learn to respond to stress with less autonomic nervous system activity and/or to recover more rapidly from a stress reaction, e.g. "fight or flight." (Note: Stress is a situation that makes it necessary for the person to readjust. However, stress is not necessarily negative, since happy as well as unhappy events may require an adjustment. In fact, people thrive on the right amount of stress. Stress becomes distress when there is a continual or intense need to readjust or adapt.)

5. Reduced skeletal muscle tension may reduce strain or pressure on pain-sensitive structures. This may relieve pain.

6. Increases confidence and a sense of self-control in coping with pain; better able to decide on appropriate action for handling the pain and avoid harmful or unproductive efforts.

7. Decreases fatigue, especially after a technique done for 5–20 minutes. This may result in a more energized feeling than taking a nap for an hour.

8. Distracts from pain, since most relaxation techniques for pain include sufficient structure and activity to prevent thoughts from returning to pain. Certain types of relaxation imagery can give the patient a sense of freedom from being confined to bed or being hospitalized.

9. Increases the effectiveness of other pain relief measures. For example, even a quick and easy technique may increase the effectiveness of an analgesic. A relaxed person may be more susceptible to suggestions or intentions of pain relief.

10. Increases subjective reports of improved mood and decreased distress, e.g. pain is more tolerable and the patient increases involvement in various activities.

11. Decreases distress or fear during anticipation of pain, e.g. desensitizes the person to anxiety-producing aspects of a painful procedure.

Some possible *limitations or disadvantages* of relaxation for the person with pain are:

1. The suggestion to try relaxation techniques may be misinterpreted by the patient as meaning that the health-care team regards the pain as being of psychological origin or "not real pain."

2. The success of relaxation may be misinterpreted by the health-care team as meaning that the pain is mainly or exclusively caused by psychological problems.

3. Others may doubt the existence or severity of the patient's pain when he/she uses relaxation because it will not look like the patient is in pain. This may discourage the use of relaxation.

4. Relaxation is not a substitute for appropriate analgesics and other methods of pain relief.

5. It does not necessarily relieve pain and certainly is not a panacea for all pain-related ailments. There are exceptions, e.g. progressive relaxation has been shown to reduce pain of ulcerative colitis.

6. It is only an adjunctive treatment for pain—rarely will relaxation alone be sufficient to treat pain.

7. Once pain becomes severe, it is difficult to use relaxation even for the person who is well trained, e.g. relaxation may help prevent a migraine but may be useless once the migraine occurs.

8. Unwanted side effects are rare, but they may occur. This is most likely with the longer, meditative techniques. For example, the patient may experience anxiety or previously denied feelings of sadness or grief (see Table 6.2).

9. Since not every relaxation technique works for everyone, with some patients it may take time to find or develop an effective technique for the individual.

10. Patient may find relaxation helpful without experiencing the traditional relaxation response (shown in the box on p. 168).

Problems	Possible Solutions
1. Falls asleep.	1. Set timer, or sit in straight-back chair. Ask about sleep patterns: especially inquire about sleep problems and medications. Patient may simply need to get more sleep.
2. Increased coughing or other respiratory problems.	2. May need to avoid deep breathing. Suggest breathing quietly, perhaps through pursed lips. To avoid changing the patient's normal breathing pattern, use a technique without a focus on breathing. Coughing is likely to be a problem with patients who smoke or have upper respiratory problems.
3. Prickly, tingling feelings, especially in the extremities.	3. Change positions; be sure extremities are not crossed.
4. Increased awareness of pain.	4. Add more distraction, such as activity, thoughts, or imagery to the technique. Avoid focusing on areas of pain. If this does not help, suggest shorter techniques.
5. Transient increase in heart rate, or increased awareness of heartbeat or breathing; eyelids flutter.	5. Assure patient this is normal. Encourage focus on other parts of relaxation technique or add external focus. Try heartbeat breathing at the beginning of the technique. If increased heart rate continues, gently suggest the patient discontinues the technique, report findings to the doctor, and see suggested solutions for item 10 below.
6. Feelings of suffocation.	6. Take a deep breath when desired. Adjust position to allow fuller expansion of lungs.
7. Restless legs (creeping or crawling sensation often of unknown cause, may result in the patient feeling the need to get up and walk around).	7. Mild cases may be relieved by keeping the legs cold; some patients report relief from heat. Otherwise, use brief relaxation techniques.
8. Increased focus on body functions and discomforts.	8. Change to a technique with an external focus, i.e. avoid a focus on the body; keep eyes open; try briefer technique.
9. Mild anxiety; fear of loss of control.	9. Reassure patient that he/she is in control and that these feelings will probably subside. Consider shorter techniques or progressive relaxation with eyes open.
10. Hallucination, "out of body" feeling, loss of contact with reality, or general increase in depression or withdrawal.	10. Gently explain need to stop technique. To avoid feelings of failure, suggest short techniques with eyes open. Report findings to the doctor, and discuss the need for psychiatric referral.
11. Sudden or increased crying, sadness, or extreme anxiety, such as perspiration, rapid respiration, and trembling.	11. Gently suggest discontinuing the technique. To avoid feelings of failure, suggest briefer techniques or progressive relaxation with the eyes open. Ask patient if he/she wishes to deal with these feelings, and report findings to the doctor. If patient wants to deal with feelings, provide time for this or consider appropriate referral.
12. Patient uses technique frequently and this is associated with increased isolation and decreased function; patient may seem to "overdose" on relaxation.	12. Patient may desperately need other methods of pain relief that enable him/her to function at a higher level. Or, patient may try to use relaxation as an acceptable way to withdraw from others. Gently try to persuade patient to reduce use of that technique, and introduce briefer techniques. Present other methods of pain relief. Report findings to the doctor and discuss the need for psychological/psychiatric referral.

NOTE: If the patient regularly uses relaxation techniques, periodically ask how he or she feels during and after the technique. Be alert to:
• *Patient reluctance to report certain problems.* He/she may believe the problem is inevitable or unavoidable. Or, the patient may feel inadequate because he/she interprets a problem as his/her own failure.
• *The patient not always considering the above to be problems,* e.g. items 10 and 12. They may be the patient's usual method of coping or they may be temporarily effective. Before suggesting solutions, note whether or not the patient considers these to be problems. Of course, sometimes intervention is indicated even when the patient does not consider his/her reactions a problem, e.g. progressive withdrawal.

Table 6.2 Relaxation: Possible Problems and Solutions.

11. In some situations for some patients, relaxation may increase pain and distress.

12. Some elderly people do not seem to benefit as much or as quickly from relaxation training but do seem to benefit from more simple and brief techniques.

13. In spite of appropriate teaching and reassurance, some patients who are motivated to use relaxation will become more distressed. For example, failure to achieve profound relaxation or unrealistic expectations of the benefits of relaxation may result in frustration.

For an overview of practical guidelines for matching relaxation techniques to patients and situations, see the box below.

RELAXATION TECHNIQUES: ACTIVE PATIENT INVOLVEMENT

Some relaxation techniques require varying degrees of patient involvement, mentally and physically. Examples of the techniques and specific instructions for teaching are in the appendix. Following is an overview of patients and situations that may be either appropriate or inappropriate opportunities to use these relaxation techniques.

Appropriate/inappropriate patients/situations

The relaxation techniques described in this chapter may be appropriate for almost any person with pain. It is very difficult to say with any certainty that relaxation in general or any specific technique is or is not

---

Practical Guidelines for Matching Relaxation Techniques to Patients and Situations

1. Consider the *amount of time* the patient will experience pain vs. the time involved in teaching and using the technique. Usually:
Use less time-consuming techniques for brief episodes of pain, e.g. for procedural or postoperative pain.
Be willing to invest more time for patients with chronic pain, e.g. for cancer pain or recurrent headaches.
Beware of introducing time-consuming techniques to patients who are already under considerable stress, even if they have chronic pain, since this may add another stressor.

2. Consider how pain, fatigue, anxiety, and other factors influence the *patient's general ability to learn or engage in an activity*. Usually:
Use brief, simple techniques or massage during severe pain, lack of concentration, or along with other pain relief measures, e.g. *Deep Breath/Tense, Exhale/Relax, Yawn*, when narcotic is given for renal colic.
Teach more time-consuming techniques when the patient is alert and comfortable, e.g. *Meditative Relaxation* when severe back pain is in remission.

Even if the patient says relaxation is not helpful during pain or the anticipated pain will be too severe to use relaxation, suggest it is used before and after pain.

3. Note if the patient has *energy that needs to be dissipated*, e.g. is restless, "up-tight," or has the "fight or flight" response (meaning that he/she has generated energy to fight or flee but has nowhere to go). Use a technique that releases energy, e.g. *Progressive Relaxation*.

4. For the *patient who misunderstands the purpose of relaxation*, use other terminology and suggest humour or passive recipient techniques such as a back rub.

5. *Consider whether the focus is inward on the body or outward on peaceful scenes.* An inward focus can increase distress about changes in body image or feelings of failure about physical limitations. Be cautious about using an exclusively inward body focus for patients who are distressed about changes in body appearance or function, severely depressed, or have difficulty maintaining contact with reality.

recommended for a certain person or a specific situation.

Examples of *patients who may be appropriate* candidates for using and benefiting from relaxation techniques requiring some active participation are children or adults who:

- Express a need or desire to use relaxation to cope with pain or have some control over the pain, or are open-minded enough to want to try.
- Understand the instructions.
- Are able to concentrate on the directions offered.
- Say they are anxious, tense, "up-tight," or mildly depressed.
- Maintain a rigid posture or are unaware that they are tensing muscles, e.g. clenching fists or teeth.
- Have sleep disturbances or increased fatigue.
- Are adolescents or young to middle-aged adults with tension or migraine headaches.
- Have pain related to ulcerative colitis, temporomandibular joint (TMJ) problems, or surgery.
- Have on-going muscle spasm.
- Have predictable pain periods.
- Have chronic pain, on-going or recurrent, especially chronic non-malignant pain.

Although research evidence of the effectiveness of relaxation for patients with pain is minimal, most pain specialists agree that relaxation is probably a significant part of a successful pain-management programme for a person with chronic non-malignant pain. When such a patient benefits from a tape-recorded 5- to 20-minute technique, he/she is usually so grateful and the technique is used so often (several times a day for months, even years) that the time required to discuss and record the technique often seems insignificant.

Patient Example

Mrs N., 38 years old, requested her doctor to refer her to someone who could help her learn relaxation. She had been diagnosed as having a form of cancer that was essentially always fatal, but she had responded to treatment and lived much longer than expected. Now she was in considerable pain and aware that her doctor had lost hope in further progress. The doctor referred the patient to a nurse and called the nurse to advise caution since the patient was prone to high achievement standards and might feel guilty if she could not relax well. The nurse and patient spent 3 hours discussing the possible benefits and limitations of relaxation, developing a personalized technique for this patient, and tape-recording it. Numerous relaxation techniques were described to her, and she was given complete control of what would be included in the tape. She chose a rhythmic breathing pattern, a detailed description of a personally peaceful scene, and a psalm. She lived 2 more years. Until 2 days before her death she functioned well at her occupation of university professor. During those 2 years, as requested by the nurse, she regularly called to report her condition and problems. Never once did she indicate that she expected relaxation to be the answer to all her pain problems. Many other alternatives for pain relief were discussed and used. According to her reports and those of her husband, for those 2 years she listened to the tape at least twice a day, saying that it decreased stress and tension. Relaxation seemed to help her maintain her self-respect by enabling her to function in areas important to her.

While there are certainly situations where relaxation is inappropriate or unhelpful, quick and easy relaxation techniques are probably devoid of significant harm. Benefits probably exceed any undesirable side effects. However, use of those relaxation techniques that require the patient's time and effort should be carefully evaluated.

Examples of patients *who may be inappropriate candidates for relaxation techniques*, especially those that are *lengthy* (more than a few seconds) and *introspective or meditative* (focusing inward and excluding external stimuli) are children or adults who:

- State they do not want to try relaxation.
- Have a psychiatric history of hallucinations, loss of contact with reality, or delusion. Meditative or internally focused techniques may cause a loss of contact with reality and may be particularly troublesome, but such patients, if they are motivated, should be encouraged to try other brief or externally focused techniques, such as humour or jaw relaxation.
- Are significantly depressed. Time-consuming techniques, especially meditative or internally focused, may increase depression, rumination, or withdrawal.
- Are presently in extremely stressful situations and have no time or energy to devote to learning relaxation (practising a relaxation technique may simply add another stressor).

- Have cardiac problems. Cardiac patients may be at increased risk of arrhythmias due to stimulation of the vagus nerve. Therefore if the technique involves muscle contraction, e.g. traditional active progressive relaxation, warn such patients not to tightly tense muscles. If a hypotensive patient practises any type of relaxation regularly, monitor blood pressure.
- Some elderly people, since they do not seem to benefit as much or as quickly from relaxation training. However, they do seem to benefit from more simple and brief techniques, such as jaw relaxation.

Nursing-care guidelines for selecting, developing, and using relaxation techniques

Common elements of relaxation techniques

This chapter provides only a small sample of the many available relaxation techniques. Numerous ones are offered on tape. Most relaxation techniques for patients with pain have certain elements in common (see below). However, a technique may be effective without including all the items listed.

IMMEDIATE HELP FOR RELAXATION

Time involved: Reading time, 5 minutes; implementation time, 5–7 minutes.

Sample situation: The patient is not only in pain but also in considerable distress about the pain. While you and/or others are trying to do something more to relieve the pain, you want to help him/her relax to relieve some of the distress about the pain.

Possible solution: The patient may be willing to try one of two or three methods of relaxation that you intend to suggest.

Expected outcome: The patient will feel his pain is acknowledged and someone cares. He/she will experience less distress with pain.

Don'ts

1. Do not expect or suggest that relaxation will substitute for appropriate pain relief, e.g. adequate analgesic prescriptions.
2. Do not tell the patient "Just relax and it will be all right." Help him/her relax and make assurances that you are searching for appropriate pain relief methods.
3. Do not convey that the pain is largely due to anxiety.
4. Do not say that there is nothing else anyone can do.
5. Do not tell the patient he/she has to learn to live with this.
6. *Never* tell the patient the pain is not as bad as he/she thinks.
7. If relaxation helps, do not abandon the search for appropriate methods of pain relief.

Do's

1. Take a deep breath outside the patient's room and relax a little yourself. Plan on 2–5 minutes with the patient.

2. When you enter the room, tell the patient you know he/she hurts.
3. Tell the patient you are still hoping (searching) for a better alternative, but that meanwhile relaxation may be helpful.

To convey points 2 and 3 above, you might say "I know that hurting this much often makes people feel frightened and anxious, and I know that the best way to relieve that anxiety is to relieve the pain. But since that isn't possible at the moment, maybe I can at least help you find a way to relieve some of the anxiety."

4. Tell the patient you have a few moments to help him/her learn a brief technique.

If the patient is receptive to the idea of relaxation, try deep breath/tense (see appendix).

If the patient is not receptive to the idea of relaxation, ask him/her to try to remember and concentrate on something peaceful that happened to him/her, suggesting recollection of being with a loved one, especially a child or parent. Or, if available, suggest relaxing music.

5. Tell the patient when you will try to return; give yourself leeway. It's better to return early than late.
6. When you return, ask the patient how the relaxation worked.
7. If the patient says the relaxation did not help, express your regrets, and say you admire the willingness to try the technique.
8. If the relaxation helped, praise the patient's willingness to try it and encourage him/her to continue relaxation at least at intervals while you continue to try to find something to relieve the pain.

Common Elements of Effective Relaxation Techniques

Relaxation techniques often include one or more of the following:

- *Mental device* to reduce distracting thoughts, e.g. rhythmic breathing.
- *Passive attitude*, i.e. let it happen, it cannot be forced, worrying that it won't happen only creates more tension.
- *Quiet environment*, e.g. phone off hook, use headset to listen to tape.
- *Comfortable position*, e.g. lying down with support for neck and legs, not crossing extremities.
- *Behaviour already conditioned* to produce relaxation: Deep breath (big sigh following a stressful event is often paired with relaxing on exhalation) Yawn (paired with sleep) Abdominal breathing (paired with sleep) Peaceful images (patient reacts to pleasant, relaxing memories with same feelings experienced previously).
- *Repetition or practice* (using what the patient has already found helpful or selecting a technique and practising it daily helps develop conditioning).
- *Patient controls* whether or not and when and where he/she performs the technique.

Specific suggestions for teaching patients

The following suggestions for teaching patients about relaxation techniques are not necessarily indicated when a technique is used only once or a few times for quick, "on the spot" assistance with relaxation. However, the more time and effort required of the patient, the more important the following points become:

1. Emphasize that the reason for using relaxation is to reduce the distress caused by pain, not necessarily to reduce the pain. Be careful to avoid implying that the pain is caused by stress or psychological factors. Take care not to mislead the patient into thinking that the pain will go away if he/she relaxes.
2. Select terminology carefully. If the patient reacts negatively to or lacks understanding of the term "relaxation," select words from the patient's vocabulary.
3. Ask the patient if he/she has used any relaxation method in the past. If so, he/she may still be conditioned to it, so time and energy will be saved by using or building on that technique.
4. Be relaxed yourself when you talk with the patient about relaxation. Use a quick and easy technique, e.g. Deep Breath/Tense, etc. (see appendix), before entering the patient's room.
5. Live, in person, assistance (your presence and voice) with relaxation is probably the most effective, but since it is time consuming, try to tape record instructions. This saves your time, and the patient may use the tape whenever he/she wishes rather than rely on your availability.
6. Demonstrate and practise the relaxation technique with the patient. Allow for a return demonstration if time permits.
7. Anticipate the need for the patient to use relaxation. Explain and teach relaxation prior to the patient being in pain or distress, e.g. preoperatively or prior to a course of chemotherapy.
8. Consider giving the patient and family copies of patient/family teaching points about preparing for and using relaxation techniques.
9. Offer to include and teach close friends and family members. They too may benefit from relaxation. In fact, sometimes the patient is under too much stress to learn relaxation but family or friends may be appropriate candidates.
10. If several patients in the hospital or clinic setting need to learn relaxation techniques, teach patients in groups.
11. Individualize the content of the relaxation technique by asking the patient to suggest changes. Whenever possible, let the patient select the technique after he/she has been exposed to several choices.
12. Inform others (health-care team, family) of what the patient will be doing, when, and why. This may decrease the patient's self-consciousness about doing something different, avoid ridicule from those who do not appreciate the value of relaxation, prevent others from discounting pain as simply anxiety, and minimize disruptions when the patient uses the technique. Others may also help by reminding the patient to use relaxation, but *caution them not to suggest relaxation as a substitute for other appropriate pain-relief measures.*

13. Identify the need for additional pain relief before, during, or after the technique is used. Relaxation usually does not decrease pain, but it tends to enhance the effectiveness of other pain-relief measures.

14. In selecting and recommending relaxation techniques, consider the specific situation as well as the characteristics of the specific patient. The techniques described in the chapter along with indications for use are summarized in the box on the opposite page, and practical guidelines for matching techniques to patients and situations are listed in the box on p. 172.

15. Give the patient a choice of closing his/her eyes or focusing on an object. Explain that this helps avoid disturbing sights. Do not insist that he/she closes the eyes. Some patients fear loss of control or object to the degree of passivity inherent in closing their eyes.

16. If the patient indicates unwillingness to try relaxation, never insist that the patient perform a technique against his/her will. This could result in severe side effects such as marked increase in depression or loss of contact with reality. Also, some patients endure pain with less distress by using muscle tension, i.e. relaxing may make the pain worse or less tolerable.

17. To evaluate the effectiveness of relaxation, simple measures include:
    a. Pulse rate before, during, and after relaxation. This is a type of biofeedback.
    b. Pain and distress scales e.g. Visual Analogue Scales (see Chapter 2) before and after relaxation.
    c. Gentle movement of body parts by nurse or others to determine any signs of tension before, during, or after relaxation. For example, carefully support the patient's arm or leg, and slowly flex or rotate the extremity. This too may provide the patient with biofeedback about the existence or absence of tension.

18. If pain is anticipated, e.g. with a procedure, especially if the patient is fearful of it, suggest that the patient mentally rehearse the procedure while in a relaxed state, i.e. after using a relaxation technique. This may desensitize the patient to frightening aspects of the procedure.

19. Plan to provide regular reinforcement for the patient's use of relaxation. Patients using relaxation may be easily discouraged since relaxation is not consistently or dramatically effective, and it may use energy and time that are already in short supply. Indeed, for some patients, the benefits of relaxation do not warrant the time and effort required.

Serious or undesirable side effects from relaxation are not common but may occur in some patients. Relaxation lowers a person's defences. Various unexpected, and sometimes unwanted, feelings or thoughts may emerge. This is more likely to occur with meditative techniques.

As a general guideline, if any problems are not quickly resolved, gently ask the patient to stop using that particular technique. To avoid feelings of failure, suggest the patient tries a briefer technique with eyes open and/or a more structured or externally focused one. Certain problems may require referral or consultation. Table 6.2 lists problems most likely to occur with relaxation and suggests some possible solutions.

If your time is limited, consider the following three-part time plan for time-consuming techniques that involve tape-recording a meditative or progressive relaxation script:

Part 1. Plan 10–15 minutes for: discussion of the benefits of learning relaxation skills, general description of techniques you are able to provide, time for the patient to ask questions, and a specific description of the technique the patient chooses. Leave a copy of the script with the patient if he/she can read. Set a time with the patient for the next 15-minute visit, and ask the patient to provide a tape recorder with microphone and a blank cassette tape (unless these are already available). If possible, plan a way to tape record the relaxation technique with slow, non-lyric music in the background.

Part 2. Plan about 15 minutes for: review of potential benefits and limitations of relaxation and time for patient to ask questions or make changes in the relaxation technique previously selected. Record the technique. Ask the patient about his/her reactions to the technique, when he/she intends to listen to it, and to let you know if any problems arise.

Part 3. Contact the patient within 3 days and ask if the technique has been used. If not, determine why. If he/she has used the technique, ask him/her how he/she felt during and after the technique. If there are problems, consult Table 6.2. Encourage the patient appropriately. Emphasize the positive and avoid any tension or urgency in relation to relaxation.

Patient/family teaching points for general use of relaxation techniques

For brief relaxation techniques, very little teaching or explanation may be required. However, for patients who are regularly using relaxation techniques that last 5 minutes or longer, the teaching points in the appendix should be discussed with the patient and family. These suggestions are stated in the exact words that may be spoken to the patient, or the patient/family teaching point may be duplicated and given to the patient who can read.

Patient/family teaching points for specific relaxation techniques with active patient involvement

Characteristics of specific relaxation techniques and indications for their uses are outlined below.

Patient/family teaching points on individual techniques are presented in a sequence that roughly approximates the amount of time usually required for the nurse to teach the patient and for the patient to perform the technique or learn the skill (see appendix). Naturally, the more experience and knowledge the nurse has about relaxation and the more time that is devoted to individualizing the technique for the patient, the better the outcome is likely to be. However, a longer technique is not necessarily a more effective one for the individual patient. In reality the amount of time and energy available to both the nurse and patient may be a significant factor in determining which technique is chosen.

The directions for each relaxation technique are stated in the exact words the nurse might say to the patient. If the patient can read, the appropriate patient/family teaching point(s) may be duplicated and given to the patient and family.

RELAXATION TECHNIQUES: THE PATIENT AS PASSIVE RECIPIENT

All the family/patient teaching points on relaxation require the patient's active participation to some extent, and for the most part, are techniques the patient can learn to do for him/herself. However, some patients are simply unable to participate actively in achieving relaxation and need to have something done for them to help them relax; examples of this include massage, handholding and warm foot soaking.

Characteristics of Specific Relaxation Techniques and Indications for Use (see appendix)

Deep Breath/Tense, Exhale/Relax, Yawn
This takes only a few seconds; is easily learned by patient; is appropriate to introduce when patient is already tense and in pain, e.g. during a procedure, or may be taught prior to brief painful procedures or preoperatively.

Humour
This takes very little of the nurse's time to suggest to patient; patient may spend as much time as is wished using it. It may be appropriate for patients who are elderly; who resist or misunderstand the idea of relaxation; who are depressed or easily lose contact with reality; who have little time or energy for learning the skill of relaxation; or who are from a different culture (assuming a tape from the appropriate culture can be obtained). It may be used to relieve boredom of prolonged pain under confining circumstances; also appropriate for brief procedural pain.

Heartbeat Breathing
The nurse may have to teach the patient how to find and count the radial pulse, and some patients may have difficulty with this. If not, it takes very little of the nurse's or patient's time. Heartbeat breathing has an internal focus but is used only briefly. It may relieve a sudden, sharp increase in fear or anxiety and may be used without others noticing. It may be very helpful to patients who are aware of a sudden increase in heart rate during stress.

Progressive Relaxation Instructions
This also usually takes a minimum of three contacts with the patient for a total of 35 minutes or more. The first two contacts take about 15 minutes. The second usually involves tape recording the technique. The third is a follow-up and may take only a few minutes, unless problems have occurred.
Its potential advantages are that it involves physical activity that gives a sense of "doing something," e.g. muscle contraction, dissipates energy, is focused inward without the necessity of keeping the eyes closed, does not rely exclusively on mental activity, and easily gets the patient's attention by asking him/her to perform specific tasks.

Give this *priority* for patients with prolonged pain who exhibit signs of moderate to severe anxiety or "fight or flight," especially if they cannot engage in their customary physical exercise. They need to get rid of that muscular energy. Later they may benefit from a more meditative approach.

INDIVIDUALIZED NURSING-CARE PLAN

Patient Who May Benefit from a Brief Relaxation Technique

Patient Description: Ms P., age 47, is admitted for a cholecystectomy the following day.

Preoperative teaching and postoperative follow-up include the following.

Assessment	Potential Nursing Problems	Planning/Intervention	Evaluation/ Expected Outcomes
Identify: • Ability to understand and follow directions. • Previous use of relaxation. • Desire or willingness to try a brief relaxation technique following surgery. • Possibility of including family or friends in relaxation teaching.	Pain, related to impending surgery. Fear related to outcome of surgery and pain. Sleep pattern disturbance before and after surgery related to hospital environment and to the pain and stress of surgery.	Describe one or two brief relaxation techniques and let the patient choose. Teach the relaxation technique by including the following: • Detailed explanation (consider patient/family teaching tools). • Provide demonstration and period for patient to practice (include family or friends if possible). • Encourage practise again before surgery. • Review technique with patient as soon as feasible following surgery. Emphasize that learning a simple relaxation technique may have the following benefits: • Aids sleep periods and decreases fatigue during day. • Reduces distress of hospitalization, surgery, and discomfort. • Reduces strain on the incisional area, thereby reducing some pain. • Enhances the effectiveness of pain-relief measures such as analgesia. • Facilitates a return to comfort following an uncomfortable activity such as deep breathing or turning. Teach the patient to try to remember to use relaxation at the following times: • Before, after, and if possible during painful activities. • Before pain occurs or increases. • Along with, not instead of, pain-relief measures, such as analgesia. Inform health-care team members about patient's use of relaxation and the need to forewarn patient of pain so relaxation can be used preventively.	Patient reports one or more of the following occur when she uses relaxation: • Less discomfort during a painful activity. • More rapid return to comfort following a painful activity. • Less distress following a painful activity. • More rapid onset of analgesia following medication. • Greater pain relief from analgesics. • Improved ability to return to sleep when awakened during the night. • Decrease in fatigue during the day. • Ability to decrease incisional pain. Patient appears to feel pride and a sense of control in relation to using relaxation.

INDIVIDUALIZED NURSING-CARE PLAN

Patient Who May Benefit from Regular Daily Use of a Relaxation Technique

Patient Description: Mr C., age 34 years, is recuperating at home following a work-related back injury 6 weeks ago. He has ongoing pain from muscle injury and spasm. He comes to the clinic for physiotherapy three times a week, in addition to performing daily exercises at home, sees the doctor once or twice a week for trigger point injections, and with the clinic nurse once a week to review his progress and coordinate his care. Medications include muscle relaxants and non-narcotic analgesics.

Assessment	Potential Nursing Problems	Planning/Intervention	Evaluation/ Expected Outcomes
Identify: • Level of pain and distress. Consider teaching patient to use pain and distress scales. • Use of medications and their effectiveness. • Sleep disturbance. • Fatigue or excessive undirected physical energy. • History of psychiatric disorders and current level of depression. • Ability to understand and follow directions. • Time available to patient for use of relaxation. • Desire for personal control of distress, pain and fatigue. • Previous use of relaxation. • Desire or willingness to try relaxation. • Possibility of including family or friends in relaxation training.	Pain, potentially chronic, related to back injury. Anxiety, moderate, related to pain and lack of control over ability to progress and return to work. Sleep pattern disturbance related to pain and distress.	Emphasize belief in patient's pain and in the primary cause being related to work injury. Describe benefits, limits, and types of relaxation available. Unless contra-indicated, encourage use of techniques lasting 3 minutes or longer. Allow patient to choose technique. Teach relaxation technique by including the following: • Give more detailed description of technique. • Ask if patient wants any changes. • Provide demonstration and/or period of patient practice. • Provide relevant patient/family teaching points and/or tape recording. • List ways to prepare to get the maximal benefit from the use of relaxation, e.g. positioning. • Emphasize learning skill by practising the same technique daily during periods of minimal pain and stress. • Include family member or close friend during instructions. If patient desires objective evidence or record of achieving relaxation, suggest use of pain and distress scales or pulse rate before and after using technique. If available, someone can test extremities for tension during or after use of the technique. Emphasize use of relaxation preventively and as an addition to, not as a substitute for, other appropriate treatment. Suggest use of relaxation before and after distressing or painful activities, and at bedtime and if awakened during the night. Plan a time within the next 3 days to check with patient regarding his response during and after use of relaxation. Plan regular follow-up to determine if any problems occur and to provide reinforcement, including assurance that immediate and dramatic effects are not expected.	Patient reports one or more of the following: • Less distress from daily discomfort and from pain related to physical therapy exercises, perhaps indicated as a lower number on the distress scale. • Less sleep disturbance. • Less fatigue. • Generally improved mood. • Better pain relief from nonnarcotics and muscle relaxants when he uses relaxation at the time he takes the medications. • Sense of control over his progress. If patient reports problems with relaxation and suggested solutions are not effective, gently explain that the technique should be discontinued and obtain appropriate consultation or referral.

Appropriate/inappropriate patients/situations

Examples of *appropriate patients* are those who are:
- Debilitated or acutely ill, i.e. limited physical or emotional energy.
- Babies and young children; elderly.
- Confused or agitated.
- In acute or sudden distress or pain.
- Extremely fatigued or sedated, e.g. immediate postoperative period.
- Those with families or friends who would like to do something to help the patient and who can learn to perform these relaxation techniques for the patient.

Examples of *inappropriate patients* are those who:
- Are uncomfortable with physical touch.
- Dislike feelings of passivity or dependence.

Nursing-care guidelines and patient/family teaching points for specific techniques

The patient/family teaching point for simple touch, massage, or warmth includes information for all caregivers and may be duplicated and given to the patient, family members, or friends.

For additional information about massage and for a teaching guide that can be duplicated and given to the patient/family, see Chapter 5, Cutaneous Stimulation, on superficial massage, and "Patient/Family Teaching Point: Massage of Body, Hands, or Feet," (see appendix).

Imagery

DEFINITION OF IMAGERY FOR PAIN RELIEF

Imagine not having pain. In a way, that is what imagery for pain relief is—the use of one's *imagination* to control pain. This involves mental images or internal representations. Imagining is a form of thinking that most people use rather regularly. It is commonly referred to as "trying to picture" something, visualizing, daydreaming, or fantasizing.

Imagery techniques for physical healing date back hundreds of years. Recently, imagery has been used in the treatment of medical conditions such as cancer, hypertension, acne, alcoholism, arthritis, and in the management of symptoms such as depression, anxiety, and nausea and vomiting, as well as pain related to cancer, backache, and headache.

The box below summarizes common uses of imagery or imagination in relation to pain.

Common Uses of Imagery or Imagination in Relation to Pain
1. Imagery may be used for *distraction* from pain, resulting in increased tolerance for pain.
2. Imagery may be used to produce *relaxation*, resulting in decreased distress associated with pain.
3. Imagery may be used to produce an image of pain relief, *resulting in a decrease in the perceived intensity of pain.*

Many structured pain-relief imagery techniques are preceded by a relaxation technique or involve a relaxing image. These imagery techniques may result in relaxation and distraction in addition to decreased pain. In other words, there may be considerable overlap between imagery techniques for pain relief, distraction from pain, and relaxation.

> **KEY POINT:** Caution! Are people saying any of the following about your patient's pain? "It's just his imagination." "It's all in her head." "It's psychogenic." "He just thinks he hurts; it isn't that bad." If so, this is not the chapter you need to read. Look up pp. 20–21 on misconceptions in Chapter 2 on assessment.

Imagery for the purpose of pain relief may be *defined* as using one's imagination to develop sensory images that decrease the intensity of pain or that become a pleasant, more acceptable, or nonpainful substitute for pain, e.g. numbness or coolness. In other words, imagery may act as an analgesic or anaesthetic. Images may vary from brief, such as those used in ordinary conversation, to lengthy, such as those developed systematically for the individual. The latter is often referred to as therapeutic guided imagery. The purpose is to use it for pain relief. The patient deliberately or purposefully imagines something about pain that will provide pain relief, rendering this activity therapeutic, or helpful. The nurse may assist the patient in doing this by guiding him/her through the use or development of an imagery technique.

BENEFITS AND LIMITS OF PAIN-RELIEF IMAGERY

The use of imagery for pain relief is based in part upon *two interrelated beliefs*:

1. Images may affect the functioning of the body in ways over which we ordinarily have little or no control. Mental images or representations may be a key to partial control over body functions that we do not usually consciously control by rational thoughts.
2. The body may react to images (or memories of an event) in a manner very similar to its functioning or response during the actual event. For example, even when a person remains physically inactive, imagining jumping can increase heart and respiratory rates or imagining bending the arm can result in minimal but measurable muscular activity. However, simply imagining watching rather than performing these activities may produce few if any effects. Likewise, trying to increase heart rate simply by desiring it to happen has little or no effect (Jacobsen, 1930; Jones and Johnson, 1980; Mast, 1986).

When conflict exists between imagination and the will, it has been said that imagination always wins. A simple example experienced by many people is the fear of speaking in front of a large audience. As you wait to give your speech you may find that your hands and knees are trembling and your heart is pounding. You may very much want to stop the trembling and pounding, but your will is not as strong as the threat or danger you imagine in relation to public speaking. Your imagination has won over your attempt to will your body to act in a different manner.

The potential benefits of imagery are perhaps best appreciated by seeing imagery in the context of a total situation. Imagery occurs naturally in relation to many everyday events as well as health-care situations. Imagery may be conceptualized as *occurring within a sequence of events*:

1. An object or event is sensed, e.g. seen, felt, or heard. Example: the patient feels back pain.
2. An emotional response to the event or objects occurs. Example: the patient is afraid the back pain

will not be relieved and will interfere with plans to go to work.
3. Plans or images such as a mental rehearsal are evoked, sometimes only for a split second. Example: the patient thinks about taking an analgesic that never works very well, imagines him/herself at home alone instead of going to work, and wonders how he/she will pay the rent that month.
4. The body responds, i.e. a physiological response occurs, such as increased heart rate and increased muscle tension. Example: the patient feels the back muscles tighten and the heart pounds.

The power of imagery is considered by some to be primarily the image's physiological effect on the body. For this reason, some view imagery as a potential self-healing technique. With regard to pain control, imagery may decrease pain by altering the physical cause of pain.

However, imagery may be beneficial without affecting the physiological aspects of pain, i.e. the cause of pain or the physiological response to it. Imagery may be used to render a painful sensation more acceptable, e.g. changing burning pain to a warm sensation. Imagery may also be beneficial without either altering the pain sensation or reducing the intensity of pain. Like relaxation, imagery may at times simply reduce the distress associated with pain.

Admittedly, the scientific basis of imagery is elusive, and health professionals are obliged to be cautious about what cannot be explained or understood. However, the professional literature refers to imagery as a useful technique that is within the realm of nursing practice. Not every nurse will feel comfortable helping patients with imagery, but every nurse can encourage and respect the use of it.

The following discussion of the specific, potential benefits and limitations or disadvantages for patients who use imagery to relieve pain is especially relevant to more involved imagery techniques. Subtle, conversational images may have some of the same benefits or limitations, but this use of imagery is initiated by the nurse, is brief, and should occur naturally. Hence, as long as these are positive images, there is little danger in using them, and the benefits may range from being great for a susceptible patient to being negligible for others.

Potential benefits of pain-relief imagery for the person with pain may include one or more of the following:

- Forms and strengthens a close, trusting nurse–patient relationship.
- Assists expression of feelings about pain and associated problems.
- Encourages exploration and understanding of personal beliefs about illness and may alter erroneous or harmful ideas about pain.
- Increases confidence in and ability to control or heal the painful experience. Imagery techniques tend to capitalize on the patient's strengths such as creativity and ability to concentrate. When imagery is successful, the patient may feel very proud.
- May increase the effectiveness of other pain-relief measures. For example, imagining increased warmth at an injection site may increase circulation to the area, cause faster absorption of an analgesic, and result in quicker onset of pain relief.
- Decreases intensity of pain or changes the pain sensation into one that is more acceptable.
- Dramatic and long-lasting pain relief from imagery has occurred in some patients. However, effectiveness remains highly unpredictable.

Possible limitations or disadvantages of pain-relieving imagery techniques are:

- The suggestion to try an imagery technique may be misinterpreted by the patient as meaning that the health-care team regards the pain as being imaginary or "not real".
- The successful use of imagery for pain relief may be misinterpreted by the health-care team as meaning that the pain is primarily imaginary or caused by psychological problems. Or, they may conclude the pain is not severe or significant if it can be controlled with a non-traditional method.

- Successful use of imagery is rarely a substitute for other appropriate pain-relief measures. In the majority of cases, imagery is only an adjunctive treatment for pain.
- Some patients and health-care team members inaccurately regard imagery as unscientific and may scoff at the nurse or patient who uses it. The possibility that imagery may effectively relieve pain may be contrary to their belief systems.
- Unwanted side effects may occur, especially with the longer, meditative imagery techniques (see Table 6.4). Some side effects may be similar to those that may occur with relaxation (see Table 6.2). Other side effects may be a result of the specific image, e.g. imagining cold may decrease the blood supply to an ischaemic area and contribute to increased pain.
- Imagery does not work for every patient with pain, even when the patient believes in its effectiveness and is highly motivated to use it.
- It may take time to find or develop an effective technique for the individual.
- Occasionally, the actual use or development of imagery is not only time-consuming for the nurse but also an emotionally exhausting experience.
- Imagery that focuses on the pain sensation may increase pain or distress.
- Unsuccessful use of imagery for pain relief may lead to feelings of failure in the patient.

IMAGERY TECHNIQUES FOR PAIN RELIEF

Numerous imagery techniques for pain relief have been developed and used successfully. However, in keeping with the purposes of this book, this chapter includes only selected examples that appear to be reasonably

KEY POINT: Possible Effect of Imagery:

Person feels pain.

Person responds emotionally, e.g., fear, helplessness.

Person responds physiologically, e.g., increased muscle tension.

*Person imagines what will happen, e.g., no relief, increasing pain.

* Imagery may interrupt the process here to change the image of what will happen, thereby changing the physiological response. A positive image may result in a helpful physiological response.

effective with appropriately chosen patients, are minimally time-consuming, low risk, and do not require knowledge or skills beyond those expected of the professional nurse with basic education.

Overview of types of imagery and indications for their use

There are four basic types of imagery. These are summarized and discussed in detail in Table 6.3.

Appropriate/inappropriate patients/situations

For subtle, conversational images and for some of the simple symptom substitution or release techniques, there are few restrictions or dangers. These may be used or suggested by the nurse in a casual manner that ensures that the patient will simply reject the idea if it is inappropriate. The more involved the development and use of imagery becomes, the more important are the following guidelines for selecting appropriate patients and situations and avoiding patients who are inappropriate.

Examples of *patients who may be appropriate candidates for use of the more involved imagery techniques for pain relief* include a child or adult who:

- Requests imagery or desires non-traditional approaches to health care (in addition to traditional methods).
- Has repeated contacts with the nurse over a long period, e.g. patients in long-term care facilities or home care.
- Understands the instructions.
- Is able to concentrate on the image.
- Has acute or chronic pain, especially a patient at the beginning of potentially long-term pain problems.
- Has artistic abilities, e.g. draws or paints pictures,

writes stories, or is an actor/actress.
- Uses imagery in conversation, reads a lot, or admits to or talks about daydreaming or intense concentration during an activity.
- Is a verbal child, especially between the ages 8 and 11 years.
- Has strong religious beliefs.
- Has used non-traditional health care, e.g. studied transcendental meditation, or attends yoga classes.

> **KEY POINT:** Imagery techniques for pain relief may be helpful to patients who have pain of clearly defined physical origin.

The nurse whose educational background is limited to basic preparation or who has not specialized in mental health, counselling, or psychotherapy should probably avoid using meditative, lengthy, or intense imagery with certain patients, mainly because of possible adverse effects therewith. However, health professionals who are specially trained in counselling or psychotherapy may be able to work with the following patients in the use of imagery. *Patients who may be inappropriate for the more involved or lengthy imagery techniques* are children or adults who:

- State they do not want to try imagery.
- Have severe emotional problems.
- Have a history of psychiatric illness.
- Report hallucinations for whatever reason, e.g. psychosis, drug reaction, or sensory restriction of ICU.
- Have no time or energy to devote to using lengthy imagery. Patients may use imagery for pain relief successfully for a while but finally become exhausted and unable to continue to use it.

Techniques	Possible Uses
1. Subtle, conversational.	1. Routine explanations of how pain-relief measures work or how and when recovery takes place.
2. Simple, brief symptom substitution.	2. Brief, painful experiences or procedures.
3. Standardized imagery techniques.	3. Brief or prolonged pain in a patient who wants to use imagery, but the nurse lacks time for or experience in development of individualized imagery techniques.
4. Systematically individualized imagery techniques.	4. Brief or prolonged pain in a patient who wants to use imagery, and the nurse has time for and experience in (or a willingness to attempt) development of imagery.

TABLE 6.3 Imagery Techniques and Indications for their Use to Relieve Pain.

- Cannot concentrate.
- Are or recently have been exposed to the unfortunate experience of health-team members discounting their pain or failing to provide appropriate and effective pain relief. An exception may be made if the nurse is absolutely positive that he/she has communicated to the patient that he/she believes what the patient says about the pain felt and wants to help the latter find relief in spite of what others say or do.

Sometimes the nurse's inappropriate attempt to get a patient to use imagery is related to well-meant but misguided enthusiasm. Be alert to your own motivation to have the patient try imagery for pain relief. Occasionally, the nurse's successful use of imagery for his/her own pain or with other patients will result in an overly optimistic view that imagery can be effective for almost anyone if he/she will only try it. The nurse should carefully monitor the personal motivation or purpose in suggesting imagery for pain relief to a patient. The following quotes from Steven Levine (1982) serve as helpful guidelines:

"This offering [imagery for pain relief] should not be accompanied by even the subtlest suggestion that if those in pain use these techniques they will be "doing the right thing", that if they accept your advice they are good and that if they don't they are weak.

As I offered this alternative, I watched closely for any quality in myself that wished her to be in any state other than the way she was, any desire that might in some subtle way motivate me to be "selling" her something that I imagined was best for her".

> **KEY POINT:** Imagery techniques for pain relief are merely *offered* to the patient as one way of dealing with pain. Never force or even strongly suggest imagery to a patient.

Nursing-care guidelines for developing and using imagery techniques

For the use or development of any type of pain-relief imagery, ranging from brief conversational to lengthy individualized techniques, the following are useful *general guidelines:*

1. If you feel uncomfortable or unsure about imagery techniques, avoid trying to help a patient with pain-relief imagery. If you think the patient is an appropriate candidate for imagery, try to find someone else to assist him/her. If this is not possible and if the patient has asked you for help with pain-relief imagery, admit your feelings but encourage him/her to try on his/her own.

2. Always acknowledge the reality of and your belief in what the patient says about the pain felt. Before you introduce imagery techniques for pain relief, try to be sure that the patient knows you believe that most or all of the cause of the pain is physical, and you believe what is said about the nature of the pain sensation.

3. If the patient discounts the pain in any way, e.g. suggests that maybe he/she is imagining the pain or must be mad to hurt when others can find no reason, tell the patient that you seriously doubt that he/she is mad or is imagining the pain.

4. Listen for and incorporate the patient's spontaneous use of images. Use the positive, helpful images, but try to rephrase negative, unhelpful images. For example, the patient may comment that it feels like the muscles in his/her back are in knots. If you later give a muscle relaxant, suggest that this will help untie those knots in the back muscles. Pain relief and/or recovery may be impeded if the patient maintains an image of the pain or an image that causes pain.

5. Images need not be anatomically or physiologically correct to be useful. For example, the patient may imagine that incisional pain is a red, hot, hard square that, as it begins to hurt less, becomes a pale pink, cool, soft circle. On the other hand, the next guideline is also important.

6. Consider the potential effect of an image if it is taken literally. Images may affect the functioning of the body. For example, avoid using anything patients are allergic to, e.g. picturing themselves in a field of wheat if they are allergic to wheat. Consider the effect of the image on circulation, e.g. warmth may increase peripheral circulation, whereas coolness may decrease it. Therefore, if a sensation of cold is suggested in the imagery, consider whether or not applications of cold would be contra-indicated for a particular patient. Another example of the need for caution might be the patient who has a cardiac condition that requires complete bed rest and reduced oxygen needs. Heart and respiratory rate may increase if an image is used that involves imagining running as fast as possible to escape pain.

7. Consider using the patient's religious or spiritual beliefs or practices, if any. Many religious writings and practices involve imagery that can be helpful in relieving pain.

8. Consider using the patient's artistic ability and interest, if any, e.g. drawing or painting pictures. For example, musicians or painters may more easily relate to or create auditory or visual images, respectively. Perhaps a connoisseur of fine wines would relate best to the taste or smell of pain.

9. Use the individual patient's preferences, if any, for sensory descriptors. The person may use several sensory modalities when describing pain, but one modality may be predominant or specific words may be used repeatedly. For example, the patient may describe pain using mainly visual descriptions such as the colour, size, and shape of the pain. "Screaming" pain is an example of an auditory description. "Bitter" pain is related to the gustatory (taste) and olfactory (smell) senses. "Writhing", "fast", and "crawling" are kinesthetic (movement) descriptions; "rough", "burning", and "hard" are tactile (touch) descriptions.

10. Stress to the patient the importance of developing personal images and that they may be either vague or clear. When standardized images or systematically individualized images are used, examples of what others have done may be helpful, but avoid giving the patient specific images of his/her own pain sensation or methods of pain relief. However, to help patients develop their own images, offer to answer any questions they have about their pain and methods of relief.

11. Try to focus more attention on soothing and positive descriptions of pain than on the word pain or on disturbing aspects of the pain. For example, rather than limiting your remarks to saying that pain in the legs is getting less and less, it may be more effective to focus more on the leg becoming more comfortable and relaxed with accompanying soft, smooth, healing sensations.

12. If the patient has difficulty imagining a method of relieving pain, use imagery involving the desired result or state. Images may be either or both of the following:

    a. *Process image*, a method of achieving the desired result, e.g. imagining how the pain is relieved.

This usually involves focusing on the pain and the pain relief measure. Not all patients can imagine this. Further, a focus on pain may increase pain.

    b. *Final state image*, a representation of the desired state, e.g. the body without pain. The dying patient may remember his/her body without pain or imagine the effective result of a pain-relief measure. A recovering patient may imagine his/her body at a future time, relieved of pain by some pain relief measure, or healed and without pain. The patient need not focus on the pain nor have any idea of how the process of healing or pain relief will take place.

13. Use permissive directions and suggestions when you discuss or guide imagery. Simply offer the image rather than force it upon the patient. Use words and phrases such as "Perhaps...", "If you wish you may...", or "You might like to...".

14. If the patient seems easily frustrated or overly anxious to succeed, suggest that he/she sneaks up on the image instead of trying to imagine it immediately. For example, a relaxation technique prior to the image may help the patient calm down and concentrate better. Or, if he/she has chosen to achieve warmth by imagining him- herself sunbathing at the beach, suggest starting by imagining getting ready to go to the beach. Another method is to work with an image over time. The patient may imagine the pain felt as a red-hot poker and want to try to relieve it by imagining a stream of cool water flowing over it. The patient might practice this two or three times a day for days, starting with a small trickle of warm water that gradually becomes a cooler and larger stream.

15. Provide additional pain relief if needed, e.g. an analgesic in addition to imagery.

16. When imagery effectively relieves pain, be sure the patient is also assessed and treated appropriately for the underlying cause of the pain.

17. Inform others (health-care team, family) of what the patient is doing, when, and why. This may decrease the patient's self-consciousness about doing something different, avoid ridicule from those who do not appreciate the potential value of imagery, and minimize disruptions when the patient uses the technique. Others may also help by reminding the patient to use imagery for pain relief, especially

preventively. But, *caution others not to suggest imagery as a substitute for appropriate pain-relief measures.*

18. Be alert to problems that may result from the use of pain-relief imagery and their possible solutions, summarized in Table 6.4 (see also problems related to relaxation, Table 6.2).

Subtle, conversational imagery

Subtle imagery may be contained in the nurse's usual statements and questions to the patient. This need not take any additional time if images are already a natural part of the nurse's thinking and conversation. Many

Problems	Possible Solutions
1. Reports problems with working out the logic of the specific imagery, e.g. unable to work out how to move healing energy in or out of a certain area.	1. The patient may observe some rules of logic when using the imagination. Offer to listen and try to help solve the problem. If this fails to help, remind the patient that anything is possible in one's imagination. If the patient continues to dwell on the problem, gently explain that this is not achieving the desired goal of pain relief and suggest that he/she try another imagery technique or stop using imagery.
2. Increased pain.	2. Most likely to occur if a process image is used because of focus on pain. Try changing the image of how pain is relieved. If this fails, suggest switching to a final state image, i.e. focus on a pain-free image from the past or future, not on the pain sensation and how it will be relieved.
3. Increased distress, e.g. anxiety, depression, withdrawal..	3. Suggest that the patient tries an entirely different image, explaining that sometimes a person chooses what he/she thinks is a pleasant or desirable image but which may contain unidentifiable sources of conflict or emotional disturbance.
4. Feels drowsy, sluggish, or tired afterwards.	4. The patient may simply be fatigued and need more sleep or rest. Or, try shortening length of imagery technique. Add a technique that slowly ends the imagery with suggestions of being rested and alert, e.g. count slowly from 1 to 5 while feeling more alert and beginning slight body movements, starting at the feet and progressing up to the head.
5. Fear that imagery will be so effective that it will eliminate pain as a useful warning signal, i.e. fear that bodily harm will occur without his/her awareness.	5. Be sure imagery is not being forced on this patient. If the patient does want to use imagery, explain that it can be restricted to a specific area or pain, that the patient may retain some of the pain if so wished, and that numbness rarely results and can be deliberately avoided.
6. Very difficult to arouse following imagery.	6. This is rare if imagery is used with the patient's full consent and the patient has been fully informed of the content of the imagery technique, especially if he/she has participated in developing the imagery. This is most likely to occur when imagery is guided by someone. The patient usually will spontaneously become aroused within a short time, e.g. may go to sleep and awaken refreshed. To arouse sooner, try asking the patient, "Why don't you want to be fully awake?" Then deal with the answer. If the patient says he/she is sleepy, suggest awakening now and to plan to sleep later, giving a specific and appropriate time. When the patient is alert again, gently explain that drowsiness could be bothersome and that it is best if you do not conduct this imagery again. The patient may be able to conduct imagery on his/her own without extreme drowsiness, or drowsiness may be an indication of a severe, underlying mental or emotional disturbance.
NOTE: If any of the above problems are not easily resolved, gently explain to the patient the need to stop using imagery and consider a consultation from a professional therapist.	

TABLE 6.4 Imagery for Pain Relief: Possible Problems and Solutions.

nurses already automatically use images in their routine discussions with patients, e.g. patient teaching or discharge planning.

To develop your ability to use images more naturally in conversation with patients for the purpose of assisting with pain relief, *specific guidelines* are:

1. Identify a specific pain-relief measure and try to explain how it relieves pain by using words that paint a mental picture or create sounds or tactile–kinesthetic feelings.

Example: When you administer an analgesic you might say, "Now it's as if the medication is slowly

IMMEDIATE HELP FOR IMAGERY

Time involved: Reading time, 5 minutes; implementation time, 10 minutes.

Sample situation: Patient is in pain and probably will continue to be for about 30–45 minutes while you and/or others are trying to do something more to relieve the pain, e.g. obtain appropriate analgesic prescriptions.

Possible solution: Patient may be willing to try a simple type of imagery or use personal spiritual beliefs.

Expected outcome: Patient will feel that the pain is acknowledged and someone cares. He/she finds the sensation of pain is relieved by becoming less intense or by changing to a more acceptable sensation. Or, he/she merely finds the pain more tolerable because the imagery distracts him/her momentarily. The patient may note a feeling of less anxiety.

Do's

1. Take a deep breath outside the patient's room and relax a little yourself. Plan on spending up to 10 minutes with the patient. You are about to discuss something the patient may find strange; you need to be relaxed and confident.

2. When you enter the room tell the patient you know he/she hurts. Be certain that you have assured the patient that you consider the pain real, not imaginary, and that you believe it is just as intense as is claimed.

3. Tell the patient you are still hoping (searching) for a better alternative, but that meanwhile you would like to *offer* the opportunity to try a technique that may ease the pain for just a little while.

4. Explain that you are going to describe a method of using concentration and imagination to help with pain for a brief time. Tell the patient that this may sound strange and he/she may not want to try it. If so, that is perfectly acceptable, but you want to offer it just in case it turns out to be something he/she wants to try and finds helpful.

5. Ask the patient if he/she daydreams or has a good imagination, or if prayer or any kind of faith helps with pain or illness.

If a negative reply is given, say the patient may be better at it than is thought. Ask if he/she remembers a bedroom from his/her childhood (progress to any bedroom he/she remembers). Ask how many windows it had and how many doors. If the patient can answer with confidence, point out that this is a result of

memories that are mental pictures of some sort and not a result of storing numerical information. It is one example of how people who do not even have vivid mental pictures still use their imagination, e.g. images from the past. If the patient cannot answer these questions, admit that you might be wrong about the appropriateness of this method. Ask if he/she wants you to continue. If so, try either of the following.

If the patient gives a positive reply to daydreaming or a good imagination, use simple symptom substitution (p. 188), stressing that you are hoping that this will at least reduce unpleasant aspects of the pain for a short time. If the patient cannot concentrate well, try providing another sensation, e.g. cold, to focus on.

If he/she gives a positive reply to some type of faith, use the *Ball of Healing Energy*, suggesting that he/she substitutes personal faith for the healing energy and that this may reduce the pain.

6. Tell the patient you will return to find out if he/she decided to try this and if it helped. Tell the patient when you will return, but give yourself leeway. It's better to return early than late.

7. When you return, ask the patient what was decided about the imagery.

If the patient says he/she did not try the imagery, say that you appreciate it being considered.

If it did not work, tell the patient you admire willingness to try the technique, reassuring him/her that it does not always work.

If it did help, tell the patient you do not expect him/her to rely on it as the only source of pain relief.

8. In all cases, continue to explore and explain other plans for pain relief.

Don'ts

1. Do not expect or suggest that imagery will substitute for appropriate pain relief, e.g. adequate analgesic orders.

2. Do not attempt to present imagery for pain relief if you feel unsure or uncomfortable about it. *Or,* admit these feelings before you proceed, and explain why you think it's worth a try.

3. Do not say there is nothing else anyone can do.

4. Do not tell the patient that he/she must learn to cope with pain on his/her own. (The patient may learn to do this, but not in 10 minutes.)

5. Never tell the patient the pain is not as bad as is claimed.

floating through your body to find your pain and make it smaller and smaller, leaving feelings of comfort and healing."

2. Use words and phrases that tend to convey relaxing, pain-relieving images.

   Examples:

   - Floating
   - Smaller
   - Softer
   - Melting
   - Dissolving
   - Smooth
   - Lighter
   - Quieting
   - Releasing
   - Slowly leaving
   - Healing
   - Cool or warm
   - Letting go
   - Soothing
   - Less and less
   - Loosening

   Notice when you use these words naturally. Practice using them more often in relation to pain relief.

3. Notice when a patient is given an image of what is causing the pain, and try to make sure he/she is also given an image of how the pain will subside or be relieved.

   Example: The doctor may explain how he/she will make an incision in a certain place and remove or repair something internally. The nurse may then add one or more of the following:

   - Afterwards a soft comfortable dressing will be in place.
   - A well-wrapped, lightweight cold pack may be placed over the area to make it feel soothingly cool.
   - Medication (narcotic) will help the brain feel fewer nerve impulses from the area.
   - Another medication (non-narcotic) will go to the area to help soothe any swelling or irritation.
   - As you rest and take in nutrients the area will begin repairing and healing itself.
   - Within a week (or whatever period of time is reasonable) you will feel healed and healthy again.

4. Use only those images or descriptors that feel natural to you. You need to be at ease and comfortable with what you describe to the patient.

Simple, brief symptom substitution

Helping a patient develop an image that substitutes a more acceptable sensation, or perhaps a pleasant sensation, for pain for a brief period of pain, need not take much of the nurse's time. *Specific guidelines* are:

1. When pain is known to the patient because it is present or an impending painful procedure has been experienced before, the nurse's conversation with the patient may include the following:

   - Ask the patient, "How would you describe this pain?"
   - Note any words that seem more acceptable or less uncomfortable than the actual sensation, such as stinging versus knifelike. Suggest "Perhaps it would help if you try focusing on just that feeling and try to ignore the total discomfort for a little while." Or the nurse could say "You might try pretending for a little while that this is what is happening instead of the actual discomfort."

2. When pain is anticipated but not previously experienced by the patient, the nurse may describe what the sensation usually feels like to other patients, being careful to use descriptive words that are not necessarily unpleasant or very bothersome sensations.

   Examples of what the nurse might say:

   - If burning pain is typical, suggest to the patient "This procedure may hurt less (or be less troublesome) if you concentrate on or try to imagine the pain as being simply warm instead of burning. Maybe you can imagine the sun shining on you and warming the area."
   - If a procedure involves cleansing with an antiseptic, suggest to the patient "When you feel the cool sensation of the area being cleaned, try to focus on that coolness and try to ignore some of the other more uncomfortable sensations."

3. For any type of brief pain, known or unknown to the patient, the nurse may try to help the patient substitute a sensation by actually providing a separate sensation for the patient to focus on. The nurse may say "I can give you a cube of ice to hold in your hand and you can try for a while to concentrate on the extreme cold rather than the discomfort in the rest of your body. You may even try to imagine the numbness in your hand transferring to numbness in the areas that hurt."

> **KEY POINT:** Suggestions for symptom substitution are probably best used for brief pain (a matter of minutes, not hours) and should merely be offered to the patient as possible alternatives.

The remainder of the pain-relief images are more time consuming. The specific images and some overall considerations are explained in the patient/family teaching points (Appendix). They are suitable for copying and giving to the patient. It may be appropriate to offer to tape record these lengthier images for the patient. If so, and if your time is limited, you may wish to consider the three-part time plan, as suggested in the box on p. 176 for taping relaxation techniques.

Patient/family teaching points for general use of imagery for pain relief

This chapter includes two types of imagery for pain relief that require at least a moderate amount of patient involvement: (1) standardized imagery and (2) systematic, individualized imagery. These techniques may be used in a concentrated manner for several minutes or more. The patient is asked to consider the content, approve or disapprove of what is included, and perhaps suggest specific content. The patient may also devote time to practising the imagery or may use it fairly often.

For the above types of imagery, the patient/family teaching point Using Imagery for Pain Relief may be used. If the patient is able to read, it may be duplicated and given to the patient.

Comparison of hypnosis and imagery

Some patients will ask about possible similarities between imagery and hypnosis, either because of unfounded fears of hypnosis or because of a desire to try hypnosis. In either case, the nurse needs to provide accurate, reassuring information:

- Hypnosis is a broad concept and has been used for numerous purposes. Therapy with hypnosis (hypnotherapy) involves the use of many techniques, one of which is imagery.
- There is no single, accepted definition of hypnosis. However, it is generally believed that all hypnosis is self-hypnosis (sometimes directed by another person, e.g. psychologist) and that hypnotic thinking is a state of alertness and intense concentration, very similar to normal, everyday thinking. Concentration is not only intense but also narrowly focused with

diminished peripheral awareness. Hypnosis is not loss of consciousness nor is it mind-control initiated by someone else.

Patient/family teaching points for specific images for pain relief

The specific imagery techniques for pain relief covered in this section are presented in a sequence that roughly approximates the amount of time usually required for the nurse to teach the patient and for the patient to perform or learn the technique. The least time-consuming techniques are presented first.

The more experience and knowledge the nurse has about imagery and the more time can be devoted to individualizing the technique for the patient, probably the better the outcome. However, some of the standardized techniques are permissive and vague enough that the patient may interpret or individualize them as he/she listens. Further, although research evidence is lacking, clinical experience has demonstrated that the standardized techniques selected for this chapter have a reasonable success rate.

The directions for each imagery technique are stated in the patient/family teaching points in the exact words the nurse might say to the patient and family. Following are four image techniques. Three are standardized images for pain relief: (1) *Emptying the Sandbag,* (2) *Breathing Out Pain, and* (3) *Ball of Healing Energy* (Levine, 1982). The fourth technique is comprised of questions and suggestions for helping a patient create highly individualized imagery for pain and its relief using Imagery for Pain Relief (Appendix). If the patient is able to read, the directions for any of these techniques may be duplicated and given to the patient.

If you talk to guide the patient through the technique or if you tape record it for the patient, speak slowly and quietly in a monotone, pausing at regular intervals. Usually there is a pause at the end of each sentence, between paragraphs, and wherever you see "..." within a script.

If you are teaching a standardized pain-relief image to a group of patients, use the phrase "area of discomfort" instead of the specific body part that hurts—unless they all have pain in the same area.

INDIVIDUALIZED NURSING-CARE PLAN

Patient Who May Benefit from a Pain-Relief Imagery Technique

Patient Description: Ms M., 23 years old, is 8 months pregnant with her first child. Over the last 6 weeks she has experienced increasing low back pain of mild to moderate intensity with the most discomfort in the evening and at bedtime. Daily physical exercises plus a cold pack for 30 minutes several times a day have reduced her pain during the day, but she has requested additional assistance with pain relief due to difficulty sleeping at night. She wants to avoid medications because of their potential harm to her unborn child.

Assessment	Potential Nursing Problems	Planning/Intervention	Evaluation/Expected Outcomes
Identify: • Interests/abilities in art, non-traditional health care, religion. • Ability to understand directions and concentrate. • Mental picture or image of pain. • Use of sensory descriptors of pain and non-painful terms. • History of emotional or psychiatric disorders.	Pain, related to strain on back muscles. Sleep pattern disturbance related to low back pain. Knowledge deficit related to non-pharmacological methods of pain relief.	Emphasize belief in patient's statements about pain and in the cause of pain being related to muscle strain. Describe the benefits, limits, and types of imagery techniques available. Help patient choose imagery technique, explaining difference between final state and process images. Help the patient develop own pain relief imagery by using the Patient/Family Teaching Point: using Imagery for Pain Relief (Appendix) and include the following: • Use permissive directions and suggestions. • Offer to answer any questions patient may have about imagery or the cause and relief of pain. • Emphasize need for patient to develop own image, using memories of actual experiences if possible, and focusing on one image rather than several. • Explain that images need not be "medically correct" or vivid. • Incorporate patient's spontaneous use of positive images or non-painful descriptions of pain or its relief, as well as any spiritual aspects desired by patient. • Consider potential effect of images if taken literally. • Suggest use of a brief relaxation technique prior to imagery. • Offer to provide written instructions and/or tape recording of technique. Encourage patient to use imagery early before pain becomes severe. Suggest patient selects one brief part of the imagery technique to focus on if she awakens during night or is bothered by pain while busy during day. Suggest simultaneous use of other pain-relief measures, e.g. positioning, cold pack. Plan a time during the next 3 days to check with patient regarding effects of imagery, and ask if any problems occurred. Plan regular follow-up to assess continuing effects of imagery and any changes in pain.	Patient reports one or more of the following: • Decreased intensity of pain. • Pain sensation becomes a different and more tolerable sensation. • Improved sleep, e.g. gets to sleep quicker, able to fall asleep readily if awakened, feels more rested in the mornings. • Pride or increased confidence in ability to handle discomfort. If patient reports problems with imagery and suggested solutions are not effective, gently explain that the technique does not always work no matter how hard one tries and that it should be discontinued while other pain-relief measures are explored. Obtain appropriate consultation, if needed.

SELECTED ANNOTATED REFERENCES THAT CITE RESEARCH OR GIVE CLINICAL SUPPORT

Distraction

Many of the noninvasive pain-relief measures, such as distraction, have not yet been adequately researched. This sometimes makes it difficult to document or justify the use of these techniques. The following brief, annotated list provides some clinical or research support for use of distraction as discussed in this chapter:

Clum, GA, Luscomb, RL, and Scott, L: Relaxation training and cognitive redirection strategies in the treatment of acute pain, *Pain* **12**:175–183, 1982. Cognitive redirection, consisting of focusing on pleasant images, during laboratory infliction of ischaemic pain significantly reduced the perception of pain, whereas relaxation training did not.

Cogan, R, Cogan, D, Waltz, W, and McCue, M: Effects of laughter and relaxation on discomfort thresholds, *J Behav Med* **10**: 139–144, Apr 1987. Two experiments were conducted in a laboratory setting using human subjects to measure pressure induced discomfort thresholds before and 10 minutes after listening to 20-minute long audio tapes. The first experiment compared effects of laughter-inducing, relaxation-inducing or dull-narrative audio tape, and of no tape. Discomfort thresholds were higher for the laughter and relaxation tapes. The second experiment compared effects of laughter-inducing, interesting narrative, or uninteresting narrative audio tapes, completed multiplication tasks, or no intervention. This showed that only laughter significantly increased discomfort thresholds. In conclusion, it appears that laughter is more effective than other types of distraction and that the effects continue for at least 10 minutes after the laughter subsides.

Dalton, JA: Education for pain management: a pilot study, *Pat Educ Counsel* **9**:155–165, 1987. An experimental study of cancer patients taught to use distraction, massage, and relaxation showed the greatest behavioural change was in the use of distraction. The distraction technique taught was almost identical to "Active Listening to Recorded Music" on p. 177 of this chapter.

Eland, J: Personal communication, University of Iowa, Iowa City, Iowa, 11 Feb, 1987. Use of patient-selected music via headset, similar to "Active Listening to Recorded Music" on p. 177 of this chapter, in 94 patients from paediatric, oncology, and burn units for brief, painful procedures such as bone marrow aspiration, was found helpful by all patients. Only one patient refused to try it.

Fritz, DJ: Noninvasive pain control methods used by cancer outpatients, *Oncol Nurs Forum* (suppl) p 108, 1988 (abstract). An itemized questionnaire about self-initiated, noninvasive pain control measures was administered to 53 oncology out-patients. Patients rated laughter as the most effective of these measures in relieving pain.

Schultz, DP: Sensory restriction: effects on behavior, Academic Press, New York, 1965. Presents findings of many studies regarding the effects of boredom on pain, e.g. boredom increasing attention to pain, and studies that show the critical importance of physical exercise in reducing the effects of boredom.

Scott, DS, and Barber, TX: Cognitive control of pain: effects of multiple cognitive strategies, *Psychol Rec* **2**:373-383, 1977. Very brief instructions, including examples of distractions, raised average pain tolerance 100% in a group of laboratory subjects. Pain intensity, however, did not change. They concluded it was much easier to change tolerance of pain than to change perception of pain.

Relaxation

Many of the noninvasive pain-relief measures, such as relaxation, have not yet been adequately researched. This sometimes makes it difficult to document or justify the use of these techniques. The following brief, annotated list provides some clinical or research support for use of relaxation as discussed in this chapter.

American Nurses' Association. For statements on generic and specialty nursing practice, including use of relaxation and suggestive therapies, write: ANA, 2420 Pershing Rd, Kansas City, MO 64108.

Bruya, MA, and Stevertsen, B: Evaluating the effects of music on electroencephalogram patterns of normal subjects, *J Neurosurg Nurs* **16**:96–100, Apr 1984. Electroencephalogram (EEG) responses of 47 adult volunteers were compared while they listened to music by Chopin and by the new age composer Steven Halpern. Brain-wave activity did not support the claim that Halpern's music puts subjects into a state of relaxed, alert consciousness. The study raised many questions and no conclusions were possible. However, some subjects said that they found Halpern's music disturbing and irritating.

Ceccio, CM: Postoperative pain relief through relaxation in elderly patients with fractured hips, *Orthopaed Nurs* **3**:11–19, May–June 1984. Patients aged 56–89 years were taught jaw relaxation prior to surgical repair of fractures and compared to a control group that was not taught relaxation. Pain and distress scores after the painful activity of turning during which the experimental subjects used jaw relaxation showed significantly lower pain and distress compared to the control group. Overall intake of analgesics was also lower. Other studies (e.g. Flaherty and Fitzpatrick, 1978) have also demonstrated that relaxation taught preoperatively can reduce pain and analgesic intake postoperatively.

Cleeland, CS: Nonpharmacological management of cancer pain, *J Pain Sympt Manag* **2**:S23–S28, Spring 1987. This overview emphasizes that relaxation is never a substitute for other appropriate therapies such as analgesics for the patient with cancer; it is most clearly indicated for patients without significant prior psychiatric history. Successful use of relaxation should never be misunderstood as indicative of the pain being psychogenic.

Clum, GA, Luscomb, RL, and Scott, L: Relaxation training and cognitive redirection strategies in the treatment of acute pain, *Pain* **12**:175–183, 1982. A laboratory study using ischaemic pain showed that relaxation training appears to reduce distress attendant upon experiencing pain, but does not reduce pain perception during the actual infliction of pain.

Graffam, S, and Johnson, A: A comparison of two relaxation strategies for the relief of pain and its distress, *J Pain Sympt Manag* **2**:229–231, Fall 1987. This study compared the effectiveness of taped transcripts of guided imagery and progressive muscle relaxation in 30 oncology patients. The patients' pain and distress ratings before and after listening to each tape showed that both strategies were equally effective in reducing pain and distress. However, most patients preferred the progressive muscle relaxation technique, some saying it was difficult for them to clear their minds to visualize the peaceful scene described in the guided imagery tape. Although the authors did not mention this, it seems possible from the patients' comments that the progressive muscle relaxation may have served as a distractor from pain. Thus distraction, either instead of or in addition to relaxation, may have produced pain relief.

Horowitz, BF, Fitzpatrick, JJ, and Flaherty, GG: Relaxation techniques for pain relief after open heart surgery, *Dimens Crit Care Nurs* **3**:364–371, Nov–Dec 1984. This study compared the effects of jaw relaxation with those of generalized passive relaxation in patients following open heart surgery. Generalized passive relaxation was more effective than jaw relaxation, significantly reducing distress postambulation. There was no apparent effect on pain sensation in either group. Both techniques apparently were effective to some extent, e.g. both reduced systolic blood pressure on postambulation.

Kulich, RJ, and Warfield, CA: Relaxation in the management of pain, *Hosp Pract* **20**:117–121, Dec 15, 1985. This excellent overview of benefits of relaxation training for chronic non-malignant pain emphasizes relaxation, not as pain relief but as adjunctive treatment and only as partial rather than perfect control. It gives specific ideas about teaching relaxation, including contraindications and problems.

Lapp, JE: Music vs. biofeedback for migraine headache, unpublished paper, Calif. State Univ., Fresno, Calif., 1986. Patients with migraine who were taught relaxation and imagery skills and listened to self-selected, non-lyric, "easy-listening" music reported significantly fewer and less intense migraine headaches 1 year later than did those who used biofeedback instead of music. This difference was probably due to the fact that the music group practised significantly more, stating that music heard randomly throughout the day served as a stimulus to practice.

Mast, D, Meyer, J, and Urbanski, A: Relaxation techniques: a self-learning module for nurses: Unit III, *Cancer Nurs* **10**:279–285, 1987. This article includes specific instructions for teaching the patient deep breathing, passive muscle relaxation, and relaxing imagery. An example of a relaxation log is included.

Mogan, J, Wells, N, and Robertson, E: Effects of preoperative teaching on postoperative pain: a replication and expansion, *Int J Nurs Stud* **22**:267–280, 1985. Preoperatively one group of patients was taught a relaxation technique consisting of rhythmic breathing, pleasant imagery, and generalized muscle relaxation. Equal time was spent with a control group. Following elective abdominal surgery, the group taught relaxation reported less distress caused by the pain, but the pain sensation itself did not seem to be affected.

Peveler, RC, and Johnston, DW: Subjective and cognitive effects of relaxation, *Behav Res Ther* **24**:413–419, 1986. This study shows that passive muscular relaxation with pleasant mental imagery and meditation was as effective as simple information when both were conducted by a therapist, but that in solo practice relaxation was much more effective. Based on this study and a review of the literature, the suggestion is made that regular practice of relaxation can make adaptive thoughts more accessible, i.e. if relaxation improves mood, there may be greater likelihood that positive, helpful thoughts will emerge. It is noted that the beneficial effects of relaxation persist well beyond the period of practise of the technique.

Turner, JA, and Chapman, CR: Psychological interventions for chronic pain: a critical review. I. Relaxation training and biofeedback, *Pain* **12**:1–21, 1982. Based on this extensive review of the literature up to 1981, the authors conclude that the efficacy of relaxation techniques has only been shown for headache and to some extent for temporo-mandibular joint pain. They also find that evidence to date indicates that biofeedback is not more effective than relaxation training for headaches. They suggest that relaxation could be a valuable therapeutic tool for patients with chronic non-malignant pain if it is taught as a coping skill to assist in learning better ways of responding to life stresses that trigger or exacerbate pain. A later review (Turner and Romano, 1984) arrived at the same conclusions. An even more recent review (Roberts, 1987) again concluded that biofeedback has not been shown to be essential or to be superior to other treatments for chronic pain and may even exacerbate pain in some patients.

Imagery

Many of the noninvasive pain-relief measures, such as imagery, have not yet been adequately researched. This sometimes makes it difficult to document or justify the use of these techniques. The following brief, annotated list provides some clinical or research support for the use of imagery for pain relief, as discussed in this chapter.

Barber, TX, Chauncey, HH, and Winer, RA: Effect of hypnotic and nonhypnotic suggestions on parotid gland response to gustatory stimuli, *Psychosom Med* **26:**374–380, 1964. This study suggests that an image may exert more control over physiologic response than does the actual stimulus. When subjects were told to imagine that water applied to their tongues was sour, measures of saliva showed a significant increase. When subjects were asked to imagine that citric acid applied to their tongues was tasteless, measures of salivation showed a decrease as compared to salivation during baseline treatment with citric acid.

Burish, TG, and Lyles, JN: Effects of relaxation training in reducing adverse reactions to cancer chemotherapy, *J Behav Med* **4:**65–78, 1981. This study suggests that relaxing imagery can decrease distress without changing the physiological response. Experimental subjects who engaged in therapist-guided relaxation and imagery showed significantly lower systolic blood pressure and reported significantly lower anger, anxiety, and nausea before and after chemotherapy than the control subjects. However, there was no difference in the frequency of vomiting in the two groups.

Harano, K, Ogawa, K, and Naruse, G: A study of plethysmography and skin temperature during active concentration and autogenic exercise. In Luthe, W, ed: *Autogenic training*, pp 55–58, Grune & Stratton, New York, 1965. This study suggests the superiority of imagination over will or desire. Each subject was asked to focus on the idea of his/her arms being warm and repeat to him-herself "My arms are warm". This thinking and imagining resulted in the sensation of warmth, an increase in surface temperature, and an increase in blood volume in the arm. However, these changes did not occur when the subject tried to raise the temperature without thinking or imagining that the arm was warm.

REFERENCES AND SELECTED READINGS

Distraction

Blitz, B, and Lowenthal, M: The role of sensory restriction in problems with chronic pain, *J Chronic Dis* **19:**1119–1125, Nov–Dec 1966

Brody, R: Music medicine, *Omni* **6:**24, 110, 1984

Chaves, JF, and Barber, TX: Cognitive strategies, experimenter modeling, and expectation in the attenuation of pain, *J Abnorm Psychol* **83:**356–363, 1974

Cook, JD: Music as an intervention in the oncology setting, *Cancer Nurs* **9:**23–28, Feb 1986

Cousins, N: Anatomy of an illness (as perceived by the patient), *N Engl J Med* **295:**1458–1463, Dec 23, 1976

Davis-Rollans, C, and Cunningham, SG: Physiologic responses of coronary care patients to selected music, *Heart Lung* **16:** 370–378, July 1987

Dolan, MB: A drug you can't overuse, *RN* **48:**47–48, Nov 1985

Glynn, NJ: The therapy of music, *J Gerontol Nurs* **12:**6–10, Jan 1986

Hanswer, M, Larson, SC, and O'Connell, AS: Music therapy-assisted labor: effects on relaxation of expectant mothers, *Birth Psychol Bull* **4:**2, 1983

Herman, EP: Music therapy in depression. In Podalsky, E, ed: Music therapy, Philosophical Library, New York, 1954.

Herth, I: The therapeutic use of music, *Supervisor Nurse* **9:**22–23, 1978

Isen, AM, Daubman, KA, and Nowicki, GP: Positive affect facilitates creative problem solving, *J Pers Soc Psychol* **52:**1122–1131, 1987

Jacob, S: Bring on the music, *Am J Nurs* **86:**1034, Sept 1986

Lavine, R, Buchsbaum, MS, and Poncy, M: Auditory analgesia: somatosensory evoked response and subjective pain rating, *Psychophysiology* **13:**140–148, 1976

Locsin, R: The effect of music on the pain of selected postoperative patients *J Adv Nurs* **6:**19–25, 1981

McCaffery, M: *Nursing management of the patient with pain*, ed 2, pp 89–116, JB Lippincott, Philadelphia, 1979.

McCaffery, M: Relieving pain with noninvasive techniques, *Nursing* **10:**55–57, Dec 1980

McClelland, DC: Music in the operating room, *ARON J 1979* **29:**252–260, 1979

Melzack, R: Pain perception, *Percept Disord* **48:**272–285, 1970

Melzack, R, Weisz, AZ, and Sprague, LT: Strategies for controlling pain: contributions of auditory stimulation and suggestion, *Exp Neurol* **8**:239–247, 1963

OR patients tune in as they tune out, *RN:***12,** Jan 1987

Osterlund, H: Humor: a serious approach to patient care, *Nursing* **13**:46–47, 1983

Raber, WC: The caring role of the nurse in the application of humor therapy to the patient experiencing helplessness, *Clin Gerontol* **7**:3–11, Fall 1987

Ruxton, JP, and Hester, M: Humor: assessment and interventions, *Clin Gerontol* **7**:13–21, Fall 1987

Scott, DS, and Barber, TX: Cognitive control of pain: four serendipitous results, *Percept Mot Skills* **44**:569–570, 1977

Snyder, M: Independent nursing interventions, John Wiley & Sons, New York, 1985.

Wiener, CL: Pain assessment on an orthopedic ward, *Nurs Outlook* **23**:508–516, Aug 1975

Ziporyn, T: Music therapy accompanies medical care, *JAMA* **252**:986–987, 1984

Relaxation

Bailey, LM: Music therapy in pain management, *J Pain Sympt Manag* **1**:25–28, Winter 1986

Barsevick, A, and Llewellyn, J: A comparison of the anxiety-reducing potential of two techniques of bathing, *Nurs Res* **31**:22, 1982

Bayuk, L: Relaxation techniques: an adjunct therapy for cancer patients, *Semin Oncol Nurs* **1**:147–150, 1985

Benson, H: *The relaxation response.* William Morrow, New York, 1975.

Benson, H: *Beyond the relaxation response.* Times Books, New York, 1984.

Blanchard, EB, Andrasik, F, Evans, DD, and Hillhouse, J: Biofeedback and relaxation treatments for headache in the elderly: a caution and a challenge, *Biofeedback Self-Regul* **10**:69–73, Mar 1985

Bresler, DE: *Free yourself from pain.* Simon and Schuster, New York, 1979.

Brown, BB: *Stress and the art of biofeedback,* Bantam Books, 1978, New York.

Cogan, R, Cogan, D, Waltz, W, and McCue, M: Effects of laughter and relaxation on discomfort thresholds, *J Behav Med* **10**: 139–144, 1987

Copp, LA: The spectrum of suffering, *Am J Nurs* **74**:491—495, Mar 1974

Davis-Rollans, C, and Cunningham, S: Physiologic responses of coronary care patients to selected music, *Heart Lung* **16**:370, July 1987

DiMotto, JW: Relaxation, *Am J Nurs* **84**:754–758, June 1984

Donovan, MI: Relaxation with guided imagery. In Donovan, MI, ed: *Cancer care: a guide for patient education,* pp 242–256, Appleton-Century-Crofts, New York, 1981.

Donovan, MI: Relaxation with guided imagery: a useful technique, *Cancer Nurs* **3**:27–32, Feb 1980

Dossey, B: A wonderful prerequisite, *Nursing* **14**:42–45, Jan 1984

Fakouri, C, and Jones, P: Relaxation Rx: slow stroke back rub, *J Gerontol Nurs* **13**:32–35, Feb 1987

Flaherty, GD, and Fitzpatrick, JJ: Relaxation technique to increase comfort level of postoperative patients: a preliminary study, *Nurs Res* **27**:352–355, 1978

Freedberg, PD, Hoffman, LA, Light, WC, and Kreps, MK: Effects of progressive muscle relaxation on the objective symptoms and subjective responses associated with asthma, *Heart Lung* **16**:24–30, Jan 1987

Graffam, S: Report of survey of untoward reactions to relaxation strategies, *Pain Res Nurs Forum* **3**:3, Mar-Apr 1983

Hanswer, M, Larson, SC, and O'Connell, AS: Music therapy assisted labor: effects on relaxation of expectant mothers, *Birth Psychol Bull* **4**:2, 1983

Heide, FJ, and Borkovec, TD: Relaxation-induced anxiety: mechanisms and theoretical implications, *Behav Res Ther* **22**:1–12, 1984

Herman, JA: The effect of progressive relaxation on valsalva response in healthy adults, *Res Nurs Health* **10**:171–176, 1987

Kaempfer, SH: Relaxation training reconsidered, *Oncol Nurs Forum* **9**:15–18, Spring 1982

Kutz, I, Caudill, M, and Benson, H: The role of relaxation in behavioral therapies for chronic pain, *Int Anaesth Clin* **21**: 193–200, Winter 1983

Lapp, J: Music hath charms to soothe a throbbing head, *Psychol Today* **21**:14, Feb 1987 (as reported by P Chance)

Larson, B, Daleflod, B, Hakansson, L, and Melin, L: Therapist-assisted versus self-help relaxation treatment of chronic headaches in adolescents: a school-based intervention, *J Child Psychol Psychiatry* **28**:127–136, Jan 1987

Levin, RF, Malloy, GB, and Hyman, RB: Nursing management of postoperative pain: use of relaxation techniques with female cholecystectomy patients, *J Adv Nurs* **12**:463–472, July 1987

Longworth, JCD: Psychophysiological effects of slow stroke back massage in normotensive females, *Adv Nurs Sci* **4**:44–61, July 1982

Lyles, JN, Burish, TG, Krozely, MG, and Oldham, RK: Efficacy of relaxation training and guided imagery in reducing the aversiveness of cancer chemotherapy, *J Consult Clin Psychol* **50**:509–524, Aug 1982

Mast, D, Meyer, J, and Urbanski, A: Relaxation techniques: a self-learning module for nurses: Unit I, *Cancer Nurs* **10**:141–147, 1987

Mast, D, Meyer, J, and Urbanski, A: Relaxation techniques: a self-learning module for nurses: Unit II, *Cancer Nurs* **10:**217–225, 1987

McCaffery, M: *Nursing management of the patient with pain,* pp 137–155, JB Lippincott, Philadelphia, 1979.

McCaffery, M: Relieving pain with noninvasive techniques, *Nursing* **10:**55–57, Dec 1980

Miller, KM: Deep breathing: a pain management technique, *AORN J* **45:**484–488, Feb 1987

Newman, RI, Seres, JL, Yospe, LP, and Garlington, B: Multidisciplinary treatment of chronic pain: long-term follow-up of low-back pain patients, *Pain* **4:**283–292, 1978

Registered Nurses as Providers of Relaxation and Suggestive Therapies: A position statement. California Nurses Association, San Francisco, Mar 1982.

Restless Legs Syndrome, *Harvard Medical School Health Letter* **12:**2–3, Aug 1987

Roberts, AH: Literature update: biofeedback and chronic pain, *J Pain Sympt Manag* **2:**169–171, Summer 1987

Shaw, L, and Ehrlich, A: Relaxation training as a treatment for chronic pain caused by ulcerative colitis, *Pain* **29:**287–293, 1987

Snyder, M: Progressive relaxation as a nursing intervention: an analysis, *Adv Nurs Sci* **6:**47–58, Apr 1984

Snyder, M: *Independent nursing interventions.* John Wiley & Sons, New York, 1985.

Stuckey, SJ, Jacobs, A, and Goldfarb, J: EMG biofeedback training, relaxation training, and placebo for the relief of chronic back pain, *Percept Mot Skills* **63:**1023–1036, 1986

Swinford, P: Relaxation and positive imagery for the surgical patient: a research study, *Periop Nurs Q* **3:**9–16, Sept 1987

Trygstad, L: Simple new way to help anxious patients, *RN* **43:** 28–32, Dec 1980

Turner, JA, and Romano, JM: Evaluating psychologic interventions for chronic pain: issues and recent developments, *Adv Pain Res Ther* **7:**257–296, 1984

Wortz, E: A yawn a day, *Psychol Today* **21:**8, May 1987

Imagery

Achterberg, J, and Lawlis, F: Imagery and health intervention, *Topics Clin Nurs* **3:**55–60, Jan 1982

*Barber, J, and Gitelson, J: Cancer pain: psychological management using hypnosis, *CA-Cancer J Clinic* **30:**130–136, May–June 1980

Barber, TX, Spanos, NP, and Chaves, JF: *Hypnosis, imagination, and human potentialities.* Pergamon Press, New York, 1974.

Bresler, DE: *Free yourself from pain,* pp 347–396, Simon and Schuster, New York, 1979.

Crowther, JH: Stress management training and relaxation imagery in the treatment of essential hypertension, *J Behav Med* **6:**169–187, 1983

Donovan, MI: Relaxation with guided imagery: a useful technique, *Cancer Nurs* **3:**27–32, 1980

Greene, RJ, and Reyher, J: Pain tolerance in hypnotic analgesic and imagination states, *J Abnorm Psychol* **79:**29–38, Feb 1972

Grinder, J, and Bandler, R: *The structure of magic,* II, pp 6–12, Science & Behavior, Palo Alto, Calif, 1976.

Horan, JJ, Layne, FC, and Pursell, CH: Preliminary self-regulation of chronic pain, *Am J Clin Hypn* **20:**106–113, 1977

Jacobsen, DE: Electrical measurements of neuromuscular states during mental activities. II. Imagination and recollection of various muscle acts, *Am J Physiol* **94:**22–34, 1930

Jones, GE, and Johnson, HJ: Heart rate and somatic concomitants of mental imagery, *Psychophysiology* **17:**185–191, 1980

Kroger, WS, and Fezler, WD: *Hypnosis and behavior modification: imagery conditioning.* JB Lippincott, Philadelphia, 1976.

Lankton, S: *Practical magic: a translation of neurolinguistic programming into clinical psychotherapy,* pp 18–19. Meta Publications, Cupertino, Calif, 1980.

Levine, S: *Who dies? An investigation of conscious living and conscious dying.* Anchor Books, Garden City, NY, 1982.

Lyles, JN, Burish, TG, Krozely, MG, and Oldham, RK: Efficacy of relaxation training and guided imagery in reducing the aversiveness of cancer chemotherapy, *J Consult Clin Psychol* **50:**509–524, Aug 1982

Mast, DE: Effects of imagery. *Image J Nurs Scholarship* **18:** 118–120, Fall 1986

McCaffery, M: *Nursing management of the patient with pain,* pp 156–183, JB Lippincott, Philadelphia, 1979.

Pearson, BD: Pain control: an experiment with imagery, *Geriatric Nurs* **8:**28–30, Jan–Feb 1987

Peterson, GH: *Birthing normally: a personal growth approach to childbirth,* pp 57–73. Mindbody Press, Berkeley, Calif, 1981.

Raft, D, Smith, R, and Warren, N: Selection of imagery in the relief of chronic and acute clinical pain, *J Psychosom Res* **30:**481–488, 1986

Sachs, LB: Feuerstein, M, and Vitale, JH: Hypnotic self-regulation of chronic pain, *Ann J Clin Hypn* **20:**106–113, Oct 1977

Samuels, M, and Samuels, N: *Seeing with the mind's eye: the history, techniques and uses of visualization.* Random House and The Bookworks, New York and Berkeley, Calif, 1975.

Schwartz, GE, Fair, PL, Salt, P, Mandel, MR, and Klerman, GL: Facial muscle patterning to affective imagery in depressed and nondepressed subjects, *Science* **192:**489–491, 1976

Scott, DS, and Barber, TX: Cognitive control of pain: effects of multiple cognitive strategies, *Psychol Record* **2:**373–383, 1977

Sheikh, AA: *Imagery: current theory, research and application.* John Wiley & Sons, Inc, Somerset, NJ, 1983.

Simonton, OC, Simonton, SM, and Creighton, JL: *Getting well again.* Bantam Books, New York, 1978.

Sodergren, KM: Guided imagery. In Snyder, M: *Independent nursing interventions,* pp 103–124. John Wiley & Sons, New York, 1985.

*Spiegel, D: The use of hypnosis in controlling cancer pain. *CA-Cancer J Clinic* **35:**221–231, July-Aug 1986

Swerdlow, B: A rapid hypnotic technique in a case of atypical facial neuralgia. *Headache* **24:**104–109, Mar 1984

White, KD: Salivation: the significance of imagery in its voluntary control, *Psychophysiology* **13:**196–203, 1978

*Free reprints available through American Cancer Society. Professional Education Publication (Spiegel, 85-50M-No. 3344-PE; Barbar and Gitelson, 80-50M-No. 3385-PE).

7

Chronic Non-Malignant Pain

Special Considerations

Relevant Patient/Family Teaching Points (see Appendix):
• Overall Daily Plan
• Pace Yourself
• Planning for the Future — Review of Pain-Relief Measures

The saddest story in all of pain management may well be about chronic non-malignant pain. There is more chronic non-malignant pain than any other kind of pain. The person who has it has suffered a long time, sometimes for years. The health professionals providing care for the patient have most likely felt helpless as they repeatedly failed in their efforts to help the patient.

Perhaps no aspect of pain control is as humbling for both sufferer and caregiver as chronic non-malignant pain, sometimes referred to as chronic benign pain. However, it is far from being benign; it may be devastating, not only for the person with the pain but for family, friends, and caregivers. Chronic non-malignant pain is capable of driving a destructive pathway through the lives of all it touches. By definition, chronic non-malignant pain is prolonged because it has not responded to whatever treatment has been tried. It exacts a high price from sufferers, their families and from caregivers and the cost to society in general in the United Kingdom is thought to be on the increase. In 1982 chronic low back pain led to the loss of over 33 million days in output at work and cost the NHS approximately £156 million (Wells, 1985). By 1990 it was suggested that back pain alone accounted for some 45 million certified days off work, and cost the NHS approximately £193 million in that year (Rigge, 1990). There is an obvious lack of more general

statistics covering diseases other than chronic back pain and more research in this area is needed.

KEY POINT: By definition, chronic non-malignant pain continues in spite of efforts to relieve it. This pain is not benign – it is destructive.

DEFINITION OF CHRONIC NON-MALIGNANT PAIN

A truly satisfactory or generally agreed upon definition of chronic non-malignant pain simply does not exist. In fact, some professionals do not use the phrase, preferring other terminology, such as chronic benign pain or chronic intractable benign pain syndrome. It encompasses diverse types of pain that may occur in virtually any area of the body and vary in intensity from mild to excrutiating. The cause either may or may not be known. The characteristics of the pain may fit a well-known pattern, or the patient may be told that the type of pain felt makes no sense.

A review of the literature shows that there is strong disagreement among health professionals in almost every area of managing chronic non-malignant pain. This is not surprising since this type of pain covers such an enormous variety of conditions and people. What to call it, what it encompasses, and how to treat it remain areas of controversy. To try to settle these differences or even offer a comprehensive definition of chronic non-malignant pain would be truly presumptuous. Thus, for this chapter, we have merely chosen from among the currently used terms, defined how the terminology is used, and identified the general conditions it covers.

Our decision to use the terminology chronic *non-malignant* pain rather than chronic *benign* pain is because the word benign is potentially misleading. Benign suggests a mild condition, which is rarely true of any chronic pain, regardless of its intensity. In oncology, malignant refers to conditions that are potentially life-threatening. Thus we have chosen non-malignant because this chapter focuses on types of pain that result from causes that are not life-threatening.

Working definition

For the purposes of this chapter the *working definition* of chronic non-malignant pain is: *pain that has lasted 3 months or longer, is ongoing on a daily basis or recurs on a regular basis, is due to non-life-threatening causes, has not responded to currently available treatment methods, and may continue for the remainder of the patient's life.* To some extent the patient must live with this pain, but hopefully certain strategies or approaches will effectively manage or control the pain. To the maximum extent possible, the patients themselves are enabled to control their own pain. (Basic differences between acute and chronic pain along with a review of types or causes of chronic pain and general recommended approaches are presented in Chapter 2)

Examples of chronic non-malignant pain, somewhat overlapping and of various origins, that either may or may not be under control or managed are:

Low back pain
Headaches
Rheumatoid arthritis
Osteoarthritis
Neck pain such as whiplash
Causalgia
Neuralgia
Phantom limb pain
Peripheral neuropathy
Postherpetic neuralgia
Trigeminal neuralgia

Fibrositis or diffuse myofascial pain
Vascular diseases of the limbs such as Raynaud's disease
Crohn's disease
Irritable bowel syndrome
Chronic pancreatitis
Ankylosing spondylitis
Burning mouth syndrome
Reflex sympathetic dystrophy.

The above examples make it clear that chronic non-malignant pain may very well have an identifiable physical or organic cause. Some of these diseases may even be cured with proper diagnosis and treatment, e.g. sympathetic nerve blockade for classic causalgia. The intensity may be just as severe as any other type of pain. What distinguishes this pain from other types of pain is that it is ongoing because a cure for it is unknown and that the cause has more or less stabilized, i.e. no additional injury or healing is occurring.

Many of the suggestions in this chapter for controlling chronic non-malignant pain are covered elsewhere in this book and, certainly, are appropriate for other types of pain as well. To say that the suggestions are inappropriate for other types of pain is inaccurate. Rather, it is important to realize that there is lack of agreement about approaches to chronic non-malignant pain, that different approaches are recommended for different types of pain, and for the individual patient the type of pain may not clearly fit one category. In general, more conservative approaches aimed at self-management are usually indicated when it is obvious that the patient has a normal life expectancy but will also have continuous pain that is not life-threatening and is due to causes that have stabilized.

Perhaps more important than a definition of chronic non-malignant pain is a reminder to the reader that this chapter is written in keeping with our philosophy of believing what the patient says about pain felt, or at the very least giving the benefit of the doubt, and working with the patient in the context of full disclosure, always being honest and conveying as much information as the patient can receive.

The health-care team sometimes fails to appreciate what the person with chronic non-malignant pain experiences. Following are examples of both a doctor's and a patient's views of chronic non-malignant pain.

A health-care team member's view of chronic non-malignant pain

It was in the middle 1970s, and a neurosurgeon and nurse were discussing their concerns about the difficulties of relieving prolonged pain. The doctor's patients had chronic non-malignant pain; the nurse's patients had cancer pain and many were terminally ill. Both told stories of patients who continued to hurt despite their efforts. The doctor said "I give them analgesics and they say the pills don't work but they want more anyway. I tell them not to take the pills if they don't help. Lots of them still go to work so you know they aren't hurting all that much. I tell them they're doing OK and don't need any more pills. Then there are those I know are hurting badly—discs protruding, muscles in spasm. But how many laminectomies can you do? And I don't want to keep giving them narcotics and make addicts out of them. So I tell them for their own good that they just have to learn to live with this". The doctor concluded the conversation by saying to the nurse "At least your patients usually die". As uncaring as it may sound, this statement probably reflects the doctor's genuine distress over seeing the same patients month after month without being able to help them. In truth, he wants to end the patient's pain, not the patient's life.

Fortunately, since this scenario, due to increased knowledge about chronic non-malignant pain attitudes have begun to change.

However, through the years some of the remarks heard about patients with chronic non-malignant pain seemed angry and derogatory. Many were no doubt borne out of the frustration of seeing so many efforts fail and not knowing what else to do. Following are examples of some of the statements that have appeared in the literature and have been heard in clinical settings about people who suffer from chronic non-malignant pain:

Uses the pain
Addicted
Enjoys his/her drugs
Drug-dependent
Wants only drugs for pain relief
Uncooperative
Non-compliant
Plays pain games
Malingering
Exaggerates the pain
Hypochondriac
Controls others with his/her pain
Psychological overlay
Psychogenic pain
Imagines the pain
Not willing to learn to live with the pain
Low pain tolerance (a somewhat sophisticated way of suggesting that the patient is a wimp)
Doesn't want to get better
Wants to keep the pain
Secondary gains
Makes a career out of pain
Has a Bachelor's or Master's Degree in pain
A professional pain patient
A pain-prone person
Wishes to occupy the "sick" role
Unmotivated
Dependent on the health-care system
A "crock".

The above remarks suggest a lack of respect or a degree of dislike for the patient with chronic non-malignant pain, whether or not they are intended to do so. The attitudes potentially conveyed by such phrases serve no useful purpose in the relationship with the patient. As the years have gone by, it is increasingly recognized that collaborating with and working with the person with chronic non-malignant pain has the potential for far superior results than does being in an adversarial position and waging a war with the patient. There is still a tendency, however, to discount patients' descriptions of pain when it is chronic as opposed to acute. There seems to be an assumption that the emotional problems found in chronic pain patients confound the quality of information they give about pain (Tearnan and Dar, 1986).

A composite of the patient's view of chronic non-malignant pain

The previously mentioned conversation between the doctor and nurse reflects the health-care team's view of patients who are probably similar to the patient in the following example. Her remarks present the patient's view:

A woman with chronic non-malignant pain said, "I've lived with this pain every day for over 5 years. I've had doctors tell me I couldn't be hurting this much, that I was addicted, that I should be strong enough to learn to live with this, and all sorts of things. I take these pain-killers but they don't really help. Oh, they do help a little though, and I'm afraid the doctor will stop prescribing them so I only take them when I really need them. I've tried to keep going to work and take care of my family, but no one believes I hurt any more. I know people at work think I'm lazy when I go home early once in a while. They just don't know I barely made it there in the first place. My husband says it's just my nerves, and maybe it is. Sometimes I think I must be crazy. How could I hurt this much? I try to ignore it and just do all the things I used to do, but then I end up hurting so much I'm knocked out for a day or so. I'm so irritable and tired all the time. I feel so ashamed when I can't do what I used to do. Inadequate, like a bad person. I feel guilty. You know, I think about those hospice patients with pain and sometimes I envy them. At least they know they'll die soon. And because they're dying, lots of doctors will give them all the pain-killers they need".

How can you help this patient feel worthwhile again? You can't take away the pain right now, maybe never, but you can begin to help her by treating her with respect and by believing her.

PURPOSE AND LIMITATIONS OF THIS CHAPTER

By definition, in this chapter we are dealing with pain that has not responded to our best efforts to eliminate it. Therefore approaches suggested in this chapter are not expected to put an end to chronic non-malignant pain. Rather, the hope is to suggest ways the health-care team can assist the patient to learn to manage the pain.

The patient, family, friends, and health professionals no doubt wish they could get rid of the pain—find a cause and cure it. However, pain has now become a chronic condition that requires daily management, very much like other chronic illnesses such as diabetes or hypertension. The goals of patient care now become twofold: (1) decreasing the pain intensity to the maximum extent possible, but not expecting that it will disappear, and (2) helping the patient obtain an optimal quality of life and level of function.

To accomplish these goals, the purposes of this chapter are:

- To improve the quality of interaction between the nurse and the person with chronic non-malignant pain by addressing the common misconceptions that hamper this and suggesting some approaches to collaborating with, or working with, the patient.
- To present guidelines for establishing realistic goals and identifying appropriate nursing interventions for helping the patient with chronic non-malignant pain in various settings under limited circumstances (i.e. not within a structured rehabilitation programme), including helping the patient learn self-management techniques for dealing with the pain.
- To identify professional and self-help resources the nurse may suggest for the patient with chronic non-malignant pain, including pointers on selecting a pain-management programme.

This chapter will not, however, include the nurse's role in structured in-patient or out-patient pain-management programmes designed to rehabilitate the person with chronic non-malignant pain, nor will guidelines for establishing a pain-management programme be discussed. References at the end of the chapter will enable the nurse to pursue these interests.

MISCONCEPTIONS ABOUT CHRONIC NON-MALIGNANT PAIN

Nurses often admit that caring for a patient with chronic pain is frustrating. Typically the patient with chronic non-malignant pain returns again and again to the health-care setting, whether it is the doctor's office, the Accident and Emergency department, or an orthopaedic ward. The patient's diagnosis, or cause of pain, may not be clear, such as is often true with low back pain. The patient's report of pain, such as a migraine headache, may not be objectively verifiable by a physical examination or by X-ray; and although the patient may report severe pain, the patient is not always acting like he/she is in pain since there has been pain for so long. However, the patient may be depressed and there may also be signs of anxiety. Nevertheless, the patient may be smiling when asking for narcotic analgesics. He/she may also know the names and doses of the analgesics and related medications along with how often they are needed, watching the clock and reminding the nurse well in advance of when they are due.

Nurses may say they feel like they have lost control in such situations, failing to realize they never had control in the first place. Only the patient knows when and how much he/she hurts. Therefore the patient is in control, i.e. the final authority about the pain felt. Further, in any chronic illness, optimal results depend on the patients themselves learning how to manage their illness. In fact, in programmes for chronic pain management, an attitude of self-control and control over pain is fostered. If a patient with diabetes or chronic hypertension knows all about the medications and when they should be taken, this is viewed as desirable. When the patient with chronic pain has the same information and has learned to use it to manage the pain, ironically this can upset the health-care team.

One study of 268 registered nurses' responses to descriptions of patients with various types of pain showed that many nurses have a negative stereotype of the patient with chronic pain. They tend to believe that pain is less intense in patients with chronic vs. acute pain, especially if there are no signs of pathology. Nurses are particularly likely to have negative attitudes about patients with chronic low back pain as compared with their attitudes toward patients with headache or joint pain. There is also a tendency for nurses to believe that pain-relief measures are less effective when the patient is depressed, failing to appreciate that pain may cause the depression (Taylor, Skelton and Butcher, 1984).

Patients seem to be aware that expressions of depression may be viewed negatively. They may defend themselves against the possibility of their pain being psychologically interpreted by making a great effort to represent themselves as cheerful and nondepressed. Thus patients are in a no-win situation. If they act like their pain is emotionally disturbing, they may be diagnosed as having "mental problems", and their pain may be labelled as largely psychogenic. If they do not appear depressed, the intensity of their pain may not be believed.

KEY POINT: The health-care team's reaction to a patient with chronic non-malignant pain may present an impossible dilemma for the patient. If the patient expresses his/her depression, the health-care team may believe the pain is psychogenic or is largely an emotional problem. If the patient tries to hide the depression by being cheerful, the health-care team may not believe that pain is a significant problem.

Misconceptions that hamper assessment and treatment of patients with pain are especially difficult to correct when the patient has chronic non-malignant pain. (Many of the reasons for failing to believe the patient when saying there is pain of any sort have already been reviewed in Chapter 2). This time we are faced not only with the fact that pain is subjective and cannot be proven or disproven, but also that it is not going away. It continues or returns. Further, we are also often dealing with the chronic or repeated administration of narcotics, drugs about which we have many exaggerated fears (see reasons for under-treatment with narcotics, p. 76).

For all catastrophic events there seems to be the final question of "Why me?" How do we explain this? Uncertainty is very difficult. A bad reason may be better than no reason at all. When pain is chronic, has no clear cause, and is not life-threatening, the question of blame arises, probably because we would rather have a reason for the suffering than believe that our lives might be determined by an arbitrary and uncontrolled force. Thus with chronic non-malignant pain sometimes the patient blames him/herself and feels inadequate and depressed. Then, unfortunately, as if having the prolonged pain were not enough, the health-care team may blame the patient or fail to believe him. Shown in the following box are some of the misconceptions that surround these and other issues about chronic non-malignant pain.

KEY POINT: Health-care team members have many misconceptions about the cause and treatment of chronic non-malignant pain. Some emotional or personality characteristic of the patient is often mistakenly blamed for the cause of chronic non-malignant pain.

No pain is imaginary, and outright fabrication of chronic pain is considered rare. Furthermore, some pain specialists believe that certain causes of pain, e.g. myofascial syndrome and sympathetic dystrophy, are commonly overlooked (see annotated references: Crook and Tunks, 1985; Fischer, 1984; Hendler, 1984; Leavitt and Sweet, 1986; Reesor and Craig, 1988).

MISCONCEPTIONS ABOUT CHRONIC NON-MALIGNANT PAIN

Misconception	Correction
The patient with chronic pain lasting for years becomes less sensitive to pain and better able to tolerate it.	Research shows that, unfortunately, as pain continues through the years, the patient's own internal narcotics, endorphins, decrease and the patient perceives even greater pain from the same stimuli. Further, most patients with chronic pain become more frightened and feel they have less control over pain as time goes by, perhaps mainly because they begin to learn how severe unrelieved pain can be. In their repeated encounters with health professionals they also may learn that their pain may not be believed, and they may not receive assistance with pain relief (see annotated reference: Kosten and Kleber, 1987).
Pain, especially chronic pain, for which there is no known organic cause, is a symptom of psychological disturbance, e.g. psychogenic pain.	Psychogenic pain is often inaccurately diagnosed simply because a physical cause cannot be found or because the patient does not respond to treatment. It is presumptuous to believe that diagnostic testing is always thorough or precise enough to identify all physical causes of pain. The health-care team's inability to identify a physical cause for the pain does not justify diagnosing the pain as psychogenic (see annotated references: Fischer, 1984; Hendler, 1984).
A patient who is very expressive about pain, i.e. "exaggerates" the pain, and/or has a greater decrease in function than can be explained by the physical cause, is consciously trying to manipulate others or obtain secondary gains.	Patients with symptomatology incongruent with the physical cause of pain may have poor, or ineffective, coping styles and may be considerably distressed by the pain. The patient's lack of adaptive coping styles may predate the onset of pain. The patient may never have been able to cope with any stressful life events very well. His/her attempts to cope, such as withdrawing or being passive, may have prolonged the problems and created others. Thus when the patient who is already barely coping with life events also experiences pain, he/she is poorly equipped to handle it and may very well be overwhelmed by it. The patient's intense reaction to pain often causes the staff to discount the pain and believe that the patient has emotional problems, forgetting that many of these patients do have significant, identifiable organic damage. When the patient senses the staff's disbelief, the patient simply increases behavioural reaction in an effort to get the staff to believe him/her. This becomes a vicious cycle that is disruptive for both patient and staff. Just because the patient's response to pain seems out of proportion to the degree of physical cause does not mean the patient hurts any less. No pain is imaginary, and outright fabrication of chronic pain is rare. Some pain specialists believe that certain causes of pain, e.g. myofascial syndrome and sympathetic dystrophy, are commonly overlooked (see annotated references: Crook and Tunks, 1985; Fischer, 1984; Hendler, 1984; Leavitt and Sweet, 1986; Reesor and Craig, 1988).
If the patient is depressed, especially if there is no known physical cause for the pain, then depression is causing this pain. The pain would subside if the depression could be effectively treated.	It is normal for some patients to be depressed because of chronic pain. Chronic pain can cause depression. Further, an additional variety of types of depression may accompany chronic pain. Some types of depression could be present prior to the onset of pain but are not likely to be the cause of pain. A pre-existing depression does, however, make it more difficult for the patient to handle chronic pain. For a patient experiencing a localized sensation of pain to be told that he/she is simply depressed is infuriating to the patient. Depression of any sort is a form of suffering (see annotated references: Ahles, Yunus and Masi, 1987; Bouckoms, Litman and Baer, 1985; Hendler, 1984; Krishnan et al, 1985, Parts I and II; Pilowsky, Crettenden and Townley, 1985). To make it even more complicated, the symptoms of chronic pain are somewhat like those of depression in general. That is, even if the person with chronic pain were not depressed, that person would still exhibit some of the same symptoms as depression, e.g. decreased involvement in activities, sleep disturbances, and difficulty concentrating. When the symptoms of chronic pain are compared with those of depression, the similarities between the two make it easy to see how they can become confused and how the patient can be mistakenly identified as being only depressed. Table 7-1 illustrates how features common to most types of depression may also be a result of chronic pain alone, while others are likely to be a result of the depression caused by chronic pain.

Misconception

If the patient's pain occurs or increases soon after a traumatic life event, e.g. divorce or death in the family, this stress is probably what precipitated the occurrence or exacerbation of pain.

Patients who are awaiting litigation after an injury or who receive compensation are very likely to exaggerate their pain for financial gain, or may be malingerers. This is sometimes referred to as "compensation neurosis".

Narcotics are totally inappropriate for all patients with chronic non-malignant pain.

People with chronic pain who have been taking narcotics for months or years are very much like street drug users or addicts.

Correction

Studies fail to show that increases in tension or anxiety are predictive of an exacerbation of pain in patients with low back pain (see annotated reference: Feuerstein, Carter and Papciak, 1987). Furthermore, this is retrospective speculation. Most people have experienced some disturbing event within the last 6 months and not all have developed chronic pain. To say that an upsetting event is the cause of chronic pain is probably neither true nor very helpful. On the other hand, it is also true that if a person is having difficulty coping with an upsetting event, and is experiencing additional pain, the person will be at a disadvantage for dealing with the pain.

Numerous studies have failed to support this view. For example, Melzack, Katz and Jeans (1985) found that patients who receive compensation do not report higher levels of pain than patients who do not receive compensation. These authors say "Compensation is not a cause of pain... This does not mean that malingerers or neurotics do not exist. It suggests instead that they may be relatively rare and unfortunate patients have been misdiagnosed, mistreated and allowed to suffer under the shroud of unfair labels instead of receiving appropriate therapy" (p. 111). (See annotated references: Dworkin et al, 1985; Leavitt and Sweet, 1986; Peck, Fordyce and Black, 1978; Reesor and Craig, 1988.)

Litigation, of course, is not limited to worker's compensation. Other types of litigation that the patient with chronic non-malignant pain may be involved with are divorce or insurance payments following a car accident. Again, there is no basis for suspecting that the patient is exaggerating the pain.

There is little evidence to support this view. However, this belief has been held for many years, and even in very recent years this opinion has been strongly stated by some pain specialists. The majority of books written for the layman with chronic non-malignant pain are biased against the use of narcotics, and many articles in professional journals express this bias. For years most pain-management programmes have considered detoxification from narcotics and sedatives as one of their major rehabilitation goals. However, patients referred to pain clinics are not typical of people in the general population who suffer from chronic pain and are not referred to these clinics.

Further, several studies have shown that prolonged narcotic therapy for selected patients with chronic non-malignant pain can be a safe and humane alternative to surgery or no treatment. Most researchers suggest that prolonged narcotic therapy for chronic non-malignant pain be considered only after other reasonable attempts to control the pain have been unsuccessful, when the pain is thought to be opiate-responsive, and only in patients without a history of drug abuse (see annotated references: Crook and Tunks, 1985; Halpern and Robinson, 1985–86; Portenoy and Foley, 1986). On the other hand, one study showed that patients with alcohol-use disorder, compared with those who had no history of this, were not more likely to be prescription medication users (Holzman and Gulliver, 1986).

Street drug users or narcotic addicts do not take narcotics to relieve physical pain, nor do they claim to need or want narcotics for pain relief unless they are trying to obtain narcotics illicitly via the health-care system, e.g. from Accident and Emergency departments. Prolonged use of narcotics for pain relief may not be appropriate for all patients, but this is not addiction since narcotics are legally and medically sanctioned for use as analgesics. Further, unlike narcotic addicts, patients who take very high doses of narcotic for weeks or months, even years in some cases, will almost always stop using narcotics when the pain stops (refer to pp. regarding differences and incidence of addiction, physical dependence, and tolerance to analgesia; see annotated reference: Halpern and Robinson, 1985–86).

Although the term "drug abuse" may appear in a patient's records, the fact that a person has used narcotics for pain relief for a long time does not necessarily mean he/she is abusing them. If the long-term use of narcotics is inappropriate, then the term *misuse* is applicable. A patient may misuse narcotics for pain relief for years because they are misprescribed by a doctor (misprescribed in the sense that for some patients another method of pain relief might be a better choice).

Misconception	Correction
When patients with chronic non-malignant pain are "non-compliant", it is probably because they do not want to give up their pain.	When patients with chronic non-malignant pain do not follow the recommendations of the health-care team and this results in a continuation of significant problems, such as lack of improvement in physical function or an exacerbation of pain, it may well be that the team's recommendations are inappropriate for the patient. Non-compliance has a negative connotation, and often patients who are non-compliant are considered "difficult". Such patients tend to take more time to treat, both per visit and over time, and to have more complications and multiple treatments. Health-care team members are understandably frustrated when the patient fails to follow recommendations that they feel would be of benefit. However, non-compliance is widespread in all chronic diseases, e.g. asthma and diabetes, and should be expected to occur with chronic non-malignant pain as well.
	It may help to reconsider the situation in terms of two features: (1) the implications of the term "compliance", and (2) reasons that the health-care team's recommendations may not be appropriate for the individual.
	First, compliance implies an undemocratic and authoritarian relationship between a knowledgeable health-care provider and an informed patient who is the passive recipient of directions. It is not likely that the use of the term compliance will be discontinued, but hopefully a different attitude can be fostered. To help patients who have any chronic condition, a more collaborative relationship is desirable. The patient must have the option of being an active member of the relationship, plan care with the health-care professional, and be given respect for opinions and goals.
	Second, why might the patient fail to follow recommendations?
	• The recommendations may be too complicated for the patient.
	• The patient may not remember all the recommendations.
	• Some may be unrealistic for the patient.
	• The patient may be overwhelmed from being asked to accomplish too many things.
	• Some recommendations may have increased the patient's pain or related problems and now need to be modified.
	• The patient may also feel that control has been taken away, and may fail to follow recommendations as a means of reasserting the right to control his/her own life.
	It may be helpful to ask the patient these questions:
	• Were the recommendations written down for you and discussed with you?
	• Were you encouraged to ask questions and suggest revisions?
	• Did you agree to each item, as well as consider the total time and effort required by all the recommendations?
	• What happened when you attempted to follow the recommendations?

NURSING-CARE GUIDELINES FOR HELPING THE PERSON WITH CHRONIC NON-MALIGNANT PAIN IN THE GENERAL CLINICAL SETTING

In general clinical settings, e.g. on an in-patient orthopaedic unit, outside a structured rehabilitation programme for chronic non-malignant pain, taking care of the patient with chronic non-malignant pain is often frustrating to nurses. Such patients are commonly referred to as difficult. However, following the guidelines below may prevent difficulties. If the patient is already angry, complaining, dissatisfied, ordering nurses around, perhaps shouting, it is still not too late

to use these guidelines. The suggestions may not result in instant success, but consistent persistence usually succeeds.

Meanwhile, remember that the patient's initial reaction to you is probably based on countless unsatisfying and perhaps adversarial encounters with caregivers. Most patients who have had a pain for a very long time have been told some of the following: "It can't hurt that much." "It's all in your head." "You're just using your pain." "You're going to get addicted." "You'll just have to learn to live with this." So the patient is likely to be upset at the outset.

Depression without Pain	Responses to Chronic Non-malignant Pain
1. Weight loss or gain.*	1. Usually weight gain, often partly due to decreased physical activity; or overeating out of boredom and inability to be involved with other desirable activities.
2. Insomnia or hypersomnia.*	2. Same. Insomnia due to unrelieved pain; or hypersomnia due to medication, or due to extreme fatigue from severe or unrelieved pain or from exerting extra energy required to perform certain activities.
3. Decreased involvement in social, sexual, and work activities.*	3. Same, but not usually due to lack of interest; usually due to decreased physical ability or increased pain from activity.
4. Fatigue and loss of energy.*	4. Same. May be related to increased energy required to adapt to pain, e.g. change life style to keep pain under control; or due to general body deconditioning from inactivity; or due to sedating medications, e.g. narcotic/sedative.
5. Difficulty concentrating.*	5. Same. Due to unrelieved pain or sedating medications, e.g. narcotic/sedative.
6. Feelings of worthlessness.	6. Same. Due to loss of ability to function as did in past; due to degrading actions of others, e.g. not believing reports of pain, suggesting patient should be able to handle pain better, avoiding patient.
7. Suicidal ideas or attempts.	7. Same. Due to belief that lack of control over present pain and/or inability to function will continue, or due to self-blame for the situation.

*Features of depression which are also common responses to chronic pain in the absence of, or independent of, depression.

Table 7.1 Features of Chronic Non-malignant Pain and Depression.

A GUIDE TO SETTING REALISTIC GOALS

A less than ideal solution for the patient with chronic non-malignant pain is often necessary when the patient is cared for in clinical settings other than those specifically designed for pain management, e.g. a pain clinic. Setting realistic goals for helping the patient in these varied settings is far from simple. However, it is essential that the goals are attainable and important for both patient and nurse. Otherwise, more harm than good may be done. Pursuing unattainable goals or expecting the patient to do something he/she does not value becomes a negative and frustrating experience for all concerned.

Three practical considerations are: (1) the patient's stage of acceptance of his/her condition, (2) the patient's ability to follow through independently with recommendations, and (3) time and available resources.

Patient's stage of acceptance

The health-care team may recognize that the patient's pain is not life-threatening and is likely to persist, possibly for the remainder of his/her patient's otherwise normal life. However, the patient may not have accepted this fact. Understandably, the patient may still prefer to find a cure for the pain. It may be years before the patient accepts that a cure probably is not realistic and that he/she needs to make plans to handle pain on an on-going, usually daily, basis. This acceptance cannot be forced on the patient. It is similar to a form of grief that must be endured and worked through gradually.

At least four stages of dealing with chronic non-malignant pain have been described (Hendler, 1984):

1. During the first few weeks or months of having pain, the patient may hope it will go away or begin seeking a cure for it.

2. During the following months, as the pain persists, the patient may wonder if he/she has been misdiagnosed or if he/she has received inappropriate or harmful treatment for the pain. Bodily concerns tend to increase. This patient is still cure oriented vs. accepting that the pain will persist.

3. As years go by the increasing realization that the pain is permanent may trigger increasing anger, resentment, and depression. This patient may vacillate between looking for a cure and looking for daily pain management techniques.

4. At some point, usually several years after the onset of pain, the patient may partially or sometimes completely accept that the pain will persist for the rest of his/her life. At this point the patient is much more likely to consider permanent alterations in lifestyle and to accept or seek strategies to help deal with the pain on a daily basis. Depression may decrease but is likely to continue to some extent. Compared with other chronic health problems such as decreasing eyesight, diabetes, or limb amputation, the patient with chronic non-malignant pain is probably more likely to encounter unsympathetic attitudes in family, friends, and caregivers, e.g. disbelieving the existence or severity of the pain. Such attitudes increase the patient's distress and reinforce feelings of inadequacy.

Obviously, patients who are less oriented to seeking a cure will tend to be more accepting of self-management techniques, such as relaxation and pacing. Patients more oriented to finding a cure may be more accepting of physiotherapy, medications, and other more tangible and health-care team directed approaches to pain management.

As long as the patient believes a cure is possible or believes that control of the pain is dependent upon medical or surgical interventions, the patient is unlikely to be very committed to self-directed strategies for pain control. They may be offered, but the patient's rejection of them is predictable, since to him/her they seem inappropriate.

Patient's ability to handle recommendations independently

Regardless of the patient's state of acceptance of chronic pain, he/she may wish to pursue certain recommendations for pain control that he/she simply is not able to do. Physical limitations such as living in an isolated area with no public transportation or living in a dangerous neighbourhood may prohibit engaging in activities outside the home. Regular supervision of exercises by a physiotherapist is hampered if the patient lives several miles away from one. Physical problems such as diminished eyesight or a memory deficit may render even the simplest medication regime difficult or unsafe.

Further, the patient's coping style of active and independent vs. passive and dependent will influence the skill with which he/she is able to implement certain recommendations. No matter how good the patient's intentions may be, if there is very little experience of taking active control of daily life, efforts may not be very successful, e.g. keeping an accurate or complete daily diary or remembering to make or keep appointments.

Time and available resources

In spite of what the patient is willing and able to do to control pain, the nurse simply may not have the time to help with all or even most of the possibilities. The nurse in the Accident and Emergency department who sees a patient return every week for injections for low back pain probably knows that this is not the best approach to helping the patient. But how much time does the nurse have to do more than this?

Further, resources such as a psychologist, a doctor specializing in pain, certain medications, or a pain clinic may not be available or affordable. Thus referral to other resources is not always a reasonable option.

Trying to identify goals that are not only a priority for the individual but also realistic is no small matter. The specific nursing-care guidelines summarized on p. 208 pinpoint some frequently relevant and important approaches, and they are listed in somewhat of a hierarchy from the most commonly and easily done to the more complex activities. Although they are admittedly not comprehensive, it often is not even possible to follow all of them. Thus realistic goals may sometimes seem not only less than ideal but also less than the acceptable minimum.

> **KEY POINT:** To set goals that are important, realistic, and attainable requires acknowledgment of limitations in the nurse, patient, and surrounding circumstances.

IMMEDIATE HELP FOR CRISIS WITH CHRONIC NON-MALIGNANT PAIN

Time involved: Reading time, 7 minutes; implementation time, 20 minutes (longer if telephoning the doctor is required or if the team meeting with the doctor is included).

Sample situation: From the morning nursing report it is obvious that a crisis is occurring in the relationship between the nurses and a patient, Mr W., who has chronic non-malignant pain and has been admitted to the hospital for an exacerbation of this pain. This is the fifth hospitalization for this patient in the last 18 months. The patient does not describe his pain as any worse or different from what it was yesterday when he was admitted, but the staff's relationships with the patient have steadily deteriorated—the patient and staff seem to be "at war". The nurses say the patient is "demanding", "uncooperative", "addicted", a "clock-watcher", "never satisfied", and sometimes verbally abusive to the nurses. The nurses say there is no known cause for his pain but they believe he does hurt. However, the nurses say he makes his pain worse by getting upset, and sometimes if they only go into his room and talk to him about football, he seems very happy. Right now, the patient is alternating between refusing to talk to the staff and yelling that he wants his pain medication changed, that it doesn't work, and that he wants to see his doctor. The doctor was informed of this by telephone at about 6:00am and would not change the prescription for analgesics. The doctor will be making rounds in the early afternoon.

Possible solution: There is no immediate, truly satisfactory solution, but there may be a temporary answer that will pave the way to a better long-range plan. Use whatever analgesics are currently available, and find a non-pharmacological method of pain relief. Defuse the situation—get the staff and patient to talk to each other, and plan a patient–staff conference involving the doctor to determine goals of this hospitalization. Focus on the most positive aspects of the staff–patient relationship. This situation encompasses long-standing misconceptions and misunderstandings on the part of both staff and patient.

Expected outcome: The immediate result, hopefully, is somewhat better pain relief within about an hour and a specific plan for determining the goals of this hospitalization. Overall, the desired outcome is that the patient feels that the staff believes that he hurts; the staff knows that chronic pain is frustrating to the patient; and all staff members acknowledge that at this time there does not appear to be any way to cure the cause of the pain, but that a plan for managing the pain is needed.

Do's

1. State the problem as clearly as possible to both staff and patient, i.e. the patient is in pain and the nurses do not know what more to do for the patient. It is frustrating to the patient to ask for help and not get it; it is frustrating to the staff to use what they can and still not relieve the pain.
2. Give whatever analgesics are prescribed as often as allowed. Set up a schedule, e.g. every 4 hours.
3. Regarding the patient's behaviour, tell the patient: You understand he hurts and is very frustrated by this. Also tell him exactly when he can expect his next analgesic as you are only able to give drugs as prescribed. If he wants more analgesic, he and you must discuss this with his doctor that afternoon during rounds. If narcotic injections have been prescribed, suggest the regular use of an oral nonnarcotic and a strong oral narcotic (see pp. on how to change from IM to oral analgesics for moderate to severe pain).

   He sounds angry and, if he is, you want him to tell you why, and also, if he wishes, you will help him tell the nurses or doctors what has upset him. (This is a lesson in assertiveness—the patient has a right to be angry, and he needs to learn how to tell others when he is angry and why without using abusive language.)
4. Consider heat, cold, or massage for pain relief and do the following:

   Ask the patient which he prefers, heat or cold, explaining that this will relieve some of the pain right now. Encourage use of cold, if possible, since it works faster and relieves more pain than heat or massage.

   Stay with him until it begins to relieve pain.

   Say that you have heard he does a good job of getting his mind off pain for a while by talking about football and suggest that he tell you about a recent game while the cold (or heat, massage) begins to work. Of course, he may prefer to be silent and relax, especially if massage is done.
5. Regarding the nurses' attitudes and observations, discuss with them and include in the nursing-care plan where appropriate:

   Arguing with the patient creates an adversarial rather than therapeutic or helpful relationship.

   You personally will not argue with the patient about his pain because no one can prove or disprove the existence of pain.

   They are correct when they say that the patient makes his pain worse when he gets upset, but explain that being anxious and depressed does not cause pain—it just makes pain more difficult to handle.

   We cannot make the pain go away right now, but we can stop contributing to the patient's anxiety and depression and help him gain control simply by ceasing to argue with him about his pain.

   Taking narcotics for pain relief is not the same as addiction.

   Clock-watching is usually a result of inadequate pain relief, particularly from a short-acting analgesic.

   The patient's anger is understandable if he came to the hospital expecting pain relief and it is not provided.

   They have identified some of the patient's strengths, i.e. he maintains an interest in outside events, e.g. football, is able to be distracted from his pain by football, and is using a lot of energy to try to keep the pain from being overwhelming. Remind them that distraction is a powerful method of dealing with pain but does not make the pain go away, and distraction should be encouraged.
6. Talk with the patient, nurses, and doctor to set a time, within the next 24 hours, for a patient–staff-conference to identify the specific goals of this hospitalization and how they will be accomplished.

Don'ts

1. Do not "take sides" by agreeing with the staff or with the patient that the other is unreasonable.
2. Do not avoid the patient.
3. Do not expect to provide immediate, satisfactory pain relief.

At the very least, the goal is to work as effectively as possible with whatever is presented in the immediate situation. This usually includes the attitude expressed toward the patient, basic assessment of any changes in the patient's condition, and appropriate use of whatever analgesics are prescribed. This involves the first eight nursing-care guidelines listed below.

For example, the Acident and Emergency nurse, mentioned above, who sees the patient with low back pain return weekly for a narcotic injection can find time to follow most of the first eight nursing-care guidelines, that is, the nurse can believe the patient, refrain from referring to him/her as an addict, not try to fool him/her with a placebo, ask about any changes in pain, discuss the cause of the low back pain, recognize that an acute exacerbation may require narcotics, avoid suggesting that the patient simply stop taking all medications, and advise the patient to take whatever the doctor has prescribed on a regular basis to help prevent back pain from escalating to the point of needing to return to Accident and Emergency.

When the nurse is able to see the patient with chronic pain over a period of days, the goal is broadened to addressing the patient's methods of handling pain on a daily basis in addition to the problems in the immediate situation. Even when the

---

**A Summary of Specific Nursing-Care Guidelines
for Helping the Person with Chronic Non-malignant Pain**

1. Never argue with the patient about whether or not the patient feels the pain he says is present.
2. Never refer to the patient as a narcotic addict.
3. Never use a placebo to try to determine if the patient has "real" pain, has a physical cause for pain, or is lying about the pain.
4. Be especially alert to any changes in the patient's condition as well as any advances in treating the patient's pain.
5. Recognize and treat acute pain or exacerbations of chronic pain differently from on-going chronic non-malignant pain.
6. Be sure the patient receives what he/she feels is an appropriate explanation from the appropriate person of why pain is present.
7. Avoid sudden withdrawal of narcotic and sedative medications.
8. When analgesics are required, give them orally, if at all possible, at high enough doses to provide satisfactory pain relief, and often enough on a regular rather than a PRN basis to prevent the return of pain.
9. Review analgesics being used for relief of chronic (vs. acute) pain, usually with the goals of avoiding narcotics, encouraging non-narcotic analgesia, and suggesting trials of appropriate classes of drugs recently found to have analgesic properties for specific conditions, e.g. anticonvulsants and antidepressants for neuropathic pain.
10. When it is obviously very likely that the patient will return for treatment of chronic pain, try to develop a summary of the present treatment and a plan for the return visit.
11. Decreasing the severity of a chronic sleep disturbance is a priority, and the appropriateness of antidepressants and/or relaxation techniques should be evaluated.
12. Offer pain-relief alternatives likely to be most consistent with the patient's coping style, e.g. active vs. passive methods of coping with pain.
13. Help the patient learn and plan to use coping strategies, especially relaxation, that avoid catastrophizing.
14. Help the patient develop his/her own daily commitment to specific activities, e.g. physical and/or social, especially a return to employment of any type, if appropriate.
15. Help those living with the patient, especially the spouse, to work with him/her to establish expectations and limitations regarding the activities of the patient and others in relation to the existing pain.
16. Review with the patient support systems, and suggest additional ones, if appropriate.
17. Consider obtaining the assistance of a physiotherapist to help the patient identify physical exercises that are appropriate, with realistic goals.
18. Review with the patient any types of help sought outside traditional medical practice, providing appropriate encouragement or suggesting precautions.
19. All recommendations to the patient regarding management of chronic pain need to be specific and detailed, in writing with a copy for the patient and health-care team, and incorporated in any other recommendations so that a picture of the total plan is readily available.
20. Evaluate the effectiveness of each specific recommendation made to the patient for pain management, with regular follow-up and possibly written, daily diaries kept by the patient.
21. Assess the need for requesting a consultation to identify and treat depression, anxiety, or post-traumatic stress disorder.
22. Assess risk of suicide.

patient is seen only briefly, if it is repeatedly but without the stress of an emergency, broader goals are also appropriate. Examples of such situations are recurrent hospitalizations, weekly home visits by a nurse, or regular patient visits to the surgery of the occupational health nurse or a doctor. Repeated or prolonged contacts allow time for gradual assessment and introduction of alternative methods of dealing with chronic pain. Several or all of the nursing-care guidelines numbered 8 to 22 may be indicated.

Specific nursing-care guidelines

The nursing-care guidelines below are one of the few places in this book where the word "never" is used repeatedly. This is probably because there are more misconceptions about the treatment of chronic non-malignant pain than with other types of pain. Nursing care guidelines for helping the patient with chronic non-malignant pain (or, at the very least, not making the situation worse) are discussed in the text and summarized in the box on the previous page.

1. Never argue with the patient about whether or not the patient feels the pain claimed to be present. Whatever the patient says about the pain, or whatever indications are given about pain, must be treated with respect. Even if the health-care team doubts some or all of what the patient is saying, the patient is given the benefit of the doubt. To do otherwise is to call the patient a liar and to begin a battle with the patient over a matter that can never be proven or disproven.

As early as the 1970s this approach was recognized as important and addressed by pain specialists. For example, at one multidisciplinary pain centre during that time, about 15 health-care team members met for their weekly discussion of the patients admitted to the in-patient unit. While a particular patient was being reviewed, a doctor began to shake his head slowly from side to side. Finally a colleague asked him to share the meaning of his reaction. The doctor said he found it difficult to believe that this patient had any pain, certainly not as much as the patient claimed. The colleague responded in a routine, matter-of-fact fashion, saying that the doctor was entitled to his personal opinion, but that professionally it was their responsibility to respond to the patient's report of pain.

2. Never refer to the patient as a narcotic addict. Pain relief is a legal, medical reason for the use of narcotics. When a patient is taking narcotics for pain, no matter for how long or how much narcotic is being used, he/she is not an addict. Even if the patient has developed tolerance to analgesia and requires more narcotic to relieve pain, or even if the patient develops withdrawal syndrome when narcotics are stopped, he/she is not an addict (see Chapter 4, pp. 76–79 for definitions and distinctions between these terms). Sometimes the words *tolerance, withdrawal,* and addiction are used interchangeably, but by current definitions they are separate entities.

Not only is it inaccurate to refer to the patient who takes narcotics for chronic non-malignant pain as an addict, it is degrading to the patient. Considerable stigma is attached to the term. In our society, to be an addict is to be a "bad" person.

3. Never use a placebo to try to determine if the patient has "real" pain, has a physical cause for pain, or is lying about the pain. Pain relief from a placebo proves nothing. It merely confirms the pharmacological fact that 33% of the time or more, placebos will provide adequate pain relief for patients with obvious physical causes of pain of moderate to severe intensity (see Chapter 2.).

4. Be especially alert to any changes in the patient's condition as well as any advances in treating the patient's pain. Note the need for additional diagnostic testing. Significant changes in the patient's condition may go unnoticed because it is altogether too easy to become accustomed to chronic reports of pain. Thus a diagnosis may be missed. It is always possible that the patient will develop additional pain problems requiring different treatment, e.g. a malignancy or myocardial infarction.

Further, the condition underlying pain may change or may be eventually diagnosed and treated as advances are made in pain management. Progress is being made in many areas of pain control. It is possible that some new treatment will be indicated for the patient's pain. For example, in recent years adjuvant analgesics (pp. 113 and 292) have been found to be effective with some types of pain, such as anticonvulsants for phantom limb pain.

5. Recognize and treat acute pain or exacerbations of chronic pain differently from on-going chronic non-malignant pain. To treat acute pain differently from chronic non-malignant pain requires careful assessment to distinguish between the two. Unfortunately, it is common for some types of acute pain to be mistaken for chronic non-malignant pain. When acute pain is prolonged, e.g. lasting weeks or months, is recurrent, e.g. weekly or monthly episodes for a few days, or is an exacerbation of chronic non-malignant pain, these situations may be misunderstood as chronic non-malignant pain. Examples of acute pain that may be erroneously treated as chronic non-malignant pain are:

• sickle cell crisis
• burn pain that lasts for weeks or months
• weeks or months of pain related to multiple orthopaedic injuries following an accident (e.g. unhealed fractures, infected wounds)
• exacerbation of neck pain from excessive strain
• postoperative pain from a laminectomy performed on a patient with chronic low back pain.

Analgesics and limited activity may be indicated temporarily for acute pain, but with on-going chronic non-malignant pain the goal is usually to increase activity. Fear of causing addiction or allowing the patient to become accustomed to the relief of stronger analgesics, especially narcotics, often results in inadequate treatment of acute pain, e.g. postoperative pain. However, narcotics are entirely appropriate for sickle cell crisis, postoperative pain, or burn tanking and debridement. High doses of oral narcotics on a regular basis are appropriate e.g. while complicated orthopaedic injuries heal or during exacerbation of musculoskeletal pain. At the same time, techniques often recommended for chronic non-malignant pain may be used, such as relaxation and pacing, e.g. taking a break before pain increases (see 'Pace Yourself" in appendix). On the other hand, for daily chronic non-malignant pain, intravenous morphine is obviously not the answer.

The difference between acute and chronic pain must be clear to both patient and health-care team. Just because pain is prolonged and not life-threatening is not justification for treating it as chronic non-malignant pain as defined in this chapter. For pain to be classified and treated as chronic non-malignant pain, it also must have failed to respond to current treatment; further medical and surgical interventions to cure the cause of the pain should not be indicated; and pain must be expected to continue indefinitely. This is not the case with the above examples. Either the pain will subside as healing takes place, e.g. orthopaedic injuries, or the pain is a time-limited episode, e.g. exacerbations of chronic non-malignant pain, postoperative pain, or sickle cell crisis.

6. Be sure the patient receives what he/she feels is an appropriate explanation from the appropriate person of why he/she has pain. Ask the patient what has been said about the cause of the pain and whether or not this makes sense. If not, identify if there is anyone in particular, such as the doctor, whom the patient would like to have explain the reason for the pain. The nurse also needs to be prepared to explain to the patient why pain is present. An explanation from the nurse may suffice or be very helpful in addition to explanations from others. The explanation need not be detailed or time consuming.

Every attempt needs to be made to provide an explanation which is understandable to the patient. This increases the patient's satisfaction with the care received and tends to reduce the patient's requests for diagnostic tests, the extent to which he/she uses health-care services, and changes from one clinic or doctor to another (Deyo and Diehl, 1986).

7. Avoid sudden withdrawal of narcotic and sedative medications. Some patients have tried the "grandstand" approach of suddenly stopping all narcotic/sedative drugs. The results are often devastating to the patient. Not only does the patient face sudden return of pain, anxiety, and other emotional disturbances but also experiences very uncomfortable withdrawal, described as "super-flu" with narcotic withdrawal, and characterized by irritability, motor tremor, and other sometimes more severe symptoms with tranquillizer/sedative withdrawal.

Suggest a gradual reduction of narcotics and sedatives for patients who wish to discontinue their use and have been on them for 3 weeks or longer. Gradual reduction over periods ranging from as short as 1 week for narcotics and longer than 8 weeks for benzodiazepines helps prevent significant withdrawal symptoms and gives the patient time to find alternate methods of dealing with pain and emotional or sleep disturbances. With benzodiazepines and barbiturates, it is best to err on the side of slow detoxification by giving larger doses for longer than may be necessary in order to avoid severe, and sometimes life-threatening, withdrawal (Busto et al, 1986).

When contact with the patient is limited, it is probably wise to decrease only one drug at a time by small amounts over a long period. Try to eliminate the drug that causes the most detrimental effects on functioning, especially a drug that causes sedation. Usually the most offensive drug is a tranquillizer or sedative, such as a benzodiazepine.

Because of exaggerated fears about addiction to narcotics, the latter are usually mistakenly thought to be the most important drug to eliminate. Narcotics do not necessarily cause much sedation after the patient has taken them for a long time. Tolerance to sedation tends to develop rapidly and to a greater extent than tolerance to analgesia. Research shows that certain patients with chronic non-malignant pain have been successfully maintained on narcotics for long periods and that use of narcotics enables patients to return to work when other approaches fail (Portenoy and Foley, 1986; Tennant et al, 1988).

8. When analgesics are required, give them orally, if at all possible, at high enough doses to provide satisfactory pain relief, and often enough on a regular, rather than on a PRN basis, to prevent the return of pain. Analgesics should never be withheld until the pain becomes severe. During an exacerbation of chronic pain, the parenteral route may be used initially to relieve severe pain quickly, but then the patient should be changed to oral analgesics as soon as possible, probably both narcotic and non-narcotic (see Chapter 4, regarding how to use oral analgesics for severe pain).

> **KEY POINT:** Either use narcotics well or use them not at all. If narcotics are prescribed, the frequency and dose must be adequate to relieve the pain.

9. Review analgesics being used for relief of chronic (vs. acute) pain, usually with the goals of avoiding narcotics, encouraging non-narcotic analgesia, and suggesting trials of appropriate classes of drugs recently found to have analgesic properties for specific conditions, e.g. anticonvulsants and antidepressants for neuropathic pain. Narcotic analgesics are not strictly prohibited in the treatment of chronic non-malignant pain, but because of side effects, such as sedation, constipation, and possible increased doses over time due to tolerance to analgesia, narcotics are avoided unless other treatment measures fail. Then, narcotics

may be considered appropriate if they enable the patient to maintain or improve quality of life or level of function, and if the pain is felt to be opiate-responsive.

Muscle relaxants constitute another class of drug that is used with caution. The effectiveness of muscle relaxants when they are taken orally is somewhat questionable. If they do produce muscle relaxation, this is often accompanied by some sedation. Thus they are usually used on a time-limited basis, sometimes for an acute injury or exacerbation, or in conjunction with active physiotherapy until the patient is able to do exercises that keep the muscles from contracting (see p. 117).

Since non-narcotic analgesics such as paracetamol or nonsteroidal anti-inflammatory drugs rarely interfere with daily function, their regular use may be indicated when analgesics are needed for a patient with chronic non-malignant pain. The most effective non-narcotic with the fewest side effects for the individual is given at the highest appropriate dose and on a regular basis (see Table 4.2, pp. 66–67).

Relatively recently certain types of neuropathic pain have been successfully treated with drugs other than the usual analgesics. Dull, aching neuropathic pain may respond to antidepressants (see pp. 115–116). Lancinating or shooting neuropathic pain may be relieved by anticonvulsants (see pp. 116–117).

Careful selection and adjustment of medications for pain relief may result in good pain control without the use of narcotics.

10. When it is obviously very likely that the patient will return for treatment of chronic pain, try to develop a summary of the present treatment and a plan for the return visit. It is especially important to identify which pain-relief measures have been effective and which have not, hopefully enabling the staff to avoid repeating any approaches that were not effective.

The goal of the following is to use the information available from this admission/clinic visit to facilitate arriving at the best possible plan for pain relief for the next attendance. Further, by involving the patient and showing respect for his/her opinion, other desirable outcomes of this interaction may be that an adversarial relationship is avoided or minimized and the patient feels less angry, anxious, or helpless when next seen. Within the constraints of time, try the following (this is an outpatient example):

- About 24 hours before discharge, make a list of all pain-relief measures used during this hospitalization, e.g. all analgesics, sedatives, muscle relaxants, and other pain-related medications administered, any non-invasive pain-relief measures used, and physiotherapy (involve the physiotherapist, if possible, or at least obtain specific information about what was done and what exercises are recommended now).
- Review this list with the patient and ask if there are any additions.
- Ask the patient to give an estimate of how helpful each item was. Use information from flow sheets (e.g. p. 38), if available.
- Based upon the patient's answers, identify with the patient what would seem to be a logical plan of treatment when he/she returns. Findings may suggest a revision of the previous plan. For example, if the patient had both narcotics and nonnarcotics ordered but they were never given together, the future plan may be to try this combination.
- Provide the patient with a written copy of the plan, and keep a copy on the ward.
- Integrate this plan with medications, exercises, and any other approaches for pain control following discharge. The patient/family teaching point "Planning for the Future: Review of Pain Relief Measures", Appendix, may be copied and used for this purpose. This form may be completed by both patient and nurse. One copy is given to the patient and another is kept in the patient's notes.

11. Decreasing the severity of a chronic sleep disturbance is a priority, and the appropriateness of antidepressants and relaxation techniques should be evaluated. Sleep disturbances are common in chronic non-malignant pain, and their continuation may have an increasingly detrimental effect on the patient's efforts to manage pain. A poor night's sleep contributes to depression, muscle soreness, difficulty thinking, and decreased motivation. Avoid sedative/hypnotic medication to which the patient may become tolerant, especially benzodiazepines and barbiturates. Tricyclic antidepressants, Chapter 4, at sub-therapeutic doses are often excellent bedtime sedatives. Also offer to help the patient learn relaxation techniques, Chapter 6, that may promote sleep and assist in sleeping on if he/she wakes during the night.

12. Offer pain-relief alternatives likely to be most consistent with the patient's coping style, e.g. active vs. passive methods of coping with pain. When the pain is brief, or acute, passive coping styles, e.g. depending on others for help, are generally more effective than active coping, and probably should be encouraged. The patient may very well recover from acute illness more rapidly if he/she decreases physical and emotional demands and allows others to care for him/her for a brief time.

However, as pain becomes chronic, maintaining quality of life and a high level of function is usually better accomplished with active coping styles, e.g. learning self-management techniques, than with passive ones. In an acute situation or when structured time with the patient is limited, it is difficult to change the patient's coping style. However, knowing the type of coping the patient uses helps determine which pain-relief measures might be most successfully offered to the patient.

Patients with passive coping styles tend to avoid physical activity and to depend on others to tell them what to do about pain control. Their coping style may consist mainly in taking medication for pain relief, accepting or requesting help from others, talking about their pain, and resting frequently. These patients might most readily accept not only medication regulation, but also use of heat, cold, and perhaps TENS, listening to music for distraction, relaxation if it is made easily available, a backrub, or group support such as maintaining contact with their church.

Patients who have active coping styles may use medication and other approaches used in the more passive coping style but they also tend to try to ignore the pain, stay busy, and engage in physical activities. These patients might most readily accept experimenting with various types of pain relief, including cutaneous stimulation (Chapter 5), or noninvasive pain relief (Chapter 6), relaxation, consulting with the physiotherapist to determine appropriate daily exercise, or contacting a self-help organization such as Self-Help In Pain (SHIP). Usually active coping styles should be encouraged, but caution patients to pace themselves (see Patient/Family Teaching Point: Pace Yourself, Appendix).

13. Help the patient learn and plan to use coping strategies, especially relaxation, that avoid catastrophizing. Catastrophizing is a form of thinking that focuses on the negative characteristics of a situation and escalates to feeling helpless to control pain and believing that the worst may happen. This prevents the patient from making realistic choices about how to keep pain under control.

A variety of coping strategies may also help the patient regain control, including silently repeating hopeful statements such as "I can handle this. I know what to do," using imagery, or performing a distraction strategy (Chapter 6). Help the patient anticipate problems and decide on a course of action in advance. Try writing down the specific problem in one column and the possible solutions in the adjacent column. This is an exercise in problem-solving, and it gives the patient something tangible to turn to when in distress and unable to think clearly.

Relaxation techniques seem particularly helpful to people with chronic pain of any type. Explain to the patient that using a relaxation technique, such as a tape or music, is a way of slowing down and calming down so that it is easier to think of ways to cope with the pain instead of becoming more upset and overwhelmed by the pain.

14. Help the patient develop his/her own daily commitment to specific activities, e.g. physical and/or social, especially a return to employment of any type, if appropriate. Physical or mental activity is important for all patients who must cope with pain daily, but it seems especially important for the depressed patient (consider using Patient/Family Teaching Point: Overall Daily Plan, Appendix, as a guide). Returning to employment is not always appropriate. The patient may be far too disabled to return to the previous employment, and re-education for a new job may not be feasible. For the very disabled patient, guidelines for simply maintaining the normal sensory environment may be appropriate (pp. 167–168). Or, the patient may have been retired from work for some years and have no desire to return. A female patient may never have worked outside the home.

However, if at all possible, for the patient who was employed prior to the onset of pain, a return to some level of employment is helpful in many ways, ranging from earning money to increasing feelings of worth. Even volunteer work without financial compensation may have many advantages such as providing one type of support system for the patient, distracting the patient from pain, and increasing feelings of being capable and

adequate because of making some sort of contribution to others.

15. Help those living with the patient, especially the partner, to work with the patient to establish expectations and limitations regarding the activities of the patient and others in relation to the patient's pain. Any person living with the patient may experience uncertainty and helplessness, even physical problems, due to activities or changes necessitated by the patient's pain. Such persons may benefit from identifying the extent to which they can realistically control the pain and daily living activities. It may be helpful to emphasize the following:

- The patient is in charge of controlling his/her own pain.
- Pain should not become the partner's or family's dictator.
- What can the patient commit him/herself to doing regardless of what the pain is like? A list of specific activities is helpful. Others close to the patient need to know what they can depend on. This also helps the patient feel responsible and adequate.
- What can the partner or family members do to help the patient without placing a burden on themselves?
- Are there things the patient does not want the partner or family to do for him? For example, the patient may feel embarrassed or "babied" by certain types of help.
- Which activities or plans include the patient but should be carried out even if the patient is unable to participate?
- Are there certain times when the patient should avoid talking about the pain felt?
- Should the patient consider using resources outside the partner or family to meet certain needs, e.g. someone else to talk to about the pain or engaging in recreational or social activities without the family? If the patient has sources of satisfaction outside the family, the family need not feel totally responsible for the patient's well-being and the patient need not feel completely dependent on the family.

16. Review with the patient existing support systems, and suggest additional ones, if appropriate. Support systems include groups or individuals to whom the patient may turn for assistance with managing pain. Family members or those living with the patient are a common support system. However, the entire burden of support should not fall on the family or partner alone. Family members need to be able to set limits on what they can do for the patient.

Other support systems that the patient can contact on a regular basis include friends not living in the home, members of the health-care team such as a psychologist or nurse, members of various groups to which the patient belongs such as church groups, people who regularly engage in activities of the patient such as volunteer projects, and co-workers if the patient is employed.

The need for a contact person 24 hours a day is especially important for the patient with severe pain and depression. It is likely to be a difficult need to meet. For reasons mentioned above, this person should not be someone living with the patient. The contact person might be a health professional such as an appropriately trained community nurse in home-care, a friend outside the home, or a member of a local organization of patients with chronic pain.

The contact person and all members of the patient's support systems need to realize that attempting to rescue the patient from pain is not the answer and that a permanent "happy ending" is not likely. It is very difficult to be the person the patient contacts when the latter needs help with unrelieved pain. By definition, there is no instant or magic remedy. The helping person must know that the pain is likely to continue.

The most important help that others can offer the patient is to believe what the patient says, not argue with the patient, and validate with the patient that it is indeed difficult to try to cope with ongoing pain. The most reassuring assistance is usually an emphasis on the patient's attempts to handle the pain and an acceptance of the fact that attempts will not always be successful. Continued attempts must be encouraged. The patient can benefit from knowing that his/her reactions to this devastating situation are understandable, that someone believes the pain is exactly what is claimed, and that someone likes him/her enough to continue a relationship.

17. Consider obtaining the assistance of a physiotherapist to help the patient identify physical exercises that are appropriate with realistic goals. Patients with chronic pain tend to become inactive and physically deconditioned. Many have an exaggerated fear that exercise will increase the pain. Thus the patient may benefit in several ways from closely supervised physical activity.

The patient needs to know exactly what exercises to do, how many repetitions, for how long, and how often. It is very important to help the patient avoid doing exercises to the point of causing pain. Hence the emphasis is on doing exercises that are appropriate, not pushing until there is pain. The patient's regime is set at a level that hopefully will not precipitate pain.

The exercises should be written down for the patient. Encourage the patient to keep a written performance record and to note any problems that arise. The daily diary (Appendix) or a modification of it may be used for this purpose. A written record helps the patient feel a sense of achievement and enables the physiotherapist to make appropriate changes.

18. Review with the patient any types of help sought outside traditional medical practice, providing appropriate encouragement or suggesting precautions. It is not unusual for patients with chronic pain and musculoskeletal problems to seek non-medical health care such as homeopathy, osteopathy, acupuncture, faith healing or various health foods. In fact, patients with pain are probably the largest group of patients utilizing these services. These non-medical modalities are not necessarily harmful and may prove somewhat helpful if they are appropriately supervised by the nurse ordoctor. Stress to the patient the importance of using these approaches in addition to rather than instead of traditional health care.

19. All recommendations to the patient regarding management of chronic pain need to be specific and detailed, in writing with a copy for the patient and health-care team, and incorporated with any other recommendations so that a picture of the total plan is readily available. To put all of this in writing is admittedly time consuming and may not seem very practical in an acute care setting. However, with any chronic health problem, the patient is likely to receive numerous instructions from various health-care team members. It is difficult for the patient to remember these, and team members are not always aware of what other recommendations have been made. It is also likely that some instructions may be incompatible or contradictory. Thus in the long run, it undoubtedly saves time for the patient and health-care team if all attempts to help the patient are organised into one plan.

It is also helpful if one person, e.g. the primary nurse, is designated as being responsible for coordinating the total plan. Then both patient and health-care team members know whom to contact when conflict or confusion occurs. To begin such a plan, spend time obtaining information from the patient, verifying this with other health-care team members, and putting it in written form. When simple problems or crises occur, this information facilitates evaluating the circumstances and deciding on a course of action, saving time and making the situation much easier for everyone.

20. Evaluate the effectiveness of each specific recommendation made to the patient for pain management, with regular follow-up and possibly written daily diaries kept by the patient. Too often the assumption is made that a recommendation is safe, effective, and useful unless the patient reports a problem. However, the patient may encounter problems following through with a recommendation and decide to discontinue it without realizing that a simple modification might enable him/her to benefit from it. Or, the patient may continue with something in spite of problems and cause a worsening of the existing condition. In either case, considerable time may be lost before the health professional is contacted and able to rectify the situation.

Whether the recommendation involves medication, relaxation, physiotherapy or some other approach, make specific plans for follow-up. This may involve making another appointment to see the patient or asking the patient to telephone in a few days to report the results.

If a period of days or weeks goes by, the patient is likely to have difficulty remembering exactly what happened in relation to the pain. Also, memory may be adversely affected by many factors, such as pain, medications, and a desire to forget or deny how severe the pain has been. When the patient is unable to give a specific or complete history of pain and its management, a daily diary is probably indicated (see appendix).

21. Assess the need for requesting a consultation to identify and treat depression, anxiety, or post-traumatic stress disorder. Anxiety and depression often accompany pain, especially prolonged pain, and may respond to various types of treatment. For example, if depression predates the onset of pain, psychotropic medication may be indicated. There is growing recognition that pain incurred as a result of unexpected trauma, e.g. an accident, may lead to post-traumatic stress disorder. This may have a paralysing effect on the patient but may respond well to therapy that gradually desensitizes the patient to fearful aspects.

However, suggesting a psychological or psychiatric evaluation may well be misunderstood by health-care team members and the patient. Try to approach this by clarifying that depression and anxiety rarely cause pain, but that pain often causes depression and anxiety that make the pain more difficult to handle. Reassure the patient that after even a few weeks of pain, it would be abnormal if no depression or anxiety were felt. It may be more acceptable to the patient and less misleading to others to refer to the frustration, rather than the depression, of dealing with pain.

22. Assess suicidal risk. Many people with chronic non-malignant pain become depressed, and it is not unusual for them to express suicidal thoughts. The risk of suicide is high in some patients, particularly those with prolonged, uncontrolled, severe pain. Remember, too, that the angry patient may also be suicidal. When a patient expresses hostility toward us for our failure to help, it is altogether too easy to withdraw and become self-protective, forgetting momentarily how devastated the patient may be.

GUIDELINES FOR USING PATIENT/FAMILY TEACHING POINTS (SEE APPENDIX)

Once as much of the pain as possible has been relieved, the major goal in assisting the patient with chronic non-malignant pain is to maintain as good a quality of life as possible on a daily basis. Many approaches discussed elsewhere in the book may be helpful. But no matter what strategies are used by the patient, it is almost always necessary to focus on how to incorporate these into the patient's daily living. Two recurring themes in helping patients accomplish this are **pacing** and **looking at the total day.** The patient/family teaching tools in the appendix address these issues. They may be duplicated and given to the patient/family.

INDIVIDUALIZED NURSING-CARE PLAN

Patient with Chronic Non-malignant Pain

Patient Description: Ms G., 35 years old, has had neck and shoulder pain often accompanied by headaches for 5 years, initially caused by lifting heavy objects at work and later precipitated by simple, daily tasks involving use of the arms. She is divorced and has three children living with her, ages 7, 9, and 12 years. None of her family live near her but she mentions several friends and she attends church one or more times each week. She is presently employed as a sales assistant in a department store, but she misses an average of 4 days a month due to pain. She cries easily and says that she is unable to do all that is expected of her and that her frequent absences from work occur when she does too much. Her history includes regular Accident and Emergency visits (about twice a month) for narcotic injections, numerous medical consultations including neurology, completion 3 years ago of a structured in-patient pain management programme in another town, a variety of analgesic prescriptions, and several physiotherapy referrals that included an unsuccessful trial of TENS. Now she has been referred to an out-patient orthopaedic clinic for on-going care. Her present prescriptions include Tylex (codeine 30mg and paracetamol 500mg) for pain and diazepam 10mg for nervousness and sleep. She reports taking diazepam once during the day, usually in the morning, and 2 at night (30 mg/day) and Tylex only on days when she really hurts, approximately 5 a day at times.

Assessment	Potential Nursing Problems	Planning/Intervention	Evaluation/Expected Outcomes
Identify: • Satisfaction with explanations given for cause of pain. • Location and intensity of present pain, using a scale of 0–10 (0 = no pain, 10 = worst pain). • Increases or changes in pain. • What has and has not been effective in relieving pain, using a modification of the form Planning for the Future, (see appendix). • Degree of sleep disturbance. • Coping style. • Regular daily activities in relation to pain and methods of pain relief, especially analgesic consumption, requesting the patient to complete the daily diary (see appendix) for 2 weeks. • Support systems. • Use of non-traditional medical care. • All current recommendations from others regarding pain management, e.g. exercises suggested by physical therapy.	Pain, chronic, related to myo-fascial problems in the neck and shoulders. Ineffective individual coping related to mostly dependent and passive approaches to pain control. Knowledge deficit related to methods of formulating a comprehensive plan for daily management of chronic pain.	(The following would be attempted over a period of several months in approximately the sequence listed.) Express belief in what she says about her pain and respect for the frustration of dealing with daily pain. Obtain a prescription for the strongest non-narcotic she can take without side effects, and instruct her in regular daily dosing (use Patient/Family Teaching Point for NSAIDS, see appendix) to relieve on-going pain and prevent increased pain. Use whichever method of cutaneous stimulation has been most effective in the past, encouraging regular use for on-going pain as well as use as soon as pain begins to increase. Encourage cold if it has not been tried. For episodes of increased pain, suggest the following: • Take Tylex as soon as pain begins to increase rather than waiting until pain is severe, and take it every 4 hours until pain begins to subside. • Continue regular doses of non-narcotic. • Use cutaneous stimulation. • Contact nurse (yourself) by phone. (Use of nurse as support system.) • Ask a friend to take care of her children for a while. (Use of friends as support system.) Further increase her support systems by encouraging her involvement with church activities and suggesting she talk with her clergyman about calling him when her pain becomes distressing.	Returns for each clinic appointment with partially completed daily diaries. Expresses increased confidence in managing pain by using prayer, relying on friends, calling the nurse, planning her total day, etc. After a few days on regular doses of non-narcotic, reports decrease in daily pain level from 5 to 3 on a scale of 0–10. Decrease in days absent from work. Reports improved sleep from antidepressant. Gradual decrease in daily dose of diazepam. When pain increases, calls nurse or clergyman, takes Tylex on a regular basis, asks a friend to help with responsibilities, and does not go to Accident and Emergency.

Continued

INDIVIDUALIZED NURSING-CARE PLAN cont'd

Patient with Chronic Non-malignant Pain—cont'd.

Assessment	Potential Nursing Problems	Planning/Intervention	Evaluation/Expected Outcomes
• Need for a consultation to treat depression, anxiety, or post-traumatic stress disorder. • Suicidal risk.		Help prevent catastrophizing by, for example, incorporating her frequent use of prayer as a relaxation strategy, encouraging her to pray regularly for about 5 minutes at least 2 or 3 times a day, especially at bedtime and when she becomes agitated or fearful of increasing pain. Introduce pacing by encouraging her to give priority to safe care of her children and going to work, spending less energy on housekeeping chores and delegating some to her children (use form Pace Yourself, Appendix). For sleep disturbance, suggest use of an antidepressant and a gradual decrease in diazepam. Avoid sudden withdrawal of diazepam. For example, suggest decreasing the total daily dose by 2.5mg every 3 weeks. Provide a written copy of all recommendations for pain management made by all health-care team members. Review this to establish feasibility of accomplishing all of it. Formulate a reasonable daily plan, incorporating recommendations of health-care team plus instructions on form Overall Daily Plan, Appendix . Evaluate all recommendations using the Daily Diary, or telephone calls if necessary, and establish regular clinic appointments, perhaps every 3 weeks.	

SELECTED ANNOTATED REFERENCES THAT CITE RESEARCH OR GIVE CLINICAL SUPPORT

Since so much controversy exists about what chronic non-malignant pain includes and how it should be treated, the content of this chapter reflects, to the maximum extent possible, the conclusions of research studies rather than the sometimes divergent opinions expressed in the literature. Following are the references most pertinent to the approaches suggested in this chapter.

Ahles, T.A., Yunus, M.B., and Masi, A.T.: Is chronic pain a variant of depressive disease? The case of primary fibromyalgia syndrome. *Pain,* **29**:105–111, 1987. The responses of 45 patients with primary fibromyalgia (PFS), 29 with rheumatoid arthritis (RA), and 31 people with no pain showed no differences between the PFS and RA groups regarding depression, although the PFS group has no known organic pathology, unlike the RA group. The data do not support the hypothesis that chronic pain in the absence of a known organic problem is a variant of depressive disease.

Bouckoms, A.J., Litman, R.E., and Baer, L.: Denial in the depressive and pain-prone disorders of chronic pain. *Clin. J. Pain,* **1**:165–169, 1985. In this study of 63 patients admitted to an in-patient centre for treatment of chronic non-malignant pain, depressive symptoms were present in 60%, but major depression in only 24%, a lower percentage than previously thought. Evidence strongly suggested developmental deficit in the childhood of 37% of these patients, but findings failed to support the diagnosis of pain-prone disorder as a masked depressive equivalent.

Crook, J., and Tunks, E.: Defining the "chronic pain syndrome": an epidemiological method. *Clin. J. Pain,* **1**:159–163, 1985. This study suggests that people suffering persistent pain attending chronic pain clinics are not typical of people in the general population who suffer persistent pain but who are not referred to such clinics. Pain clinic patients are likely to be deficient in coping skills, have greater adaptive problems with work and social roles, and suffer greater emotional distress. The authors suggest that because the pain of pain clinic patients is more often related to work injuries and there is a greater probability of litigation or compensation, the adversarial relationships may be a significant factor.

Crue, BL, Jr: Multidisciplinary pain treatment programs: current status, Clin J *Pain* **1**:31-38, 1985. In this review article the author addresses the practical problem of defining and classifying pain, suggesting that an acceptable pragmatic definition of pain is simply anything the patient says it is and that all pain is real (exclusive of the malingerer who consciously fakes pain). He explains the differences between the centralist and peripheralist concepts of chronic pain and the implications of this controversy. In brief, the peripheralist believes that chronic pain results from peripheral input; the centralist believes that the initial peripheral input no longer exists but has become some type of central "memory of pain" that now produces chronic pain. Both the peripheralist and centralist mechanisms of pain may exist and may occur together. The author traces the evolution of pain-treatment facilities and suggests what should be included in a comprehensive pain center.

Deyo, R.A., and Diehl, A.K.: Patient satisfaction with medical care for low-back pain. *Spine,* **11**:28–30, Jan–Feb 1986. In a questionnaire survey of 140 patients seen in a walk-in clinic for mechanical low back pain (70% of less than 2 weeks' duration), the most frequently cited source of dissatisfaction was failure to receive an adequate explanation of the problem. In comparison with patients who felt they had received an adequate explanation, those who did not thought more diagnostic tests were needed, were less satisfied with their physicians, and were less likely to want to see the same physician again. Explanation of symptoms has a high priority among these patients, and the data suggest that giving this explanation does not take additional physician time and might reduce future utilization of the health-care system. Patients not given an explanation seem inclined to see more physicians and request more testing.

Dworkin, R.H., et al: Unravelling the effects of compensation, litigation, and employment in treatment response in chronic pain. *Pain* **23**:49–59, 1985. The relationships among compensation, litigation, employment, and short- and long-term treatment response in a series of 454 chronic pain patients was examined. Only employment at the time of the initial evaluation significantly predicted long-term outcome, whereas compensation and litigation did not. A review of the literature confirmed that there are very few differences between patients who do and do not receive compensation and between patients who do and do not have litigation pending with respect to an organic basis for pain and psychological distress. Litigation also does not influence pain behavior. Further, there is little support for the view that patients typically resume employment when litigation is settled (Mendelson, 1982). The authors suggested that attention be directed away from concern about "compensation neurosis" and directed toward returning the patient to appropriate employment as soon as possible. The article ends with a quote made in another article over 20 years ago, suggesting that returning injured workmen to a job within the limitations imposed by their pain might maintain morale and allow sufficient time for the problem to subside (White, 1966).

Feuerstein, M., Carter, R.L., and Papciak, A.S.: A prospective analysis of stress and fatigue in recurrent low back pain. *Pain,* **31**:333–344, 1987. This study compared 33 ambulatory chronic low back pain patients with an asymptomatic control group. Both groups recorded mood states for 14 consecutive days. No mood state was predictive of pain onset, but fatigue was associated with pain 24 hours following onset. Overall the patients had a higher level of anxiety than the control group, but the results do not support the notion that negative mood states initiate or exacerbate pain.

Hendler, N.: Depression caused by chronic pain. *J. Clin. Psychiatry,* **45**:30–38, Mar 1984. The author believes that the psychogenic pain diagnosis is made far too freely, arising from the mistaken belief that chronic pain without organic disease is largely imaginary. He also notes that chronic pain almost always leads to depression and that this is normal. Four stages of pain are reviewed, from acute through the patient's acceptance of chronic pain. He notes that patients who exaggerate their pain are showing that they are devastated by their problem, not that they are imagining or faking pain. He feels outright fabrication of chronic pain is rare and that a patient's report about pain should not be challenged. He believes that the following are commonly missed causes of chronic pain: myofascial syndrome (or fibromyositis), sympathetic dystrophy, facet syndrome, and temporomandibular joint syndrome. He says there is evidence that sleep disorder contributes to myofascial syndrome.

Holzman, A.D., and Gulliver, S.: The relationship of a history of alcohol use disorder to treatment completion in chronic pain management. *Clin. J. Pain* **2**:115–118, 1986. An assessment of 104 patients referred to a pain management programme did not show that patients with a history of alcohol use disorder were more likely to be current prescription medication users. However, these patients were less likely to complete the treatment programme.

Krishnan, K.R.R., et al: Chronic pain and depression. I. Classification of depression in chronic low back pain patients. *Pain,* **22**:279–287, 1985. An association between chronic pain and depression has been recognized for a long time. This study of 71 patients with chronic low back pain revealed 31 with major depression and 8 with minor depression. In most patients the depression developed after the onset of pain; however, 10 patients had major depression preceding the onset of pain. The data suggest that there is more than one type of depression involved with chronic pain.

Krishnan, K.R.R., et al: Chronic pain and depression. II. Symptoms of anxiety in chronic low back pain patients and their relationship to subtypes of depression. *Pain,* **22**:289–294, 1985. This study of the same 71 patients with chronic low back pain (above) showed that anxious mood and other symptoms of anxiety are common, especially in patients with depression.

Leavitt, F., and Sweet, J.J.: Characteristics and frequency of malingering among patients with low back pain. *Pain,* **25**:357–364, 1986. A survey mailed to orthopaedic surgeons and neurosurgeons in six geographic regions of the United States resulted in 105 responses. The purpose was to determine if a consensus of opinion underlies clinical judgment concerning malingering in the low back pain patient. (The purpose was not to identify the actual existence of malingering.) The majority of surgeons (60%) agreed that malingering was relatively infrequent, occurring in 5% or less of patients who present with low back pain. Data suggested that high estimators of malingering (20% or more of patients) place more importance on the patient receiving compensation or having seen an attorney. (Note that numerous studies in this annotated reference section do not support a high incidence of malingering related to compensation or litigation.) The symptoms defined as most important in determining malingering were related to exaggeration, such as overreaction during the examination or disablement disproportionate to objective findings, or incongruity, such as pain complaints not following organic patterns and weakness to manual testing not seen in other activities. These opinions, of course, need validation.

Linton, S.J.: Behavioral remediation of chronic pain: a status report. *Pain,* **24**:125–141, 1986. A review of publications, especially those from 1982 and later, concerning the outcome of behavioral treatment of chronic non-malignant pain showed that relaxation training was a particularly valuable tool in decreasing reported pain intensity. However, data did not support the need to use biofeedback with relaxation.

Melzack, R., Katz, J., and Jeans, M.E.: The role of compensation in chronic pain: analysis using a new method of scoring the McGill pain questionnaire. *Pain,* **23**:101–112, 1985. A study of 145 patients with chronic low back or musculoskeletal pain revealed that, contrary to popular opinion, compensation and non-compensation patients had virtually identical pain scores and pain descriptor patterns. In fact, the patients receiving compensation had significantly fewer visits to health professionals. Apparently, receiving compensation decreases anxiety. Results for the two groups were also similar on the MMPI pain triad of depression, hysteria, and hypochondriasis.

Philips, H.C.: The effects of persistent pain: the chronic headache sufferer. *Pain,* **21**:163–176, 1985. In a survey of 360 patients with chronic headache, including migraine and tension, sleep disturbance was common, but depression was not found to be elevated.

Pilowsky, I., Crettenden, I., and Townley, M.: Sleep disturbance in pain clinic patients. *Pain*, **23**:27–33, 1985. In a study of 100 outpatients with chronic pain, only 10 reported good sleep, while 70 reported poor sleep. Patients with poor sleep had significantly more affective disturbance, especially depression, than patients reporting good sleep, and also greater pain and physical disability. Sleep disturbance may provide an index to the severity of symptoms. Possibly treatment that is aimed specifically at alleviating sleep disturbances will in turn reduce emotional and physical symptoms.

Portenoy, R.K., and Foley, K.: Chronic use of opioid analgesics in non-malignant pain: report of 38 cases. *Pain*, **25**:171–186, 1986. Although the use of narcotic analgesics for relief of chronic non-malignant pain is currently viewed with disfavour, this study shows that prolonged narcotic therapy can be a safe and more humane alternative to the options of surgery or no treatment if there is no history of drug abuse. Out of 38 patients maintained on narcotics (for 4 or more years in 19 patients), management became a problem in only 2 patients, both with a history of prior drug abuse. Patients occasionally required escalation of dose for exacerbation of pain, but doses usually returned to a stable baseline afterward. Acceptable or fully adequate relief of pain occurred in 24 patients, inadequate relief in 14. No patient underwent a surgical procedure while receiving narcotics, but there were few gains in employment or social function. Patients were on a variety of narcotics, e.g. oxycodone, propoxyphene, codeine, and for 23 patients the total daily dose was less than the equivalent of 20mg morphine IM.

The authors suggest that opioid maintenance therapy be instituted only after other reasonable attempts at pain control have failed, have been documented in the patient's record, and pain continues to be a major impediment to improved function; that a single physician with committed involvement oversees the therapy, seeing the patient monthly and determining the monthly medication requirement; and that the patient gives fully informed consent, perhaps in writing, including discussion of the risks of using alcohol and other drugs along with opioids.

The authors review three other studies that reported similar success with prolonged use of opioids for chronic non-malignant pain. Taub (1982) treated 313 such patients with narcotics for up to 6 years, with problems in only 13 patients, all of whom had prior histories of substance abuse. Tennant and Uelman (1983) treated 22 patients who failed to benefit from pain clinics with the result that all reduced medical visits and two-thirds returned to work. France, Urban, and Keefe (1984) treated 16 patients with narcotics as a part of a comprehensive pain management program, resulting in improved function.

Reesor, K.A., and Craig, K.D.: Medically incongruent chronic back pain: physical limitations, suffering, and ineffective coping. *Pain*, **32**:35–45, 1988. Forty chronic low back pain (CLBP) patients with pain and symptomatology incongruent with physical findings were compared with 40 CLBP patients without incongruent findings. Incongruent pain patients engaged in less effective coping styles, such as catastrophizing, feeling less in control, and perceiving the pain as more disturbing and debilitating, than the other CLBP patients. Those with incongruent pain also had more restricted physical functioning. Pending litigation and compensation were not associated with incongruent pain, and there was no difference between the two groups regarding medication intake.

The authors suggest that clinicians are more likely to conclude incorrectly that patients with incongruent pain symptomatology have minimal organic basis for pain and that they are malingering. This in turn may prompt the patient to display more exaggerated pain expression to convince the clinician of the reality of the pain. These results suggest, however, that these patients are most likely have problems with their coping styles and their confidence in their ability to cope with the pain.

Rowat, K.M., and Knafl, K.A.: Living with chronic pain: the spouse's perspective. *Pain*, **23**:259–271, 1985. In this study of 40 spouses of patients with chronic non-malignant pain, 83% of spouses reported experiencing some form of health disturbance attributed directly to the pain. The most frequently named source of difficulty for 40% of spouses was the sense of helplessness over how to help with their mate's pain. Uncertainty concerning management of the pain and daily family life were central to the spouses' distress. Enabling spouses to recognize what control they have over the pain and their daily lives seems an important feature of working with families where an adult has chronic non-malignant pain.

Roy, R., and Thomas, M.R.: Elderly persons with and without pain: a comparative study. *Clin. J. Pain*, **3**:102–106, 1987. This study of 205 elderly subjects who were members of an organization devoted to providing social and recreational programs for the elderly revealed that nearly 70% reported a pain problem, but that disability due to pain was virtually unknown. Firm conclusions are not possible but it appears that the lack of disability due to pain was related to an attitude of acceptance of limitations accompanying aging, a zest for living, well-planned days, and continued social integration with the community at large.

Swanson, D.W., Maruta, T., and Wolff, V.A.: Ancient pain. *Pain*, **25**:383–387, 1986. Of approximately 1000 patients evaluated for an inpatient pain program, 45 (about 4%) had pain for 25 years or more, called ancient pain. This group was compared with a group of subjects with a mean duration of pain of 6.6 years. Compared with those with pain of shorter duration, those with ancient pain used more analgesics and sedatives, with more women than men misusing drugs; had a higher incidence of face and head pain; had more frequent diagnoses of depression; and had a greater elevation of nearly all clinical MMPI scales. The importance of continuing careful medical evaluation was illustrated in one case-study of a 60-year-old man with a 40-year history of back pain who obtained limited benefit from the pain rehabilitation programme. He returned 18 months later with no change in his complaints of pain but with a fever. Evaluation revealed renal cell carcinoma. This was treated, but the patient died of the malignancy about 18 months later.

Tennant, F.S., Robinson, D., Sagherian, A., and Seecof, R.: Chronic opioid treatment of intractable, non-malignant pain. *Pain Manag.* 18–26, Jan–Feb 1988. This is a report on a pilot programme that accepted referral of 52 patients who had severe, non-malignant pain, who were already dependent upon the daily administration of opioids for pain relief, and who had unsuccessfully attempted all other acceptable pain treatments. These patients were evaluated and treated between 1979 and 1986. Almost all patients had a history of numerous Accident and Emergency visits or repeated hospitalizations. The usual reason for referral was inadequate pain relief. Four techniques were used to control pain: raising the daily dose of the patient's usual opioid; changing to a longer-acting opioid, usually methadone or oxycodone (some patients, however, got better pain relief from a short-acting opioid); combining low doses of methadone, 10–40 mg per day, with a short-acting opioid such as codeine; or supplementing the patient's usual dose with morphine or hydromorphone suppositories. Interestingly, in a few patients who complained of inadequate pain relief on large doses of opioid, plasma concentrations were low, indicating inadequate absorption from the gastrointestinal tract. They obtained relief by taking another opioid. After systematic changes in opioid dosage were done using the four techniques described above, 46 of the 52 patients achieved adequate pain control according to the patient's self-report. Further, there was a marked reduction in hospitalizations and Accident and Emergency visits. The authors conclude that chronic administration of opioid is a relatively safe and effective treatment and should be made available as a last resort to this population of patients.

REFERENCES AND SELECTED READINGS

Ahern, D.K., Adams, A.E., and Follick, M.J.: Emotional and marital disturbance in spouses of chronic low back pain patients. *Clin. J. Pain,* **1**:69–74, 1985.

Anderson, E.F., Hegstrum, J.A., and Charboneau, G.J.: Multidisciplinary management of patients with chronic low back pain. *Clin. J. Pain,* **1**:85–90, 1985.

Aronoff, G.M.: *Pain centers: a revolution in health care.* Raven Press, New York, 1988.

Auld, A.W., Maki-Jokela, A., and Murdoch, D.M.: Intraspinal narcotic analgesia in the treatment of chronic pain. *Spine,* **10**:777–781, 1985.

Brena, S.F., and Chapman, S.L., eds: Chronic pain: management principles. Clin. Anaesthesiol. 3:1–236. W.B. Saunders, Philadelphia, Jan 1985.

Brena, S.F., and Chapman, S.L., eds: *Management of patients with chronic pain.* S.P. Medical & Scientific Publications, New York, 1983.

Brown, G.K., and Nicassio, P.M.: Development of a questionnaire for the assessment of active and passive coping strategies in chronic pain patients. *Pain,* **31**:53–64, 1987

Corey, D.T., Etlin, D., and Miller, P.C.: A home-based pain management and rehabilitation program: an evaluation. *Pain,* **29**: 219–229, 1987.

Coulehan, J.L.: Adjustment, the hands and healing. *Cult. Med. Psychiatry* **9**:353–382, Dec 1985.

Crue, B.L., Jr, ed: *Chronic pain: further observations from City of Hope National Medical Center.* S.P. Medical & Scientific Books, New York, 1979.

Duckro, P.N., Margolis, R.B., Tait, R.C., and Korytnyk, N.: Long-term follow-up of chronic pain patients: a preliminary study. *Int. J. Psychiatry Med.,* **15**:283–292, 1985–86.

Dworkin, R.H., Richlin, D.M., Handlin, D.S., and Brand, L.: Predicting treatment response in depressed and non-depressed chronic pain patients. *Pain,* **24**:343–353, 1986

Edwards, P.W., Zeichner, A., Kuczmierczyk, A.R., and Boczkowski, J.: Familial pain models: the relationship between family history of pain and current pain experience. *Pain,* **21**:379–384, 1985.

Feinmann, C.: Pain relief by antidepressants: possible modes of action. Pain 23:1–8, 1985.

France, R.D.: Chronic pain and depression. *J. Pain Sympt. Manag.* **2**:234–235, Fall 1987

France, R.D., Urban, B.J., and Keefe, F.J.: Long-term use of narcotic analgesics in chronic pain. *Soc. Sci. Med.* **19**:1379–1382, 1984.

Guck, T.P., Skultety, F.M., Meilman, P.W., and Dowd, E.T.: Multidisciplinary pain center follow-up study: evaluation with a no-treatment control group. *Pain,* **21**:295–306, 1985.

Haley, W.E., Turner, J.A., and Romano, J.M.: Depression in chronic pain patients: relation to pain, activity, and sex differences. *Pain,* **23**:337–343, 1985.

Holzman, A.D., and Turk, D.C., eds: *Pain management: a handbook of psychological treatment approaches.* Pergamon Press, New York, 1986.

Jensen, J.: Life events in neurological patients with headache and low back pain (in relation to diagnosis and persistence of pain). *Pain,* **32**:47–53, 1988.

Karen, H.: *Rehabilitation research review, rehabilitation of persons with chronic low back pain*. ATA Institute, Washington, DC, 1986.

Kotarba, J.A.: *Chronic pain: its social dimensions*. Sage Publications, Beverly Hills, Calif, 1983.

Levy, A.B.: Delirium and seizures due to abrupt alprazolam withdrawal: case report. *Clin. Psychiatry*, **45**:38–39, Jan 1984.

Low back pain: what about chiropractors? *Harvard Med. School Health Letter* **13**:1–4, Jan 1988.

Mendelson, G.: Chronic pain and compensation: a review., *J. Pain Sympt. Manag.* **1**:135–144, Summer 1986.

Mendelson, G.: Not "cured by a verdict": effect of legal settlement on compensation claimants. *Med. J. Aust.* **2**:132–134, 1982.

Merskey, H.: Classification of chronic pain: descriptions of chronic pain syndromes and definitions of pain terms. *Pain*, (suppl 3):S1–S225, 1986.

Merskey, H., et al: Psychological normality and abnormality in persistent headache patients. *Pain*, **23**:35–47, 1985.

Miro, J., Garcia-Monco, C., Leno, C., and Berciano, J.: Pelvic pain: an undescribed paroxysmal manifestation of multiple sclerosis. *Pain*, **32**:73–75, 1988.

Muse, M.: Nonadversarial pain management. Clin. J. Pain 3:61, 1987.

Muse, M.: Stress-related, posttraumatic chronic pain syndrome: behavioral treatment approach. *Pain*, **25**:389–394, 1986.

Muse, M.: Stress-related, posttraumatic chronic pain syndrome: criteria for diagnosis, preliminary report on prevalence. *Pain*, **23**:295–300, 1985.

Parris, W.C.V., Jamison, R.N., and Vasterling, J.J.: Follow-up study of a multidisciplinary pain center. *J. Pain Sympt. Manag.*, **2**:145–151, Summer 1987.

Perlman, S.L.: Modern techniques of pain management. *West. J. Med.* **148**:54–61, Jan 1988.

Portenoy, R.K.: Postherpetic neuralgia: a workable treatment plan. *Geriatrics* **41**:34–48, Nov 1986.

Rigge, M.: Pain (Research on prevalance of pain in Britain). *Which? Way to Health*, April 1990, pp. 66-68.

Russel, M.L.: *Behavioral counseling in medicine: strategies for modifying at risk behavior*. Oxford University Press, london, 1986.

Sammons, E.E.: Drug use and misuse in chronic pain patients. *Clin. Anaesthesiol.* **3**:169–181, Jan 1985.

Stanton-Hicks, M., and Boas, R.A., eds: *Chronic low back pain*. Raven Press, New York, 1982.

Stimmel, G.L., and Escobar, J.I.: Antidepressants in chronic pain: a review of efficacy. *Psychophar-macol. Bull.* **22**:865–869, 1986.

Swerdlow, M.: Anticonvulsant drugs and chronic pain. *Clin. Neuropharmacol.* **7**:51–82, 1984.

Taub, A.: Opioid analgesics in the treatment of chronic intractable pain of non-neoplastic origin. In Kitahata, L.M., and Collins, D., eds: *Narcotic analgesics in anesthesiology*, pp. 199–208, Williams and Wilkins, Baltimore, 1982.

Taylor, A.G., Skelton, J.A., and Butcher, J.: Duration of pain condition and physical pathology as determinants of nurses' assessments of patients in pain. *Nurs. Res.* **33**:4–8, Jan-Feb 1984.

Tearnan, B.H., and Dar, R.: Physician ratings of pain descriptors: potential diagnostic utility. *Pain*, **26**:45–61, 1986.

Tennant, F.S., and Uelman, G.F.: Narcotic maintenance for chronic pain: medical and legal guidelines. *Postgrad. Med.* **73**:81–94, 1983.

Turk, D.C., Rudy, T.E., and Stieg, R.L.: Chronic pain and depression. I. "Facts". *Pain Manag.* **1**:17–25, Nov–Dec 1987.

Turk, D.C., and Stieg, R.L.: Chronic pain: the necessity of interdisciplinary communication. *Clin. J. Pain* **3**:163–167, 1987.

Turner, J.A., and Clancy, S.: Strategies for coping with chronic low back pain: relationship to pain and disability. *Pain*, **24**:355–364, 1986.

Urban, B.J., et al: Long-term use of narcotic/antidepressant medication in the management of phantom limb pain. *Pain*, **24**:191–196, 1986.

Wall, P.D., and Melzack, R., eds: *Textbook of pain*. Churchill Livingstone, New York, 1984.

Ward, N.G.: Tricyclic antidepressants for chronic low-back pain: mechanisms of action and predictors of response. *Spine*, **11**:661–665, Sept 1986.

Ward, N., et al: Antidepressants in concomitant chronic back pain and depression: doxepin and desipramine compared. *J. Clin. Psychiatry* **45**:54–57, Mar 1984.

Wells, N.: Back pain, Office of Health Economics. London, 1985.

Whipple, B., and Komisaruk, B.R.: Elevation of pain threshold by vaginal stimulation in women. *Pain*, **21**:357–367, 1985.

White, A.W.M.: Low back pain in men receiving workmen's compensation, *Canad. Med. Assoc. J.* **95**:50–56, 1966.

8

Pain in Children

Special Considerations

The younger the child, the more defenceless he/she is against pain. Yet it seems that the younger the child is, the less adequately is pain controlled. Problems of under-treatment of pain that adults encounter are even more extensive with children. For example, the first hospice for care of terminally ill patients in the United Kingdom was established in 1905, and the first in the United States in 1974; however, a survey conducted by Children's Hospice International in 1984 revealed that less than 10% of 1400 hospice programmes provided services to children (Martin, 1985). This has led to the concept of providing hospices specifically for children, and the first such hospice in the United Kingdom, Helen House, was established at Oxford in 1982. Incredibly some health professionals still debate issues such as whether or not the young child (especially the newborn) hurts at all, and if so, whether or not it matters.

Certainly not all children in pain receive inadequate relief. However, inadequate or inconsistent pain relief for children appears to be widespread.

■ The authors would like to thank Joann M. Eland, PhD, RN, Associate Professor of Nursing, the University of Iowa, Iowa City, Iowa, and Donna L. Wong, MN, RN, PNP, Nurse Counsellor in Private Practice, Tulsa, Okla, for their review of this chapter and for their many helpful comments and suggestions.

The causes of inadequate pain relief in the young may more likely be due to lack of knowledge than to lack of concern. Fortunately, in the last few years interest in pain control in children has increased significantly. A search of the literature published between January 1970 and August 1975 produced a total of only 1380 articles on pain, and a meager 33 dealt with pain in children (Eland and Anderson, 1977). A quick glance at the reference section of this chapter shows we have come a long way since then. Further, by the late 1980s two books devoted entirely to pain in children were published: *Pain in Children and Adolescents* by McGrath and Unruh (1987) and *Childhood Pain* by Ross and Ross (1988).

However, we are still far from a satisfactory approach to assessing and relieving pain in children. In an early study of pain in children one school-age child completed the sentence "Pain is ..." like this: "When you scream for help and nobody comes" (Schultz, 1971, p. 672). To this child we may now say that we are coming — too slowly perhaps, but we are on our way.

This chapter provides basic information and practical approaches to assessing and relieving pain in children. Specifically, the *purposes of this chapter* are:

- To apply previously discussed methods of assessment and pain relief to children from birth through adolescence.

Age Group Terminology	Approximate Age
Premature neonate or pre-term infant	Gestational age equal to or less than 37 weeks
Neonate (full term) or newborn	Gestational age approximately 38 weeks Postnatal age less than 1 month
Infant	1 to 12 months
Toddler	1 to 3 years
Pre-schooler	3 to 5 years
School age	5 to 12 years
Adolescent	13 to 18 years

*Terminology for the different age groups in the very young is not yet standardized and is probably one of the reasons for inconsistent research findings regarding assessment and relief of pain in the very young.

Table 8.1 Guide to Definitions of Age Groups*

- To add selected age-related considerations (see Table 8.1 for age-related terminology).
- To encourage the reader to explore beyond this chapter to obtain additional knowledge and to develop greater skills in caring for children with pain.

Thus throughout this chapter the reader will be referred to previous chapters and will also be introduced to new material. The level of material presented assumes that the reader has basic knowledge about the growth and development of children and about the care of children during health and illness.

However, this chapter is neither a complete nor a thorough guide to pain in children. Not only is paediatrics itself a speciality area but also there are many sub-specialities within paediatrics. *The limitations of this chapter* are:

- Specialities within paediatrics are addressed only briefly and some not at all. Separate discussions of the various speciality areas such as those related to age groups (e.g. neonatology), and those related to specific diagnostic entities (e.g. cancer, headache, or abdominal pain), are beyond the scope of this chapter.
- This chapter is an introduction to some of the many possible ways of helping children with pain and their

parents. Due to space limitations, many methods of assessment and relief that are included in this chapter are not discussed in detail.

References at the end of the chapter will guide the reader in pursuit of additional information and more depth in various speciality areas. Further, considerable research is in progress, and the reader is reminded to refer to the current professional literature for the most recent advances in the care of children with pain.

MISCONCEPTIONS

Pain in children tends to be doubted more often and to a greater degree than pain is doubted in adults. Children with pain are not only subjected to the many misconceptions that exist about pain in the adult patient but also encounter misconceptions specific to their young age. Pain in preverbal children seems especially likely to be questioned. But even when the child is verbally fluent, adults unfortunately tend to behave as if children are less credible or less accurate when they report pain.

An article published in 1968 (Swafford and Allan) illustrates the confusion that seems to have existed for some years about pain in children. These inconsistent statements appeared within the same article: "As long as the onset of remembrance of pain is unknown, the neonatal infant has the same right to analgesia and anaesthesia as older patients" (p. 132). Yet the authors also state "Paediatric patients seldom need medication for relief of pain after general surgery" (p. 133) and "Infants and children below the age of 10 years rarely require narcotics" (p. 135).

In an attempt to clarify confusion about pain and its treatment in children, some of the more common misconceptions are presented below. Each misconception is accompanied by information that corrects it.

Misconception: Young children, particularly neonates, do not feel pain.

Correction: There is more evidence to support the belief that neonates, including premature infants, feel pain than there is evidence that they do not. In any debate of this point, the burden of proof now rests with those who believe the neonate or young child feels no pain. Further, there is some evidence that younger children are more sensitive to pain than older children.

Although it is simply not yet known whether children experience more, less, or the same pain as adults, it is far from a proven fact that pain in infants and children is absent or even less than that in adults. Many years ago it was thought that the infant did not feel pain because of an immature nervous system in which the nerves were not completely myelinated. However, it is now known that myelination progresses rapidly after birth and in any case is not necessary for pain transmission.

Several recent studies clearly document that newborns and infants respond with dramatic physiological and observable behavioural changes to stimuli that adults would feel as painful, such as heel lance, immunization and other surgical procedures.* Further, an article in *The New England Journal of Medicine* (Anand and Hickey, 1987) listed 201 references pertaining to pain in the human neonate. There is little doubt that neonates and infants feel pain, or, more specifically, react to noxious stimuli with distress indicative of pain.

Several preliminary studies of children's reports of pain have suggested that there is increased pain with decreased age, i.e. given comparable stimuli, younger children may perceive a greater intensity of pain than older children (e.g. Fowler-Kerry and Lander, 1987; Haslam, 1969; Katz et al, 1982). Further, in a study of analgesic requirements of terminally ill children, those age 1–4 years required higher doses of oral narcotics than those 5–14 years old (Burne and Hunt, 1987). Infants and toddlers also seem to require higher doses of IV fentanyl for procedural pain than do older children (Billmire, Neale and Gregory, 1985; Maunuksela, Rajantieand Silmes, 1986).

Whenever pain in infants and young children is questioned by the health-care team, the above articles may be cited along with the following examples of *statements made by professional organizations regarding pain and its control in the child:*

- In a joint statement from the American Academy of Pediatrics, the chairmen of the Committee on Fetus and Newborn, Committee on Drugs, Section on Anesthesiology, and Section on Surgery state, "There is an increasing body of evidence that neonates, including those born pre-term, demonstrate physiologic responses to surgical procedures that are similar to those demonstrated by adults and that these responses can be lessened by anaesthetic

agents... (We) believe that local or systemic pharmacologic agents now available permit relatively safe administration of anaesthesia or analgesia to neonates undergoing surgical procedures and that such administration is indicated according to the usual guidelines for administration of anaesthesia to high-risk, potentially unstable patients... the decision to withhold such medication should be based on the same medical criteria used for older patients" (Poland, Roberts, Gutierrez-Mazorra and Fonkalsrud, 1987, p. 446).

- In a joint statement, presidents of both the International Pain Foundation and the International Association for the Study of Pain state, "We are appalled by the needless pain that plagues the people of the world.... We are appalled, too, by the fact that pain is most poorly managed in those most defenseless against it—the young and the elderly. Children often receive little or no treatment, even for extremely severe pain, because of the myth that they are less sensitive to pain than adults and more easily addicted to pain medication" (Liebeskind and Melzack, 1987, p. 66).

- In the publication of the proceedings of the 8th World Congress of Anaesthesiologists, Steward (1984) states, "The extent of pain perception of the pre-term infant is unknown, but it is generally accepted that pain can be felt, and therefore, that anaesthesia is indicated during surgical procedures" (p. 189).

Misconception: If a child can communicate well verbally, a denial of pain should be regarded as true.

Correction: Certain fears will cause children to conceal the fact that they have pain. Also, children with prolonged or gradually increasing pain may not be able to identify that pain is what they are experiencing.

Children may deliberately and effectively disguise or deny their pain, since admitting to pain may result in various frightening possibilities. Many children are extremely fearful of injections. If the child learns that a report of pain results in "the needle", the child may decide he/she would rather endure the on-going pain than be subjected to this method of providing pain relief. Also, many children do not comprehend the

---

* Bell and Ellis, 1987; Craig, McMahon, Morison and Zaskow, 1984; Dale, 1986; Franck, 1986; Izard, Hembree, Dougherty and Coss, 1983; Owens and Todt, 1984; Stang et al, 1988; Williamson and Williamson, 1983.

logic underlying the administration of a painful injection in the buttocks to obtain relief in the abdomen 30 minutes later. Further, the child may believe that if he/she denies the existence of pain, he/she can go home from the hospital sooner or avoid some painful procedure.

Sometimes the issue is not denial of pain but rather an inability to recognize pain, particularly chronic pain. As time goes on, the child seems to lose the basis of comparison and forgets what it was like not to have pain. Even short-term pain that has a gradual onset may be difficult for the child to identify. Pain that suddenly occurs or increases usually evokes an immediate response from even the neonate, but when pain sneaks up, the child's awareness and response may be minimal or less dramatic. Awareness of the underlying pathology, e.g. what a tumour may be compressing, and trial doses of analgesic accompanied by careful observations of the effect are important ways to uncover this type of pain. (See discussion of denial of pain and refusal of analgesics in Chapter 2.)

Patient Example

A 13-year-old with far advanced Ewing's sarcoma repeatedly denied pain. However, he was silent and withdrawn and his pathology strongly suggested that pain was present. Therefore trial doses of analgesics were administered regularly, and 36 hours later the child's behaviour had changed into that of an outgoing teenager. When he was questioned about why he had not admitted that he hurt, he replied, "I think I had been hurting for so long that I forgot what it was like not to hurt" (Eland, 1985b, p. 109).

Misconception: If the child neither reports pain nor requests pain relief, no pain is present.

Correction: Children do not necessarily know that they must report pain or ask for pain relief. Once they have done so, they may not understand the need to persist.

Obviously, the neonate or older child who cannot verbalize well will not be able to request or demand pain relief. Neonates and pre-verbal children simply have no choice about whether or not they must tolerate pain since they are unable to defend themselves.

Due to a lack of experience with pain, older children may not know the alternatives to suffering pain nor the socially expected methods of obtaining pain relief. Like some adults, they may not even know it is necessary to report the fact that they feel pain, assuming that the health professionals caring for them are aware of this and are in control of it (Stevens, 1987). Apparently, it is not unusual for the parents of a child with pain to fail to request an analgesic for the child because they think the nurse is aware of what is needed and can be given (Eland, 1988a).

Patient Example

A 17-year-old daughter of one of the authors who had an emergency appendectomy remarked, "I just lay there afraid of more pain." She was asked, "Why? Didn't you know you could tell the nurse you hurt and ask for medication to relieve it?" She replied, "I didn't know I had to tell the nurse. I thought the nurses were taking care of me. I think most teenagers would just lie there like me and think the nurses know they hurt and are doing whatever they can to stop it. I thought the nurses had done all they could do." When asked later what she thought of the situation, she answered, "Tell the nurses we're younger than adults and more scared so we need more attention." (Reported with the patient's permission.)

Misconception: If the child sleeps, plays, or can be otherwise distracted from pain, there is not much pain present.

Correction: Children are especially talented in the effective use of distraction and physical activity to handle pain, and they may also sleep or pretend to do so as a method of handling pain. The child, like the adult, need not act like he/she is in pain to be in pain (see Chapter 2). Further, the coping mechanisms of distraction, physical activity, and sleep cannot be used indefinitely.

Children are perhaps even better able than adults to use distraction to make pain more bearable. Children also seem to make greater use of physical activity to cope with pain. Adults in pain tend to "take to bed" but, especially for young children, physical activity is often an effective coping strategy. A toddler usually becomes more, not less, active when in pain. This, coupled with the belief that if the toddler gets out of his/her room and keeps moving he/she may avoid painful procedures, results in a big incentive for early ambulation in this age group.

Playing may provide both distraction and physical activity as well as give the child a sense of control. Many children in pain play until they almost drop from exhaustion. Escape to the playroom is especially likely since it serves the dual purpose of removing the child from his/her room and providing the opportunity for play.

On the other hand, children may sleep or pretend to do so to withdraw from pain or procedures. The child may fake sleep, hoping to avoid or delay a painful procedure, e.g. burn debridement. Or, a child may close the eyes to block out a distressing environment, e.g. monitors and tubes. Even a baby may use sleep as a coping strategy. In response to postoperative pain following circumcision, healthy newborns may sleep quietly without eye movement rather than fuss and cry, as do older infants. When they are aroused, some are irritable. Others are lethargic and difficult to arouse (Marshall et al, 1980). This behaviour may persist for up to 24 hours. Thus many of the child's effective coping strategies preclude expressions of pain. If the child is pretending to be asleep or playing and laughing to distract him- herself from pain, he/she cannot at the same time show expressions of pain such as crying.

Misconception: Children are able to tolerate pain better than adults.

Correction: The above misconception is the culmination of several previously discussed mis-conceptions, e.g. that children often do not act like they are in pain since they may play, engage in physical activity, or sleep, and may not report pain or ask for pain relief.

Actually, to some extent children may be able to use certain coping strategies, such as distraction and physical activity, better than adults. Thus at times the child may be better able to tolerate pain than the adult, but the adult's overall ability to cope with pain is considerably greater than the child's. The adult with pain usually has more control over the situation, including more knowledge about pain-relief measures such as medications or complementary therapies, more outside sources of help such as friends to telephone, and more ability to persist in obtaining pain relief such as asking the doctor to increase a dose or requesting a consultation.

The child's apparent tolerance for pain may also depend upon which painful experience is being observed, e.g. how distressing that type of pain is for the child and which coping strategies the child is permitted

to use. During a venepuncture, the adult may simply talk and seem to ignore it, but a child may protest or scream. On the other hand, following a herniorrhaphy, an adult may walk bent over for a week, but a child may be playing actively within a few hours. One study showed that children who were not afraid did not always demonstrate behavioural distress even though they reported pain (McGrath, de Veber and Hearn, 1985).

Further, as the duration of pain increases, some children, like adults, seem to have less tolerance for pain, e.g. they may scream with greater forcefulness (Katz, Kellerman and Siegel, 1980; Savedra, 1976). It is difficult to know if this is because perception of pain increases or because the child feels more distress.

However, most children probably tolerate pain simply because they cannot or do not pursue pain relief as well as adults. As discussed above, older children, may assume that "the nurse is taking care of me and knows when I hurt and what I need."

Misconception: The potential side effects of narcotics make them too dangerous to use to relieve pain in children.

Correction: If the pharmacokinetics are understood and the child is properly observed, narcotics may be used safely in children, even in newborns, premature infants, and children being weaned from a ventilator (e.g. Bell and Ellis, 1987; Lynn, Opheim and Tyler, 1984; Lynn and Slattery, 1987).

All drugs have potential dangers, but this does not preclude the use of narcotics since the most dangerous side effects, such as respiratory depression, can be easily monitored. Further, should respiratory depression or any other life-threatening side effects occur from narcotics, the effects are almost always easily and quickly reversed by the antidote naloxone.

Misconception: Narcotics should be avoided or used sparingly in teenagers because they are at high risk of developing narcotic addiction. Indicators of abuse or addiction in teenagers are when they enjoy themselves after narcotic injections, prefer the "needle" to a tablet, or ask for narcotics before they are due.

Correction: The risk of narcotic addiction in adults being treated with adequate doses of narcotic for pain relief is considerably less than 1%, and there is no reason to suspect it is any greater with children. When a person's pain is relieved, it is natural and even desirable for them to enjoy being free of pain. A preference for

227

injections instead of oral narcotics is most likely related to the fact that a dose of narcotic given IM provides 2–6 times more pain relief than the same dose given orally. Requesting narcotics frequently is usually a sign of inadequate pain relief; and some studies indicate there is considerable variation in morphine pharmacokinetics among individual children (Nahata and Miser, 1985). All of the above misconceptions about addiction are discussed in greater detail in Chapter 4.

Further, research on children fails to support fears that addiction will result from use of narcotics to treat severe pain. In one study of 38 children and adolescents with sickle cell crisis, 76 episodes were treated with continuous IV narcotic infusion, and no addictive behaviour was observed in any of the children (Cole, Sprinkle, Smith and Buchanan, 1986). Similarly, in three adolescents using IV PCA for sickle cell crisis pain, no evidence of abuse was noted (Schechter, Berrien and Katz, 1988).

On the other hand, physical dependence (withdrawal) may occur after a course of narcotics. Parents and children as well as health-care team members need to understand that this is not the same thing as addiction.

The increase in substance abuse during the 1980s, especially among adolescents and young adults, has resulted in increased concern about narcotic addiction in this age group when their pain is relieved with narcotics. Not only does this probably contribute to under-treatment of pain in children on a daily basis in many clinical areas, but also it prevents research efforts. Deeply entrenched beliefs about the addiction proneness of adolescents with sickle cell disease resulted in the medical staff of one hospital withdrawing previously granted approval to perform research on the use of IV PCA (patient controlled analgesia) in these adolescents (Schechter, Berrien and Katz, 1988, p. 112).

Misconception: Pain is not life-threatening and has no lasting effect on infants and young children, and they will not remember it anyway.

Correction: Pain may have adverse and even life-threatening consequences in the neonate. The onset of memory is unknown, and absence of conscious memory of an event is not evidence that it has no physical or psychological effect on the person.

While some argue that the neonate cannot feel pain, others fear that pain in neonates may be life-threatening, especially if the baby responds with crying and decreased oxygenation, which may in turn cause intraventricular haemorrhage, a major cause of death among premature infants (Beaver, 1987). Heel lance is considered a relatively benign procedure, yet research has shown that it causes increased heart rate and blood pressure and decreased transcutaneous oxygenation in premature infants (Beaver, 1987). Neonates with various physical causes of pain have been noted to be agitated, cyanotic, bradycardic, hypoxic, and hypercapnic (Bell and Ellis, 1987).

Regarding the onset of memory of pain, a study of behavioural responses of infants in an immunization clinic strongly suggests that by 9 months of age some infants cry in anticipation of an immunization based on having had one 6 weeks earlier (Levy, 1951, 1960).

Very little data exists on the later effects of past experience with pain, but one study of adults revealed that those who had more pain during childhood had greater sensitivity to pain and less tolerance to pain as adults (Collins, 1965). A study of children showed that those who had endured extensive periods of pain were developmentally retarded or regressed (Quinton and Rutter, 1976).

COMMUNICATING WITH THE CHILD AND PARENTS

One of the ways that assessment and relief of pain in the child differs from the adult scenario is that additional communication skills are necessary. Involvement of the parents or family is usually more essential in the care of the child than in the adult. Further, communication with the child requires an appreciation of the cognitive abilities and concerns of the various age groups along with the usefulness of play as a communication tool.

Talking with the parents

When the patient is an infant or child, the rights to which a patient is entitled are essentially transferred to the parents. As guardians of those rights, the parents need information that will enable them to make decisions about the care of their child. Further, the child's family can be a great asset in the assessment and relief of the child's pain.

Family members other than the parents may also be important and helpful resources. The child's grand-parents or brothers and sisters may offer valuable information and assistance. And of course, the parents are not always the key carers. For convenience, however, the key carers are usually referred to in this chapter as parents.

Talking with the parents provides not only an opportunity to obtain helpful information about assessing and relieving the child's pain and to show respect for the parents' knowledge about the child but also an avenue for increasing the parents' sensitivity to their child's pain and increasing their ability to be involved in providing pain relief. Regarding assessment and relief of a child's pain, important topics to discuss with the child's parents are:

- Their priorities in the current situation. The parents may have more immediate concerns than pain and may not be able to focus on identification and relief of pain until other matters have been settled. Try to sit down with them in a quiet place to discuss this, and offer to talk and to answer questions then and later. Decreasing the parents' fears usually also decreases the child's apprehension. Even the very young child tends to assimilate the parents' attitudes about painful or distressing events.

- Clarification of what is meant by the word *pain*. Many adults associate the word with discomfort that is excruciating and intolerable. Identify the words the parents use to refer to pain, e.g. *uncomfortable* or *hurting*, and try to use these terms in the discussion. Also, ask them what words the child uses for pain.

- The child's previous experiences with pain. A history of the child's pain experiences may be very helpful, including types of pain, how the child reacts to pain, and what the parents do for the child (Hester and Barcus, 1986). Talking with the parents about the child's past pain experiences and reactions to them may help improve their ability to detect pain in their child. In particular, it may help to review the differences in the child's behaviour when pain is sudden and when it is on-going.

- Their assessment of the child's current pain. The parents have the potential for understanding their child better than anyone else by virtue of having spent more time with the child under a variety of circumstances. They possess a wealth of information about the child. Remember, however, that the parents may be at a disadvantage in some situations. The parents may never have seen the child in as much pain before, or they may be upset about the illness or surrounding circumstances. Parents may have emotional reactions of helplessness, fear, or guilt that may prevent them from admitting to themselves that the child has pain, e.g. guilt over allowing an accident to happen. Or, they may need to feel in control of the child's behaviour or need to feel that the child is being brave.

- The need to inform the health-care team whenever they think the child is hurting. Remind the parents, as well as the child, that the team does not necessarily know when the child is hurting.

- How the Continuous-Assessment Sheet (see Figure 8.1) may be used to identify the safety and effectiveness of pain-relief methods. Ask for the parents' help in devising an assessment sheet specific to their child. For example, even when the child is pre-verbal, the nurse and parent may use the assessment sheet together to titrate analgesics. A continuous IV infusion of morphine was successfully given for several days in a 10-month-old child with prolonged cancer pain simply by the mother and nurse making independent pain ratings based on observation of various types of behaviour, such as sleep and crying (Dothage, Arndt and Miser, 1986). Examples of how the assessment sheet may be modified for a young child are shown in Figure 8.1.

- How they feel about staying with the child while he/she is in pain, especially during painful procedures. Explain that no matter how old they are, children often want their parents with them when they are hurt and scared. Pre-school children in particular fear abandonment. Help the parents recognize the value of their presence when the child is in pain. This is difficult for many parents. To help the parents feel more comfortable, offer to answer questions about the child's condition and care. The more frightening the circumstances, the more important the parents' presence may be. Therefore, for example, during a visit to Accident and Emergency, allow the parents to sit near the child and to touch him/her. Prior to surgery, let parents stay during induction of anaesthesia. Allow and encourage parents to visit the intensive-care unit. When the parents and other family members must be absent, encourage them to bring toys or pictures from home. If possible, have the family make tape recordings for their child, e.g. conversation over dinner or bedtime stories.

- What they usually do to relieve the child's pain or to comfort the child. Ask them what is most effective and what they would like to try now. Also, ask parents if they know how far in advance the child wants to be informed about painful events. Children

between 5 and 12 years of age have greatly different preferences for the timing of information about pain (Ross and Ross, 1984).

- Their interest in learning new ways to comfort the child and relieve the pain, e.g. non-invasive techniques for pain relief such as helping the child distract him- herself with a favourite story or by blowing bubbles.

CONTINUOUS-ASSESSMENT SHEET FOR PAIN

Age: 6 Mo

Patient *Jim*   Date *13/4*

*Pain rating scale used *Behaviours indicating pain: cry, whimper, restlessness, frowning or angry looking face, inability to sleep, parent unable to elicit smile.*

Purpose: To evaluate the safety and effectiveness of the analgesic(s).

Analgesic(s) prescribed: *Paracetamol 60mg.*

Time	Possible Pain rating behaviours	Analgesic	R	P	BP	Level of arousal	Possible Other† comfort behaviours	Plan and comments

CONTINUOUS-ASSESSMENT SHEET FOR PAIN

Age: 6 years

Patient *Joy*   Date *29/5*

*Pain rating scale used *Faces* (0 = no pain, 5 = worst pain)*

Other common pain behaviour is crying easily and wanting to be held.

Purpose: To evaluate the safety and effectiveness of the analgesic(s).

Analgesic(s) prescribed: *Codeine 30mg + Paracetamol 240mg*

Time	# of face Pain rating	Analgesic	R	P	BP	Level of arousal	Other† Pain behaviours	Plan and comments

Fig. 8.1 Examples of how the continuous-assessment sheet from p. 38 can be adapted for infants and young children.

* See Figure 8.2 for illustration of the "faces" rating scale.

KEY POINT: For the benefit of both the child of any age and the parents, allow the parents to be with, touch, and hold the child to the maximum extent possible without causing undue distress for either.

Parent interview. The topics discussed above may be formulated as statements and questions to use in on-going discussions with parents about assessing and relieving pain in their child, presented in an interview format on pp. 232–233. A copy of this form along with a copy of the assessment sheet on p. 38 may provide an efficient and fairly complete approach to obtaining information. As mentioned previously, it may also be a useful format for teaching the parents about assessment and relief of pain in their child and involving them in this process.

Thus the *purposes* of the "Parent Interview Regarding Child's Pain/Hurt" are:

1. To obtain information from the parent(s) regarding assessment and relief of a child's pain, especially if the child is reluctant or has minimal or no ability to communicate the information him- herself.
2. To increase the ability of the parent(s)'s to assess and relieve pain in the child.
3. To involve the parent(s) in providing comfort and relief for the child.

Ideally, the interview is conducted with the nurse and both parents present. Of course, a formal interview with a written record of the responses is not always possible or desirable. It is probably most important for those children with prolonged or frequent hospitalizations or illnesses. The questions may be discussed with the parents without actually using the written tool, or the tool may be used as a guide to discussions without making a written record of the parents' responses.

Further, the interview is an on-going process, and certainly need not be completed at one sitting. Not all the questions need to be asked of all parents. Simply begin with the questions that seem most relevant. When time is limited, give priority to identification of verbal and non-verbal behaviours that indicate pain so that a meaningful assessment sheet can be implemented to evaluate pain relief measures. In some instances the parents might wish to keep a copy of the interview and make their own notations on it to share with the nurse later.

Talking with the child

Even when a child has no verbal ability, such as is the case with the infant, talking to the child may convey at least an attitude of caring. Remember, too, that the child's ability to understand what is said is almost always greater than the ability to communicate verbally. Non-verbal communication, such as some form of play or physical contact, may be an important aspect of interacting with a child of any age.

General guidelines for communicating with infants and older children (adapted and expanded from Whaley and Wong, 1989) are:

- Allow the child time to feel comfortable with the nurse.
- Avoid sudden or rapid advances.
- Talk to the parent initially if the child is shy.
- Try talking through objects such as dolls or puppets before directly questioning a young child.
- Give the older child an opportunity to talk without parents or friends being present.
- Assume a position that allows for eye contact but do not force eye contact or maintain it for long periods.
- Speak in a quiet, unhurried voice.
- Use simple words and sentences, but avoid upsetting terms such as "needle" instead of injection or "deaden" instead of numb.
- Offer physical contact. Once an infant or toddler makes eye contact and shows no fear, hand the child a toy and gradually increase physical contact, eventually holding him/her. A similar approach may be used with the older child, beginning with handing him/her a toy or touching the arm or shoulder, eventually offering physical comfort such as an arm around the shoulder or holding a hand.
- Be honest, especially about the possibility of pain occurring.
- Give the child an opportunity to express concerns and ask questions. Ask open-ended questions, wait for answers, and do not interrupt. Avoid "putting words in his/her mouth".
- Use actual equipment or pictures in explanations. Demonstrate on self or doll, or use figure drawings (e.g. p. 32 or p. 241). Be sensitive to the older child's desire not to be treated childishly.

Parent Interview Regarding Child's Pain/Hurt

Child: Parent/caregiver: Date:

I. Total Current Situation
What are your major concerns (unrelated to pain), if any, about the current situation/hospitalization in general, e.g. finances, care of other children, cause or seriousness of illnesses?

What are your child's major concerns (unrelated to pain), if any, about the current situation/hospitalization in general, e.g. being separated from parent; sleeping in a different bed or room; missing a birthday party; school work, etc?

II. Child's Previous Experiences with Pain/Hurt
What types of pain has your child had before? Include descriptions of cause, duration, severity, frequency, and other important aspects.

What words, if any, does your child use for pain or hurt?

How does your child usually act when *suddenly* hurt, e.g. falls down?

How does your child usually act when he/she has been *hurting for a long time,* e.g. with a sore throat or earache?

III. Assessment of the Child's Current Pain
Since no one but the child knows if he/she hurts, the health-care team needs your help in finding out when your child is hurting and whether or not efforts to relieve the pain are working. What behaviour indicates that your child is or is not in pain at the present time? For example, can you get your child to smile at you?

A written record, called a Continuous Assessment Sheet can be very helpful. What do you suggest is recorded on this sheet?
List types of behaviour that probably indicate pain:

List types of behaviour that probably indicate comfort:

■ May be duplicated for use in clinical practice. From McCaffery, M; Beebe, A; and Latham, J (ed.): *Pain: Clinical Manual for Nursing Practice*, London, 1994, Mosby, an imprint of Times Mirror International Publishers Ltd.

Continued.

IV. Comforting the Child and/or Relieving the Pain

When your child hurts, what do you usually do to comfort your child or relieve the pain? What work best? What could you do now?

When your child hurts, what does the child do for him- herself that seems to help? How can we help the child help him-herself?

Considering the pain your child now has or will have, what are your concerns about being with your child while he/she is hurting or is undergoing a painful procedure?

What would you like to learn about how you can soothe or distract your child during pain?

If painful procedures are performed, do you wish to be with your child? If this varies, during which procedures do you wish to be present and which ones would you rather avoid?

Do you have any ideas about how far in advance your child would like to be informed about a painful procedure?

Other Comments

Is there anything special we should know about your child and pain? Is there anything disturbing to the child that we should *not* do?

Specific guidelines for discussing assessment and relief of pain with the child are:

- Talk with the child about previous hospitalizations and painful experiences. Note the exact words the child uses for pain. Children may not know the names of body parts or the meaning of the word pain. Pain is actually a difficult concept that includes numerous different sensations as varied as pricking from a needle, deep aching visceral pain, headache, and indigestion.

- Regardless of age, remind any child who has verbal ability, even the adolescent, to tell the health-care team when pain is present. Explain that nurses and doctors cannot always tell when the child has pain and that we need his/her help.

- Establish the child's understanding of time. For example, can he/she tell time using a clock or watch? Use this information to help the child understand when pain will occur and how long it will last and how long before analgesics take effect. A timer may be set to illustrate the passage of time before the analgesic relieves pain or the length of time it takes to perform a certain procedure. Ask the child if he/she has any preferences about when he/she would like to be told about an impending painful event, e.g. the day before or an hour before.

- Give the child choices in relation to pain, whenever possible. For example, allow the child to choose which buttock or thigh will receive an injection. Offer two or more methods of handling pain, e.g. holding your hand, looking at a pop-up book, breathing slowly and deeply. Adolescents are particularly resistant to rigid rules and tend to respond well to mature reasoning and explanations.

- State directions firmly and positively along with the exact time an event will occur, especially something painful. Toddlers, preschoolers, and even older children are likely to try to postpone a painful procedure, but after appropriate choices have been given, it is important to proceed. Give one direction at a time and wait until the child has responded; e.g. instruct the child to lie down, then wait until he/she has done so before directing him/her to turn on his/her side. Praise the child for doing what is requested, e.g. "that's right," "very good".

- Perform painful procedures outside the child's room, whenever possible, and never in the playroom. The child needs to feel that bed, room, and playroom are safe places. For example, take the child to the treatment room for painful suture removal or a lumbar puncture. If there is a playroom, post a sign on the door to remind health-care team members that it is off limits for all painful procedures.

- Express a positive attitude toward injuries, procedures, pain, and blood. Keep wounds clean and neat, and comment on any progress or good prognosis, e.g., say that an incision looks good. Explain the need for procedures. If the sight of blood cannot be avoided, assure the child that it is normal, perhaps remarking that it is a good red colour. Let the child know when a procedure is over or when bleeding has stopped. Explore any misconceptions about pain or blood, e.g. indications that the child will die or be disfigured or that all of his/her blood could run out of a hole made by an injection. Discuss when the child will look just like he did before or be able to return home or go to school.

- Discuss with the child what he/she does and does not want done to relieve the pain, and why. Two useful items to ask about are the presence of a parent and the use of plasters. Regardless of age, most children want a parent, especially the mother, present when they hurt. If this is not possible, talk with the child about his/her family, friends, and pets. As for plasters, they seem to have a magic power for very young children, and even an adolescent may want a plaster to shield a wound from sight or to avoid seeing a drop of blood from an injection. For on-going pain or following a painful procedure, the younger child may want a plaster not only on him- herself but also on a doll or some other object.

Patient Examples

Plasters seem to help in a variety of painful circumstances. Young children who have pain under a plaster cast that has been applied to a broken limb may request that a plaster be placed on the cast. Following open heart surgery, one young child seemed distressed and would not co-operate with procedures until the nurse complied with his request to use plasters to cover the transparent dressing over his incision. Another child, 3½ years old, was terminally ill and being cared for at home, receiving morphine at various doses over 100mg/hr. The mother reported to the nurse that her daughter was fully alert and comfortable and had requested that a plaster be placed on the infusion pump because "that's where the feel good comes from" (Wiley, 1988).

- Discuss with the child his/her reactions to pain. Explain that during procedures it may be necessary for the child to help by being very still, but that he/she can usually cry or scream if wished. In spite of the fact that adults are often disturbed by behaviour such as screaming or crying, some children find it helpful and perhaps need permission to act that way without being considered a sissy. However, be alert to the possibility that the child may want very much *not* to cry or scream, and explain tactics such as deep breathing that may help to avoid crying.

- Praise the child's responses to pain and offer a symbol of courage. During or after the procedure, you may say, "You help so much by trying to be still," or, "You are really able to scream and let us know when it's hurting." Offer to let the child keep any clean and safe articles involved in the procedure, e.g. a cotton ball or a syringe without the needle.

- Carefully observe the neonate's, and especially the pre-term infant's, responses to eye contact, touch, or being talked to. A child this age may easily be overloaded with sensory stimuli even from simple manipulations such as feeding, and certainly from a painful event. Frequent rest periods may be needed to allow for recovery from stress and use of self-regulatory behaviour (Als, 1982). Painful procedures probably should be performed as quickly as possible and the premature infant allowed to recover before inflicting additional pain or stimulation. This might decrease the intensity of the physiological response, e.g. smaller increase in heart rate.

An appreciation of the prominent features of the ways children tend to think about and react to pain at different ages aids communication. The reader is referred to other resources for summaries and detailed accounts of the child's concepts of pain during the major stages of cognitive development and responses to pain at various ages.*

Play

Play is a special tool for communicating with children. In relation to pain, play may involve learning about painful procedures before and after they occur, such as handling a syringe or participating in activities such as handing tape to the nurse. Materials for play may include those actually used in the procedure; replicas available in toy stores or from speciality groups; books; pictures of equipment; or the child's doll or stuffed animal.

Play is important business for the child. Whenever possible, use play both before and after a painful experience. Prior to a painful event, play may be used as a rehearsal. After a procedure or during on-going pain, play serves to promote understanding of what is occurring or what has already happened. The possible benefits of play are (Wong and Whaley, 1986):

- Facilitates mastery over an unfamiliar situation.
- Provides opportunity to learn about parts of the body and diseases.
- Corrects misconceptions about the use and purpose of equipment and procedures.
- Provides distraction.
- Promotes relaxation by providing a means for release of tension and expression of feelings.

ASSESSMENT

Assessment of pain in children from birth through to adolescence will include a discussion of the following:

- Assumptions and beliefs about the existence of pain in children and the possible indications of pain.
- A multidimensional approach to assessment of pain.
- Specific pain scales that may be useful with children who are verbally fluent.

Assumptions and beliefs

Assessment of pain in children, especially the very young, requires active use of educated assumptions and guesses. Based on certain assumptions, guesses are made, action is taken, and the outcome is evaluated, recognizing that once again certain assumptions must be made.

*Als, 1982; Als et al, 1986; Hurley and Whelan, 1988; McGrath and Unruh, 1987; Piaget, 1930; Ross and Ross, 1988; Whaley and Wong, 1989; Wong and Whaley, 1986.

The pain sensation is subjective and cannot be proved or disproved in any age group. Thus in the absence of absolute proof, our approach to pain assessment in the child is based on the following basic assumptions or beliefs:

- All children, including neonates, have the ability to feel pain.
- Anything that causes pain in adults also causes pain in children.
- Some things that do not cause pain in adults may cause pain in children.
- Assessment encompasses responses at the moment and over time. Assessments are made at regular intervals and compared, and a written record is kept.
- In determining the presence (not absence) of pain, priority is given to any information directly communicated by the child; i.e. self-reporting of pain is the most valuable method of identifying pain.
- Self-reporting of absence of pain is viewed with suspicion and explored further if pathology or other behaviour indicates that pain might be present. Children, like adults, may deny pain or refuse analgesia for many reasons.
- Children respond to pain not only in a variety of physical and physiological ways but also without exhibiting any observable responses. Lack of response does not necessarily mean lack of pain.

In the assessment of pain in neonates, pre-verbal children, children who are not fluent verbally, and those who are reluctant to admit pain, the following additional assumptions and approaches are especially important:

- In the absence of the ability and willingness for self-reporting of pain, detection of the possibility of pain requires attention to multiple facets with special attention to *changes* in responses.
- Opinions about the child's pain are sought from parents and others.
- An on-going, open dialogue about the child's pain is encouraged in the hope that increasingly accurate assessments and insights will occur.
- There is no way to be sure that a child does or does not have pain—it is always a guess.
- There is no way to be sure that pain-relief measures are or are not effective—this, too, is always a guess.

A multidimensional approach to pain assessment in children

For those children who cannot communicate verbally about their pain, observations must be made of physiological signs and non-verbal behaviour, including vocalizations such as crying or groaning, along with knowledge of pain associated with procedures and pathological processes. Few guidelines exist for which kinds of behaviour are most indicative of pain. The meaning of the direction of change in response—e.g. increased or decreased pulse—is not always clear. Further, since most research on pain, especially in the very young, has been related to brief procedural pain such as responses to injections, very little is known about the child's response to prolonged or chronic pain that may last for hours, days, or months.

Currently, several easily used and apparently reliable and valid instruments or tools are available for assessment of pain in children aged 3 years and older. However, even in children with the ability to communicate verbally, assessment can be seriously hampered by simple problems such as failure to establish what the specific words mean to the child. Or, the child may deliberately conceal pain because he/she fears the consequences of pain; e.g. fear that an injection will be given to relieve pain or fear that pain will result in a longer hospital stay.

The need for reliable and valid tools for assessment of pain in the neonate and very young child is one of the most pressing problems in management of pain in this group. Lack of sufficient data to construct simple and accurate tools for this youngest and most defenseless group of children has probably seriously hampered development of pain-relief strategies, and even prevented an awareness of the need for pain relief.

However, *the absence of reliable and valid pain assessment tools for the very young is perhaps not as important as the willingness to believe that the very young do indeed have pain*, even if we cannot measure it with the seeming accuracy with which we measure pain in older children and adults. Despite having had tools available for several years to assess pain in adults, pain continues to be under-treated. Thus while an assessment tool for the very young is needed, the existence of one would not necessarily assure that pain would be relieved.

While assessment or measurement of pain is absolutely essential if the effectiveness of pain-relief methods is to be identified, simple awareness that the very young are capable of feeling pain may be sufficient data on which to base a systematic attempt to relieve the pain. For example, some physiological parameters (e.g. heart rate) in neonates may be measured in response to procedural pain. Regardless of the direction of change, i.e. increased or decreased rate, the fact that a change occurs may be sufficient evidence that pain is probably perceived. Based on this observation in the individual neonate, the nurse can attempt pain relief, using measures such as narcotics or a dummy, and monitor whether or not this facilitates a return to baseline observations.

However, relying exclusively on behavioural or physiological response has serious limitations. Fatigue alone, due to pain or other reasons, may diminish the intensity of the infant's response to pain. Adults may sleep in spite of severe pain—so may a child. Likewise, in adults autonomic arousal, e.g. increased heart rate, in response to pain may occur briefly but subside in a few moments—this may also happen in a child. Further, at a young age children become aware that non-verbal behaviour is a means of communication. Thus children may be observed to behave in one way when they know others are present, and in another manner when they think they are not being observed. This can easily be misunderstood as some form of attention seeking or manipulation. However, just as an adult stops talking about pain when others leave the room and are unable to hear him/her, so may a child stop crying about pain when believing he/she is alone and there is no one there to hear him/her.

> **KEY POINT:** Although research clearly shows that neonates have a specific response to pain involving crying, heart rate changes, and facial expressions, as pain increases in duration these responses are less and less useful in indicating the presence or severity of pain.

Thus with neonates and even with children who are verbally fluent, the task of assessing pain is not always straightforward. Relying only on any single measure or indication of pain, e.g. self-reporting, physiological changes, facial expression, known physical cause, or crying, may be dangerously limiting.

> **KEY POINT:** In some children assessment of pain requires a multidimensional approach.

Components of a multidimensional assessment of pain in neonates and older children are:

- Initiate discussions about pain. Include the child, if possible, parents, and other caregivers. Do not assume that the presence of pain will be spontaneously reported. Emphasize to the parents and to the child, if the child is capable of self-reporting of pain, that the health-care team members do not always know when a child is hurting. Remind the child at regular intervals that you must be told when pain is felt. Pre-school children can usually understand when they are told that their help is needed in finding out about their pain. Help the parents become sensitive to behaviour the child may use to express pain, and explain that severe pain may exist in the absence of any obvious behavioural indication, especially if pain is prolonged.

- Obtain a self-report, if possible, by talking or playing with the child. Use whatever words the child uses to denote pain. Consider using one or more of the pain scales described later, or encourage the child to make his/her own scale such as drawings of faces. This approach is obviously impossible or of no value if the child is preverbal, unconscious, or unable to speak, e.g. on a ventilator with a muscle relaxant, and some feel that self-reporting is of no value in children younger than 4 years of age (McGrath, P.J., et al, 1985). The child, like the adult, is the only authority about his/her own pain, but is not always able or willing to communicate about the pain. Because even the verbal child may deny pain, it is vital to use the following methods of assessment in addition to self-reports.

- Identify the presence of pathological processes or occurrence of procedures that are known to cause pain in others, e.g. older children and adults who are willing to report pain. Keep in mind that sensitivity to pain may be greater in younger children so that some things that do not cause pain in adults may cause pain in premature neonates or infants.

- Notice vocalizations that may indicate pain, e.g. hiccoughs or sneezing in the neonate, and crying, grunting, moaning, screaming, and breath holding at any age.

- Observe facial expressions. Those associated with pain include a wrinkled forehead, tightly closed or widely opened eyes, tightly closed or widely opened mouth, or any distorted facial expression. Although infants differ tremendously in their response to pain, a facial expression of pain seems to occur fairly consistently as an immediate response to pain. The typical facial expression of pain consists of brows lowered and drawn together, bulging forehead with vertical furrows between the brows, a broadened nasal root, eyes tightly closed, and an angular, squarish mouth (Johnston and Strada, 1986). An expression of anger (eyebrows drawn downward and inward) may occur in older infants and toddlers (Izard et al, 1983). Especially in the infant, note whether or not it is possible to elicit a smile.

- Observe body movements, e.g. splaying of hands in the neonate, clenched fists, rigid posturing, guarding of a body part, agitation, moving head from side to side, jerking or pulling back, kicking, waving arms, or curling and uncurling fingers, fidgeting, or clinging to the parent.

- Note changes in autonomical (physiological) responses, e.g. heart rate, especially an increase, although a decrease may occur in some neonates, especially an initial drop. Other changes in a child of any age may affect, for example, respiratory rate or cause apnoea, perspiring, pallor or grey-bluish colouring (especially circumoral in neonates), a rise or fall in blood pressure, etc. (The Valsalva manoeuvre occurs when neonates cry, and this increased intrathoracic pressure decreases blood flow to the heart which may cause bradycardia, preventing an increased heart rate in response to pain.)

- Ask about any changes in daily activities or behaviour, e.g., sleep disturbance, nausea or vomiting, decreased appetite, decreased activity, or increase in rest periods, irritability or low frustration tolerance, aggressive behaviour such as hitting, restlessness, or an increase or decrease in social interactions.

- Consider a trial of an appropriate dose of analgesic and note the responses, as discussed above. This may be particularly helpful when the issue arises about whether the child's response is due to pain or anxiety. Sometimes the response is clearly in anticipation of pain, occurring before anything painful is done. At other times it is unclear whether the behaviour is a result of pain or fear of pain. In a practical sense, distinguishing between the two need not be a limiting problem. Whether or not the child's reaction is due primarily to fear or pain, the child still needs help, and most approaches to pain also help decrease distress about pain. For example, distraction or narcotics may reduce the child's fear of pain *and/or* provide pain relief.

The fear and anxiety caused by pain is sometimes misunderstood as a behavioural problem. Health-team members may become upset by a child's hostile behaviour, refusal to co-operate, regressive tendencies, or constant whimpering, but overlook the possibility that the behaviour could be caused by pain (e.g. Nover, 1973). They may try to control this behaviour with rewards or limit-setting rather than persisting with efforts to relieve pain. A trial dose of analgesic may help clarify the problem; e.g. the child may co-operate and stop whimpering when the pain is relieved.

The components of a multidimensional approach to assessment of pain in children are summarized in the box below.

Components of a Multidimensional Approach to Assessment of Pain in Children

Initiate discussions about pain. Include the child (if possible), parents, and other caregivers.

Obtain a self-report, if possible, by playing or talking with the child. Consider using one or more of the pain scales.

Identify presence of pathology or occurrence of procedures that are known to cause pain in others.

Observe:
- Vocalizations
- Facial expressions
- Body movements
- Autonomic responses
- Changes in daily activities and usual behaviour.

Consider a trial dose of analgesic and note the child's responses.

Assessment tools for children with verbal communication ability

Several instruments have been developed to obtain a self-report about pain intensity from children as young as 3 or 4 years old. This section includes only those tools that are easily used in the clinical setting and readily available, e.g. those tools for which permission to duplicate, where necessary, has been granted. These tools may be considered for use with children between the ages of 3 or 4 and 18 years.

Usually the specific tool selected for the individual child is simply the one that the child seems best able to use. Thus different tools may be used for different children. However, to avoid confusing the child and to maintain consistency in assessment, for a given child the same tool is ordinarily used over time. In some instances an entirely new tool may need to be constructed for the individual child. Research may support the validity of one assessment tool over another, and there is much wisdom in resisting the temptation to develop more tools. However, in attempting to relieve pain in the individual child, it makes sense to use whichever tool the child responds to readily and seems to understand.

General guidelines

Before using any of the pain-assessment scales, talk with the child about the following:
- Find out what words the child uses for pain, e.g. ouch, *hurt*.
- Ask the child to give two or three examples of pain (to identify the child's understanding and use of words pertaining to pain). If he/she has difficulty, ask if he/she has ever fallen down, grazed a knee, hit his/her head, or had a finger pricked.
- Consider using a numerical scale only if the child can count to the highest number on the scale, e.g. 10 or 100. Verify this by asking the child to count to that number.
- Help the child practise with whatever pain assessment tool is selected by using the examples of pain given by him/her. Time may not permit this, but practice may increase the chances of a more accurate picture of the child's pain.

The specific directions given with each of the following scales are not limited to the precise ones used in research to establish the validity and reliability of the tools. Variations of the original directions are included here to foster flexibility in individualizing these tools in the clinical setting.

Numerical scales

In general, numerical scales can be used by most children by age 9–10 years. The choice of numerical scale depends on the child's ability to count and preferences. Numerical scales may range from zero (meaning no pain) to 5, 10, or 100 (meaning the worst possible pain). However, children in school may view 100 positively, associating it with a perfect test score, and view zero negatively. This possibility should be discussed with children choosing a scale of 0–100, and consideration given to reversing the usual meaning of the scores, i.e. having 100 mean feeling perfectly OK with no pain.

Most children aged 7 years or older can probably use a visual analogue consisting of a vertical line, rather than the usual horizontal line, going from 0 to 10 (see Figure 8.2). Children do not seem to easily grasp that going from left to right on a horizontal line represents an increasing intensity of pain (Beyer and Aradine, 1987).

In addition to the general guidelines given above, including a discussion of painful experiences and asking the child to count to 10, the *specific guidelines* for using the vertical visual analogue scale on p. 33 are:
1. Explain that 0 means no hurt (or whatever term the child uses for pain) and 10 means the worst possible hurt.
2. To verify the child's understanding of the scale, ask the child to point to or state a number that means the following:
- No hurt.
- The worst hurt.
- A hurt already experienced, picking one of the examples given.
- The hurt felt now (specifying which pain if more than one).
3. For future rating, note whether the child needs to point to the scale or is able to verbalize the number.

Fig 8.2 Wong/Baker Faces Rating Scale (From Wong, D., and Whaley, L.: *Clinical Handbook of Pediatric Nursing,* ed. 2. The C.V. Mosby Company, p. 373, St Louis, 1986. Printed with permission of the publisher and authors who also give their permission for this to be duplicated and used in the care of children with pain).

Wong/Baker Faces Rating Scale

The six faces shown in the Wong/Baker scale have been used to assess pain in children aged 3–18 years. Research comparing this tool with others suggests that this faces scale is well liked by the children and one of the most accurate methods of assessing pain (Wong and Baker, 1988). The faces and specific directions for using them are presented in Fig. 8.2. General guidelines stated as for analogue scales should also be used.

Eland Color Scale

The Eland Color Scale differs from many other paediatric pain assessment tools in that it yields information about the location of pain in addition to its intensity. It consists of figure drawings, back and front views, on which the child marks the location of pain. Intensity is indicated by the colour the child uses to

mark the location (Eland, 1981, 1985a, 1988a). The Eland Colour Scale seems to be a sensitive instrument for identification of pain site. On numerous occasions the colouring of the figures has identified metastasis from cancer before objective evidence could be obtained (Eland, 1986). Specific guidelines for using the Eland Colour Scale are summarized on p.242 following Fig. 8.3.

Patient Example

An 8-year-old with small-cell sarcoma identified an area in her left upper chest using the colour chosen for moderate pain. Appropriate scans and tests done at that time revealed no pathologic processes, but 2 months later lung metastasis was found in the exact area the child had been colouring (Eland, 1986).

ELAND COLOR SCALE: FIGURES

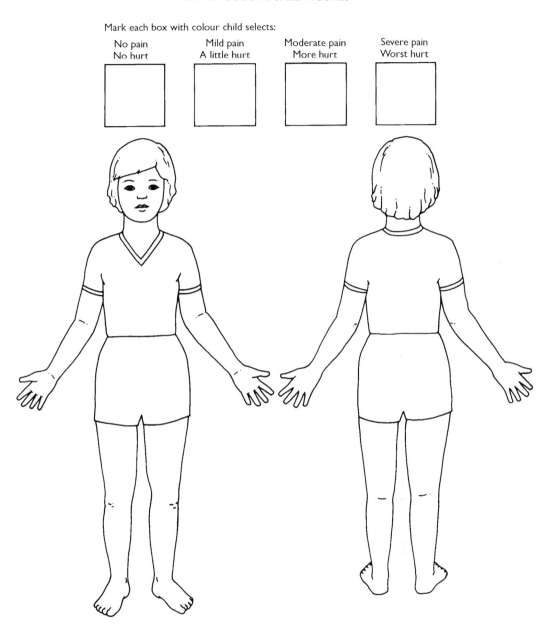

Mark each box with colour child selects:

| No pain
No hurt | Mild pain
A little hurt | Moderate pain
More hurt | Severe pain
Worst hurt |

Fig 8.3 Eland Color Scale (Printed with permission of the author, who also gives permission for this to be duplicated and used in the care of children with pain.)

ELAND COLOR SCALE: DIRECTIONS FOR USE

After discussing with the child several things that have hurt the child in the past:

1. Present 8 crayons or markers to the child. Suggested colours are yellow, orange, red, green, blue, purple, brown, and black.
2. Ask the following questions, and after the child has answered, mark the appropriate square on the tool (e.g. severe pain, worst hurt), and put that colour away from the others. For convenience, the word *hurt* is used here, but whatever term the child uses should be substituted. Ask the child these questions:
   - "Of these colours, which colour is most like the worst hurt you have ever had, (using whatever example the child has given) or the worst hurt anybody could ever have?" Which phrase is chosen will depend on the child's experience and what the child is able to understand. Some children may be able to imagine much worse pain than they have ever had, while other children can only understand what they have experienced. Of course, some children may have experienced the worst pain they can imagine.
   - "Which colour is almost as much hurt as the worst hurt (or, use example given above, if any), but not quite as bad?"
   - "Which colour is like something that hurts just a little?"
   - "Which colour is like no hurt at all?"
3. Show the four colours (marked boxes, crayons, or markers) to the child in the order he has chosen them, from the color chosen for the worst hurt to the colour chosen for no hurt.
4. Ask the child to colour the body outlines where he hurts, using the colours he has chosen to show how much it hurts.
5. When the child finishes, ask the child if this is a picture of how he hurts now or how he hurt earlier. Be specific about what earlier means by relating the time to an event, e.g. at lunch or in the playroom.

(Printed with permission of JM Eland, who also gives permission for this to be duplicated and used in the care of children with pain.)

■ May be duplicated for use in clinical practice. From McCaffery, M; Beebe, A; and Latham, J (ed.): *Pain: Clinical Manual for Nursing Practice*, London, 1994, Mosby, an imprint of Times Mirror International Publishers Ltd.

Hester Poker Chip Scale

The original tool consisted of four white chips, each representing a piece of hurt, with four pieces constituting the most hurt (Hester, 1979). This was later modified to include four red chips for levels of pain and a white chip for no pain (Molsberry, 1979). This scale can probably be used by children as young as 4 years of age.

This tool has several variations. Four or five chips may be used. All four or five chips may be the same colour to represent varying intensities of pain, with no chips equalling no pain. Or four chips may be the same colour to represent varying levels of pain and one a different colour to represent no pain. To simplify matters, the following instructions assume that four chips of the same colour are used.

In addition to the general guidelines given for other assessment tools, including a discussion with the child about his/her previous experiences with painful events, specific guidelines for using this assessment tool are:

1. Obtain four white poker chips, coins of the same size, or paper cutouts.
2. Caution: Take special care that the young ones do not swallow the chips.
3. Place the chips side by side on a surface in front of the child.
4. Using the child's terminology and any examples he/she volunteers, explain the following:
- These are pieces or chips of hurt.
- One chip means a little hurt.
- Four chips mean the most or worst hurt.
- No chips means no hurt.

5. Allow the child to handle the chips and play with them if wished. Choosing the number of chips that equals the pain must not be influenced by desire to touch or have the chips.

6. Then ask the child if he/she hurts now. If not, say that means he/she would show you no chips. If the child says he/she hurts, ask the yougster to use the chips to show you how much he/she hurts.

APPROACHES TO PAIN RELIEF

Pharmacological and non-invasive methods of pain relief discussed in detail in previous chapters for use with adults are also appropriate for relieving pain in infants and children. Much of what has already been addressed also applies to children. The purposes of this section are to present:

- Special considerations related to injections and procedural pain in children.
- Reminders of pertinent material already presented in Chapters 4–7.
- Modifications and additional considerations specific to the various age groups in children.

As was true with adults, several methods may need to be used for adequate pain relief and control of accompanying emotional states. For example, an 8-year-old child with a simple fracture of the arm may benefit from an oral narcotic, a non-narcotic, distraction, relaxation, a cold pack, and various other pain-relief methods, used at the same time or alternately.

Since assessment of the child with pain may be very complex, it is obviously difficult at times to individualize pain-relief measures for children, especially neonates and the very young. For example, adjusting the dose of analgesic and interval between doses is not as easy to do with young children who cannot communicate verbally as it is with adults who can provide numerical ratings of their pain. In spite of this difficulty, every attempt must be made to tailor pain-relief measures to the individual child.

We agree with others who have suggested that failure to try to provide pain relief for infants and children is both abusive and unethical. "Failure to relieve pain amounts to child abuse and must not be tolerated," says Rana (1987, p. 309). Stang et al (1988, p. 1511) point out that "... according to current ethical guidelines, surgical procedures cannot be performed

on research animals without using anaesthesia ... are we not morally obligated to do the same for the young of our human species?"

Avoiding injections and minimizing their effects

The most objectionable pain for children of all ages seems to be that of injections. This is evident even in the newborn when responding to the first heel lance (e.g. Owens and Todt, 1984). In a survey of 242 hospitalized children between the ages of 4 and 10 years, 49% said that the "needle" or "injection" was the worst of all the things, including surgical pain, that had hurt them during hospitalization. Some children giving this answer had multiple surgeries (Eland, 1981). Similarly, in another survey of children aged 3–18 years, the most commonly reported painful events involved needles (Wong and Baker, 1988). Since injections seem especially distressing and painful to children from birth through to adolescence, this specific type of pain is addressed separately as a special issue in pain relief for children.

Injections are frequently performed on children for two main purposes: (1) to deliver medication, including analgesics, via IV, IM, and SC routes, and (2) for diagnostic or therapeutic procedures, such as injection of a local anaesthetic or finger prick. Suggestions are made below for avoiding injections or minimizing the effects of each of these types of injections.

Alternatives to injections for delivery of medications

It is important to avoid injections for pain relief in children whenever possible. It makes little, if any, sense to a young child to have pain relieved by undergoing the painful and frightening experience of an injection. Further, the child's limited understanding of human physiology makes it unlikely that he/she will associate an injection in the buttock or thigh with pain relief in another location at a later time. Additionally, the injection of the narcotic may momentarily be more distressing to the child than the on-going pain. Many children deny pain to avoid such injections.

The following are alternatives to injections performed to administer medications:

- *Oral route, tablets or liquid.* For medication that tastes bad, ice chips or cold liquid may be used to numb the taste buds prior to taking the medication. Most non-narcotic analgesics for relief of mild to moderate pain are given orally. Remember, even severe pain may be relieved using oral narcotics if the child can swallow and if nausea and vomiting can be controlled (see p. 93).
- *Sublingual preparations.* Buprenorphine, a Controlled Drug, is currently the only commercially available sublingual preparation which has been used in school-age children in the United Kingdom. Many pharmacies in paediatric hospitals have their own unique formulations to improve compliance in children.
- Use *IV line* (not multiple venepunctures) for bolus doses or continuous infusions. Most narcotics may be administered IV.
- *SC continuous infusion* or an SC butterfly or cannula left in place and covered with a dressing for intermittent injections. Medications must be approved for subcutaneous route and the volume must be small enough not to cause irritation or tissue damage. Narcotics commonly delivered by the SC route are morphine and diamorphine, not pethidine (see pp. 96–101 regarding SC continuous infusion). An SC needle left in place for intermittent injections does not eliminate the discomfort of the medication being injected, but it does eliminate the pain of puncturing the skin—children may object more to the pain of puncturing the skin than to the pain of injecting medication. The pain of injecting the medication may be minimized by injecting slowly, and partially relieved by some of the methods suggested below, e.g. ice or cold near the site.
- The *Rectal* route may be preferable, in some cases, to IM or SC. Virtually any analgesic can be made into a suppository (see p. 95). Narcotics currently available commercially as rectal suppositories are morphine and oxycodone. Non-narcotics commercially available as rectal suppositories include paracetamol and indomethacin (in the United Kingdom, aspirin is not recommended for children under age 12, except as treatment for juvenile arthritis).

Minimizing discomfort of injections

When injections must be performed, one or more of the following steps may decrease the pricking sensation:

- *Local anaesthetic cream* (EMLA) applied under a patch is used in the United Kingdom more often than ice or ethyl chloride. It is used prior to venepuncture, but may also be used prior to SC or IM injections.
- *Ice, cold, or ethyl chloride spray* is used immediately before, during (if possible), and after the injection, e.g. being applied over the site prior to injection, then to a site adjacent to or on the opposite side during the injection, returning to the site of the injection afterwards. Ethyl chloride spray, a skin coolant, sprayed for 3–5 seconds on the injection site immediately before the injection, significantly decreases the pain children report (Eland, 1981). However, ice cubes or a cold pack are often more readily available. Be sure to explain to the child that he/she will feel something cold before the injection is given. If possible, allow the child to apply the cold pack or ice cube him- herself.
- *Offer distraction*; e.g. tell the child to "see if you can count to 20 before the injection is over," but also tell the child he/she may instead cry out, punch a pillow, or express feelings in another way as long as he/she remains still enough for the injection to be given.
- Use the *ventrogluteal site* for IM injections whenever possible. Injection into this muscle tends to hurt less than injection into the vastus lateralis muscle, rectus femoris muscle, or the posterior gluteal (dorsogluteal) muscle. The ventrogluteal site is sometimes not recommended for children younger than 3 years, but this is controversial (Eland, 1983, 1985).
- Always *be honest* with the child and forewarn him/her of the injection. Never sneak up on the child. Say the injection will hurt, using descriptive terms such as pinch or sting.
- *Allow the child to choose the site* for the injection, if possible, such as the right or left buttock or thigh.
- Offer a *"badge of courage"*, such as a colourful plaster over the injection site, especially if it bleeds. Blood can be very upsetting to the child as well as to the parents.
- Help the child *relax the muscle*. For the dorsogluteal site, have the child lie on the abdomen with legs and

toes rotated inward. For the ventrogluteal site, place the child on his/her side with the upper leg flexed and in front of the lower leg (Whaley and Wong, 1989). Asking the child to wriggle toes or take a deep breath may also help relaxation.

- To minimize the discomfort associated with actual injection of the medication itself, have the *medication near room temperature* and *inject slowly*, if possible.

To promote the child's understanding of the benefits of an injection of analgesic, a clock or timer may be used to indicate the passage of time between the injection and the probable onset of pain relief. It is extremely difficult for a child to make a logical association between the fearful and painful injection and the desired pain relief.

Minimizing traumatic procedural pain

Numerous diagnostic and therapeutic procedures that are performed on children can cause brief but significantly intense pain. Analgesics or anaesthetics are not always used to relieve this pain. If they are used, they do not always produce adequate pain relief. Children aged 7–17 years in one paediatric intensive care unit indicated that the worst stressors were painful invasive procedures (Tichy et al, 1988). This is of special interest because research shows that around the age of 7 years, there tends to be a dramatic decrease in behavioural response to painful procedures (Jay et al, 1983). Once again, we see that a lack of behavioural expression of pain does not necessarily mean a lack of pain.

Since the child's experience with the first procedure sets the tone for reactions to future ones, it is especially important that the best possible methods of pain relief are chosen initially. This includes not only pain relief during the procedure but also appropriate discussions and play before and after the procedure. In addition, if the child is very anxious and this cannot be alleviated with nonpharmacological approaches, a premedication such as midazolam should be considered. In some cases, oral premedication may be preferred, such as quinalbarbitone, chloral hydrate, or trimeprazine.

To cope with procedural pain, non-invasive pain-relief methods may be extremely helpful in addition to analgesics and anaesthetics. Some of these are discussed later in the chapter, e.g. blowing bubbles and telling the child's favourite story.

The following discussion is limited to a few suggestions for pharmacological approaches to minimizing the pain of procedures that last from a few minutes up to about 30 minutes, such as lumbar punctures, changing burn dressings, and bone marrow aspirations.

Fentanyl. IV fentanyl is recommended for a variety of brief but very painful procedures such as repair of lacerations in Accident and Emergency, reduction of fractures or dislocations, and bone marrow aspirations. Even for infants, IV fentanyl is considered by many to be a safe and ideal drug (Billmire, Neale and Gregory, 1985). It has a rapid onset (90–120 seconds), short duration of action (up to 40 minutes), and minimal side effects when it is administered in the following manner:

- Slow IV administration over 3–5 minutes, and
- Doses of 2–3 µg/kg.*

Virtually all problems with IV fentanyl, e.g. respiratory depression (including delayed respiratory depression), muscular rigidity, hypertension, and bradycardia, seem to arise from too rapid administration or large doses. When IV fentanyl is given as recommended, side effects are rare. In one study of 2000 children from 1 to 12 years of age, IV fentanyl was used during repair of facial trauma and only three apnoeic episodes occurred. Nevertheless, the child must be monitored for respiratory depression, which may not peak for 15 minutes. As with all drugs capable of producing respiratory depression, oxygen, airway equipment, and naloxone should be readily available.

Regarding suggested doses of IV fentanyl for brief procedures, it is of interest that several researchers noted that higher doses seem to be required in infants and young children than in older children. For example, using 2–3 µg/kg, to calculate doses, Billmire, Neale and Gregory (1985) found that children aged 18–36 months usually required the full dose and older children usually required less than the calculated dose. Using a broader dose range for calculation, Maunuksela, Rajantie and Silmes (1986) found that infants under 2 years of age experienced no apparent analgesia from fentanyl 5µg/kg.

Local anaesthetics—"caines". Unfortunately, many painful procedures are performed without any local

---

* or µg = microgram; 1000 µg = 1 mg.

anaesthesia. Yet infiltration of the skin with a local anaesthetic is considered so safe that there is little if any reason ever to fail to use it in a newborn or older child whenever skin must be incised, e.g. for vascular access (Stang et al, 1988; Yaster, 1987).

However, the stinging sensation of the local anaesthetic is a major reason children dislike having procedures such as lumbar puncture or bone marrow aspiration performed under a local anaesthetic. When a long-acting anaesthetic such as lignocaine is used, stinging may last up to 60 seconds. Warming the lignocaine before infiltration may help reduce the discomfort (Davidson and Boom, 1992). Topical anaesthetics, such as EMLA cream, are now widely used prior to venepuncture and cannulation (Hopkins et al., 1988; Clarke and Radford, 1986).

Anaesthetists may be helpful resources when the nurse suggests that doctors use combinations such as the above. The help of anaesthetists may also be enlisted to encourage surgeons to infiltrate surgical wounds with the long-acting bupivacaine to reduce pain and narcotic need postoperatively. This may be especially helpful in the care of children and elderly persons, since the health-care team seems particularly reluctant to use narcotics in these age groups.

Local anaesthetic patches and/or irrigation, discussed previously, is another method of using local anaesthesia in a manner that minimizes the discomfort of painful procedures such as suturing or cleansing performed on open wounds.

Ketamine. Depending upon the dose administered, ketamine may produce anaesthesia or analgesia. It has been used safely for procedural pain in children as young as 7 months and has been recommended for use during hydrotherapy and debridement for treatment of burns, laryngoscopy and other less painful procedures (Forlini, Morinand Treacy, 1987).

Ketamine anaesthesia is dissociative. The eyes may remain open, and unpurposeful movement may occur. Although the patient is awake, constant supervision is necessary.

Prior to administration of ketamine, a drying agent such as atropine is given since ketamine produces a large amount of upper airway secretions. Also prior to administration, patients must be NBM for 6 hours (4 hours for infants), which may be a disadvantage in some situations, especially if calorie intake is a priority.

At recommended doses respiratory depression is absent or minimal, and the pharyngeal and laryngeal reflexes are retained. Low doses recommended for procedures lasting 5–30 minutes, such as burn dressing changes, are as follows (Martyn, 1987):

- IV (given over 60 seconds), 0.5–1.0 mg/kg. Higher doses up to 2mg/kg may be given (Forlini et al, 1987).
- IM 1–3 mg/kg. Higher IM doses of 5–10 mg/kg may be given (Forlini et al, 1987).
- Rectally, 3–15 mg/kg.

With repeated doses, tolerance develops and larger doses are required.

Transcutaneous Electric Nerve Stimulation (TENS). For some types of localized pain accompanying procedures, TENS may be used in a manner similar to its use postoperatively (see Chapter 5). The comfortable "conventional" TENS setting may be used with the electrodes on either side of the painful area. TENS has been successfully used with children to relieve pain associated with intravenous insertion and particularly painful subcutaneous injections.

Analgesics

Do children suffer pain because of under-use of analgesics? Inadequate pharmacological management of pain in children has been suggested for many years. Most studies that compare analgesic administration in adults and children with similar painful conditions show that less analgesic is given to children than to adults, but the studies do not actually assess whether or not pain is greater in the children than in the adults (e.g. Beyer, DeGood, Ashley and Russell, 1983; Schechter, Allen and Hanson, 1986). However, based on studies in which adults do report their pain in relation to analgesic administration, it is clear that in many situations adults suffer moderate to severe pain from under-use of narcotics (see p. 76). Thus even in the absence of children's reports of pain, the analgesic record strongly suggests that children are not only under-treated for pain but also are under-treated to a greater extent than adults.

In an early study (1977), Eland and Anderson reported that 25 children aged 4–8 years, hospitalized for surgical procedures, received only 24 doses of analgesic compared with 671 doses received by 18 adults who had similar surgical procedures. Thirteen of the 25 children were given no analgesic during their entire hospitalization. Among those receiving no analgesic were children who had traumatic amputation, excision of a malignant neck mass, and repair of atrial septal defect.

Later in a survey of burn units, respondents assessed pain as the same in adults and children but choices of treatment of burn pain differed greatly for children. Some units tended to give relatively larger doses of morphine to children than to adults. However, while only 6 respondents stated they would not routinely premedicate the adult for tanking, 24 stated they would not routinely premedicate the child (Perry and Heidrich, 1982). Apparently there is a tendency to under-treat pain in children but there are also occasions when children may be treated for pain more aggressively than adults. Analgesic administration is most certainly more variable in children than in adults.

Analgesic research in children. Compared with adults, there are fewer double-blind analgesic studies in children, and the pharmacokinetics of analgesics, e.g. half-life and absorption, are not as well understood in children. Some analgesics have not yet been licensed for use in children, although that does not necessarily mean they cannot be used.

Certain warnings about using analgesics in children may unnecessarily discourage their use unless these statements are appropriately interpreted. Some drug information states that studies have shown the drug to be unsafe in children, but most state that studies establishing safety and effectiveness in children are lacking.

Physiological considerations influencing analgesic therapy in children. Maturational changes seem to have a striking effect on drug response but are still poorly understood (Stewart and Hampton, 1987). In relation to narcotic and non-narcotic analgesics, the possibility of adverse side effects, a longer duration of action, and the need for lower doses in children compared with adults may be explained in part by some of the following physiological differences in children (Pagliaro and Pagliaro, 1986):

- Renal function. In the neonate, renal blood flow is lower and glomerular filtration rate is about half that of the normal adult. Thus drugs that are primarily excreted unchanged in the urine will have a much longer half-life. However, the renal system matures relatively rapidly and reaches a state of function comparable to that of the adult by the age of 6–12 months. Recent research shows that clearance of morphine reaches or surpasses the adult level by 1 month of age (Lynn and Slattery, 1987).

- Hepatic function. Since hepatic function is not fully developed at birth, some enzymes produced in the liver and responsible for drug metabolism are reduced. Thus some drugs such as morphine will be metabolized more slowly in the neonate and have a longer duration of action (Lynn and Slattery, 1987).

- Protein binding. Many drugs bind to plasma proteins, leaving a portion of each drug circulating unbound or free. Only the free drug produces a pharmacological effect. Under the age of about 2 years, the mechanism for producing albumin, a major plasma protein, is not fully developed (Pagliaro and Pagliaro, 1986). Decreased circulating proteins potentially result in greater drug effect from higher concentrations of unbound drug, with a greater risk of toxic effects. Non-narcotic analgesics that are protein bound and likely to be associated with greater pharmacological effect include ibuprofen, naproxen, indomethacin, and piroxicam (Flower, Moncada and Vane, 1985).

- "Immature" receptors. Some drugs seem to have a stronger or weaker effect on children than on adults. It has been suggested that this could be due to some drug receptors not being fully developed in children. For example, decreased numbers of receptors or decreased responsiveness of the receptors might result in a drug having a greater effect. However, currently there is no research to support this.

Many formulas have been introduced over the years for calculating paediatric doses, recognizing that there are many physiological differences between children and adults. However, it is vital to remember that those formulas for calculating analgesic doses have not been verified with research. They are merely guidelines.

Key concepts in analgesic administration

The same key concepts that apply to adults receiving analgesics for pain also apply to the child: using a preventive approach, individualizing or titrating the dose and other aspects of the analgesic, and the patient controlling his/her own pain relief to the maximum extent possible. These are discussed extensively in Chapter 4. The following is a brief overview of these concepts along with special considerations related to their application to children:

- All analgesia is controlled by the patient to the maximum extent possible since the patient is the only person who can feel the pain being treated. Whenever possible, the patient's report of the pain is used as the reason to begin use of analgesics and then to make adjustments in the analgesic dosage so that the safest and most complete pain relief possible is provided. Obviously neonates, young children, and some older children will not be able to report pain verbally. In the absence of direct patient control over analgesia, initiation and adjustment of analgesics must be based primarily on the following:
- Non-verbal and physiological behaviour that indicate pain.
- Known pathological process or cause of pain.
- Safety.

Using the above, parent control (as opposed to patient control) of analgesia may be possible. Further, trial doses of narcotic and/or non-narcotic analgesics are indicated for children who cannot or will not report pain.

- Preventive approach. If pain is predictable, regularly scheduled doses should be instituted after determining the duration of action of the analgesic in the individual child. If an occurrence of pain can be predicted, an analgesic is given prior to the onset of pain, provided the patient's physical condition permits; e.g. if the child's condition is stable, a narcotic may be administered during surgery or in the recovery room before the child awakens. A plan to keep pain under control is particularly important in children since even the verbally fluent child may fail to report pain or deliberately conceal it. Remember that PRN orders may be implemented around the clock (ATC) if a flow sheet type of assessment indicates they are safe and needed.
- Titrate to effect. Based on the specific child's responses, the dose, interval between doses, choice of analgesic, and route of administration are individualized. When the child is unable to report pain, safety may be the major guide to titration of any of these aspects; e.g. if pain is suspected, the dose of narcotic may continue to be increased until side effects, such as respiratory depression, become a potential problem.

Non-narcotics (NSAIDs)

The specific details of non-narcotic analgesic therapy are discussed in Chapter 4, including indications, disadvantages, mechanisms underlying the effects of non-steroidal anti-inflammatory drugs (NSAIDs), adverse side effects, promising uses, and guidelines for their effective use, along with patient/family teaching tools that may be adapted for use with children and their parents. From this discussion, reminders of some important aspects that also apply to children are:

- Non-narcotics relieve more pain than most people realize; paracetamol 500mg orally relieves about as much pain as codeine 15mg orally.
- When pain is too severe to be relieved with nonnarcotics alone, continue to administer nonnarcotics along with narcotics since this provides safe, additive pain relief, and the combination of narcotic plus non-narcotic attacks pain in both the central and peripheral nervous systems. Further, the narcotic dose needed may be lower when a non-narcotic is given at the same time.
- Types of pain that seem to be especially responsive to NSAIDs such as ibuprofen are:

  Postoperative pain. Indomethacin rectally has been found effective in relief of postoperative pain in adults, and recent preliminary research suggests that IV infusion during the first 24 hours postoperatively is effective and safe in relieving pain and reducing the morphine requirement in children (Maunuksela, Olkkola and Korpela, 1987).

  Cancer pain.

  Dysmenorrhoea (painful menstrual cramps). Every adolescent girl needs to understand the value of non-prescription paracetamol or ibuprofen for this purpose.

When the child has both narcotic and non-narcotic prescriptions for pain relief, there seems to be a tendency for nurses to select the non-narcotic (e.g. Mather and Mackie, 1983). While non-narcotics relieve more pain than most people realize, they do not usually provide sufficient relief for severe pain. However, as noted above, they may be given *along with narcotics* to relieve severe pain.

For children the recommended dose for paracetamol is about 10–15 mg/kg every 4–6 hours. For practical purposes, approximate doses of paracetamol

Drug	Route	Total Daily Dose (T.D.D.) 1 month to 12 yr | over 12 yr and adult		Times Daily	Notes
Paracetamol	oral or rectal	**2–3 months** 60mg		single dose	Analgesic and antipyretic (non-opioid). Post-immunization pyrexia, repeat if necessary after 4–6 hours
suspension 120mg/5ml, 250mg/5ml. tablets 500mg, dispersible tablets 500mg. 60mg,[UL] 125mg, 250mg,[UL] 500mg.[UL]		10–15 mg/kg or **under 3 months** 10mg/kg **3 months to 1yr** 60–125mg **1–5yr** 120–250mg **6–12yr** 250–500mg	0.5–1g	single dose	Mild to moderate pain and pyrexia. Doses may be repeated every 4–6 hours. give a maximum of 4 doses in 24 hours. **When rounding doses** for convenience of administration use **lower** end of range for **younger** ages.
		Avoid large doses in liver disease – dose-related toxicity. Drug interactions include **enhanced** warfarin levels and reduced metabolism of zidovudine (with increased risk of neutropenia) in prolonged regular use. Metoclopramide **increases** absorption and cholestyramine **decreases** absorption of paracetamol.			

Notes:

1. Specific preparations listed are those used at Alder Hey Children's Hospital. For further information, please consult the pharmacist, patient's doctor, manufacturer's literature or other drug information sources.

2. [UL] indicates that the preparation does not have a UK Product Licence. It may be prepared extemporaneously in the pharmacy or purchased from a "specials" manufacturer (NHS or commerical). Consult the pharmacist for further information.

NOTE: DOSE GIVEN IS TOTAL DAILY DOSE (UNLESS STATED OTHERWISE)

Table 8.2 Doses of Paracetamol by Age and Weight (From *Alder Hey Book of Children's Doses*, 6th ed, Royal Liverpool Children's NHS Trust, 1994. Used with permission).

by age and weight are presented in Table 8.2. In the United Kingdom, the Committee on the Safety of Medicines (1986) advised that, on the evidence available, aspirin is not a suitable medication for children with minor illnesses. For ingredients and formulations of non-narcotics available for children without a prescription, see Table 8.3.

Reye's syndrome and salicylates. Since 1982 avoidance of salicylates in children and adolescents has been recommended because of the possibility that use of salicylates might lead to the development of Reye's syndrome (encephalopathy and fatty degeneration of the viscera), a rare but often fatal syndrome. Since that time, salicylate use among children has declined, as has the incidence of Reye's syndrome.

Generic Name	Ingredients
paracetamol tablets	500mg
paracetamol soluble tablets	120mg, 500mg
paracetamol oral suspension [1]	120mg/5ml, 250mg/5ml
paracetamol suppositories [2]	125mg
ibuprofen tables [3]	200mg

Notes
1. available sugar free
2. much more expensive per dose than other preparations.
3. not recommended in place of paracetamol as a **routine** analgesic for children.
   Aspirin must not be used as a non-prescription analgesic for children.

Table 8.3 Common Non-prescription Analgesics for Children.

Narcotics (Opioids)

A considerable amount of information related to narcotics has already been covered in Chapter 4, including the mode of action, forms of under-treatment, reasons for under treatment, equianalgesic doses, factors influencing selection of a narcotic, various routes of administration (e.g. oral, intermittent, intramuscular and subcutaneous injections, continuous subcutaneous infusion, intravenous spinal), and side effects, along with numerous patient/family teaching tools that may be adapted for use with children and their parents. Since narcotics are often administered parenterally, the reader is also reminded to review methods of avoiding or minimizing the pain of injections (pp. 244–245). This section presents an overview of some important aspects of narcotic administration along with special considerations for children.

Under-treatment with Narcotics

Even when the existence and severity of pain in a child is acknowledged, health-care team members may still be tempted to under-treat with narcotics because of two issues, addiction and safety.

Addiction

The exaggerated and unfounded fear of causing *narcotic addiction* has been discussed previously (see Chapter 4. and p. 227). This section focuses on how the nurse can assist parents, adolescents, and school-age children who show concern about taking narcotics and other drugs for pain relief. The following facts may help reassure them so that they can feel confident about using analgesics appropriately:

- Narcotic addiction is defined as a psychological dependence, a desire to use the drug for other than medically approved reasons. Pain relief is a legal and legitimate primary use of narcotic analgesics. Tolerance to analgesia (requiring larger doses) and withdrawal symptoms are physiological problems that are separate from addiction.
- "Depending" on narcotics or pain relievers is not the same as "drug dependency", or psychological dependence. Parents may say they don't want their child to depend on drugs, failing to appreciate that there are situations where it is appropriate to *depend* on or to use narcotics to relieve pain, just as insulin is used to manage diabetes. Emphasize that narcotics

are used to help the child feel normal or simply be him- herself. Without the narcotic the child would feel pain and be affected by it, perhaps crying and unable to sleep or eat.

- The word *narcotic* is easily misunderstood because it is often used by the media to refer to substances that can be abused. However, not all substances of abuse are pharmacologically narcotic (opioid) analgesics, or pain relievers; for example, cocaine is a common drug of abuse and is frequently mentioned in the media. Although it is legally a Controlled Drug, it is actually completely unlike a narcotic analgesic. Cocaine is classified pharmacologically *not* as a narcotic but as a local anaesthetic with a stimulant effect. Since cocaine is referred to as a narcotic and the abuse of it is often publicized, people may be unrealistically afraid of drugs that are pharmacologically classified as narcotics, e.g. morphine.
- The use of narcotics for pain relief almost never results in narcotic addiction. On the other hand, it is important to acknowledge to children and parents that drug abuse and addiction are problems in our society, and "street drugs" should be avoided. A medicine used for pain relief, however, is not a "street drug" and rarely results in feeling "high" or silly. (Referring to a narcotic as medicine instead of a drug may help make this point.)
- Narcotics are not nearly as appealing to most people as are other non-narcotic drugs such as alcohol, marijuana, and cocaine. Adolescents who are familiar with "street" drugs often say they do not like the "feel" of narcotics given for pain relief.

Safety

There is an assumption that it is safer to withhold narcotics than to give them, and there can be little doubt that narcotic administration is potentially dangerous (Cowlay and Bogs, 1992). Dealing with tiny doses of drugs and with the less physiologically stable systems in the very young may cause concerns about the immediate dangers of narcotics to over-ride concerns about immediate pain relief and complications from unrelieved pain. However, under certain circumstances, pain may be hazardous. Pain may increase the incidence of intraventricular haemorrhage in premature infants, a major cause of death in this age group (Anand, Sippell and Aynsley-Green, 1987; Beaver, 1987). Following tonsillectomy, pain may result in crying, which may precipitate bleeding (Krishnan, Tolhurst-Cleaver and Kay, 1985).

Further, under careful observation, narcotic administration is probably much safer than is usually recognized (e.g. Beasley and Tibballs, 1987). For example, in children 6 months to 15 years old receiving a total of 397 variable-rate IV narcotic infusions, respiratory rate dropped below the set minimum in only 2 patients. One responded to reduction in dose, the other required a small dose of naloxone (Dilworth and MacKellar, 1987). Research shows that infants more than 1 month old are not more sensitive to the respiratory depressant effects of morphine than are adults (Lynn and Slattery, 1987). Use of a continuous assessment sheet (p. 38) to carefully document any changes accompanying narcotic administration may reveal that physiological responses, such as respiratory function, not only remain stable but actually show improvement.

Respiratory depression is one of the most feared side effects of narcotics, but naloxone (Narcan) provides reassurance. Although narcotic administration is always accompanied by a certain amount of risk, there is an antagonist available. Naloxone reverses almost all the undesirable side effects of narcotics, including respiratory depression. Following are reminders about the appropriate use of naloxone in children:

• The individual child's respiratory rate prior to a narcotic dose should be used for comparison purposes. Respiratory rates in children vary considerably.

• The average respiratory rates at rest for children are faster than those of adults, usually 30–35 per minute in newborns and infants, 25–30 per minute in toddlers, 20–25 per minute in preschool and school-age children, and 16–19 per minute in adolescents.

• The usual recommended dose of naloxone for neonates or young children is 10mcg/kg IV given over 2–3 minutes with subsequent doses of 100mcg/kg if there is no effect from the initial dose (*Alder Hey Book of Children's Doses, 1993*). Remember that the half-life of the narcotic may be longer than that of naloxone, so infusions may be necessary in severe cases. Large doses administered rapidly may precipitate not only severe pain but also nausea, vomiting, sweating, and increased blood pressure. In children who have become physically dependent,

withdrawal syndrome may occur. Given IV, the onset of action is about 2 minutes, and slightly longer if naloxone is administered IM or SC. Naloxone may also be administered by the intraosseus route in an emergency, where venous access is difficult.

Choice of narcotics

Findings regarding narcotic use in children plus reminders from material presented in this chapter and in Chapter 4 are:

• *Pethidine* is a *poor* first choice of narcotic analgesic for several reasons. The active metabolite nor-pethidine, a central nervous system stimulant, may accumulate and lead to seizures. Since pethidine is relatively short-acting, pain relief in young children may last much less than 3 hours, necessitating administration at inconveniently frequent intervals. The older child who can tell the time may become a "clock-watcher" because pain returns long before he/she is allowed to have the next dose.

• *Morphine and fentanyl IV* have been used safely in neonates, as well as in infants and older children. Diamorphine is also used in the United Kingdom, particularly in ITU's and for terminal care. Narcotic analgesia in the neonate requires a vigilant approach. The half-life of narcotics in the neonate may be significantly longer than in the older child, and high-dose infusions or rapid administration via an IV bolus may cause seizures. Continuous IV infusion of morphine in newborns must be watched closely, even for several hours after the infusion is stopped, since the duration of action may be much longer than in older patients and the plasma concentration may continue to increase due to reabsorption of morphine (Koren et al, 1985). Nevertheless, these and other narcotics may be safely administered to neonates. Preliminary studies provide guidelines for initial and on-going dosing of narcotics in premature neonates and infants (see annotated references Beasley and Tibballs, 1987; Bell and Ellis, 1987; Hatch, 1987; Koren et al, 1985). Safe use of IV narcotics in neonates requires use of a continuous assessment sheet, gradual increases in doses, and avoidance of rapid bolus administration.

Dose

Most dosage recommendations for narcotic analgesics in children are not supported by double blind analgesic research in children. Recommendations are usually extrapolated from data on adults and appear to be based more on observations of what is safe rather than what is effective. Thus, as with adults, the initial recommended doses must be viewed merely as educated guesses. The initial dose must be immediately adjusted up or down according to the individual child's responses.

For detailed information about the use of narcotic analgesics in children, refer to the following sources:

- *Alder Hey Book of Children's Doses,* 6th edition, Alder Hey Children's Hospital, Liverpool, 1993.
- *Paediatric Formulary*, 3rd edition, Guy's, Lewisham and St Thomas' Hospitals, London, 1993.
- *Paediatric Vade Mecum,* Edward Arnold, Birmingham, 1993.

A quick guide to the usual recommended doses of morphine is presented in Table 8.4. Using this table the nurse may check a dose prescribed by the doctor against the usual recommendations. For example, if morphine 2mg IM is prescribed for a 4-year-old in severe pain and if this is not effective, the nurse may glance at the table and see at once that this dose is at the lower end of currently recommended doses. The nurse may report this information along with the child's response; e.g. "breathing well but still says he/she hurts very much," to obtain an order for an increase in dose.

Codeine is given orally, IM, or occasionally IV to young children (toddlers and pre-schoolers), rather often in some clinical settings. However, codeine is considered appropriate for mild to moderate pain, not severe pain, and tends to have dose-limiting side effects of nausea and constipation.

To control severe pain such as sickle cell crisis, the IV route is preferred, using boluses of morphine to control the pain quickly; and a continuous infusion to maintain a steady level of analgesia. Suggestions for initial doses of morphine IV and a method of fairly rapid titration are offered by Cole and others (1986, see the annotated reference for details). Pethidine is generally not recommended for pain in children, since the active metabolite nor-pethidine may accumulate and cause seizures (Howland and Goldfrank, 1986).

When tolerance to analgesia develops or when pain increases, doses of narcotic much higher than those recommended for an initial dose may be required. For example, for a 3 1/2-year-old girl with extensive metastatic cancer, the dose of morphine IV escalated from 1.8mg/hr to over 100mg/hr in a 2-week period (Wiley, 1988). In a terminally ill 4-year-old the dose of IV morphine escalated from 48mg/day to 4000mg/day over a period of only 9 days (Eland, 1988b). In a 5-year-old boy with extensive gastro-intestinal disease since birth, the safe and effective dose of IV morphine reached 225mg/hr, and several months later toward the end of his life the dose reached 1000mg/hr of IV morphine (Sentivany, 1988). Other examples of high doses given safely for relief of severe pain in children also appear in the literature (see annotated references Burne and Hurt, 1987; Rogers, 1985).

NOTE: DOSE GIVEN IS TOTAL DAILY DOSE (UNLESS OTHERWISE STATED)

Notes:
1. All initial doses must be titrated up or down according to the child's individual response by altering the dose or the dose interval.
2. Specific preparations listed are those used at Alder Hey Children's Hospital. For further information, plase consult the pharmacist, patient's doctor, manufacturer's literature or other drug information sources.
3. (UL) indicates that the preparation does not have a UK Product Licence. It may be prepared extemporaneously in the pharmacy or purchased from a "specials" manufacturer (NHS or commercial). Consult the pharmacist for further information.
4. SR = sustained release.
* Methods of calculating and administering doses of narcotic analgesics vary. Readers should be familiar with their own local guidelines and policies.
From *Alder Hey Book of Children's Doses*, ed 6, Royal Liverpool Children's NHS Trust, 1994. Used with permission.

Drug	Route	Total Daily Dose (T.D.D.)		Times Daily (divide T.D.D. by this figure)	Notes
		1 month to 12 yr	over 12 yr and adult		
MORPHINE (Controlled Drug) tablets 10mg, 30mg, 60mg (all SR); mixture 10mg/5ml (and 20mg/ml); suppositories 5mg, (UL) 15mg, 60mg.	oral or rectal	**1–12 months** 500mcg/kg **Over 1 yr** 1.2–2.4mg/kg	60–90mg	6 6 (2 for SR preparations)	Strong opioid analgesic for severe pain and sedation. **Starting dose** review regularly and adjust according to response.(A,D) For SR preparations, administer every 12 hours (increasing to three times daily if necessary).
	oral	**over 3 months** 500mcg/kg **over 1 year** 250mcg/kg		single dose	Pre-medication. (Contained in "Triatromorph").
injection 2.5mg/ml, (UL) 10mg/ml ampoules.	(I.M.)	**6–12 months** 150mcg/kg **over 1 year** 250mcg/kg	5–20mg	single dose single dose	**Respiratory monitoring mandatory.** Repeat up to six times in 24 hours.
injection 2.5mg/ml, (UL) 10mg/ml ampoules.	i.v. bolus over 5 minutes	**1–3months** 25mcg/kg **3–6 months** 50mcg/kg **6–12 months** 100mcg/kg **over 1 yr** 100–200mcg/kg	2.5–10mg	single dose single dose single dose single dose	**Respiratory monitoring mandatory.** Administer in two halves, 10 mins apart. Repeat up to four times in 24 hours. Repeat up to four times in 24 hours. Repeat up to six times in 24 hours. Repeat up to six times in 24 hours. For **sedation in ITU** a **loading dose** of 100mcg/kg is used.
	i.v. infusion	**0–6 months** 5mcg/kg/hr **6–12 months** 10mcg/kg/hr **over 1 yr** 10–50mcg/kg/hr		continuous continuous continuous	Administer i.v. bolus first as loading dose. Infuse in D5 or NaCl 0.9% at 0.1–2mg/ml. Stable for 24 hours. For sedation in ITU an infusion of 20mcg/kg/hr is used.
		10–30mcg/kg/hr		continuous	Cerebral oedema (if ventilated). Give 100mcg/kg i.v. bolus as required if autonomic reaction to stimuli present.

Causes constipation and nausea.

Avoid in moderate renal impairment or where necessary give 50–75% of dose (effects are enhanced).

Avoid in liver disease (can precipitate coma).

Drug interactions include **enhanced** sedative effects with anxiolytics and hypnotics, **antagonizes** effects of cisapride and metoclopramide. Morphine levels **increased** by cimetidine. CNS excitation or depression with MAOI's.

Can cause respiratory depression, antagonist is **NALOXONE**.

Table 8.4 Calculation of Initial Doses of Morphine for Children with Moderate to Severe Pain*(From *Alder Hey Book of Children's Doses*, 6th ed, Royal Liverpool Children's NHS Trust, 1994. Used with permission). See notes to table, p. 252.

Route of Administration

The importance of avoiding the IM or SC route, and how to use other routes of administration, especially oral or continuous IV, have been discussed (pp. 243–245). Because babies and many young children have difficulty swallowing tablets and capsules, it is best to use elixirs or dispersable tablets, when available. Tablets (except sustained-release or enteric- coated) may also be crushed and mixed with food, such as fromage frais (Hunt, 1986). This is particularly useful in children who have difficulty swallowing due to neurological disease.

Patient-controlled analgesia (PCA) is an appropriate method of administering analgesics for some children. Successful use of PCA via the IV route has been reported in children as young as 11 years (Rogers, Webb, Stergios and Newman, 1988; Schechter, Berrien and Katz, 1988). Considering the adolescent's cognitive ability and need to maintain control, PCA by any route seems appropriate to the developmental needs and abilities of this age group. IV PCA may be possible in some children as young as 6 years, or the device may be operated by the parents. Eland (1988b) reports using IV PCA with a 4-year-old child.

Physical Dependence (Withdrawal)

Physical dependence may occur in adolescents and young adults after fairly brief narcotic administration, e.g. 6–21 days. After abrupt discontinuation of narcotic therapy, withdrawal syndrome may occur within 6 to 48 hours. This syndrome includes agitation, irritability, muscular jerks, abdominal pain, diarrhoea, "gooseflesh", and itching (Miser et al, 1986). Withdrawal syndrome may also occur in the neonate when IV narcotics are abruptly discontinued. The following are essential to appropriate care:

- Be alert to withdrawal syndrome after 6 days or more of narcotic therapy.
- Reassure the patient and his family that physical dependency is not the same as addiction and does not lead to addiction. (The occurrence of physical dependence is unpredictable but is relatively frequent compared to the infrequent occurrence of addiction.)
- If pain is resolved or if spinal analgesia is begun, gradual tapering of narcotics is indicated to prevent withdrawal symptoms.

Adjuvant analgesics

Adjuvant analgesics have been discussed at length in Chapter 4, including antidepressants, anticonvulsants, so-called potentiators, and considerations in treating sleep disturbances, anxiety, depression, muscle spasms, and aching or lancinating neuropathic pain. Guidelines for the use of adjuvant analgesics are not well established and continue to be researched. Following are brief reminders of important aspects of using adjuvant analgesics:

- Appropriate indications for a trial of an adjuvant analgesic are those pain syndromes that do not respond to narcotics or non-narcotics, such as phantom limb pain.
- Adjuvant analgesics usually are not a substitute for adequate doses of narcotic or non-narcotic analgesics. Most of the time, aggressive titration of narcotic and non-narcotic analgesics are indicated before adjuvant analgesics are tried.

Cutaneous stimulation

Toddlers and older children may obtain pain relief from the types of cutaneous stimulation previously discussed in Chapter 5, including superficial massage, pressure with or without massage, superficial heat or cold, ice massage, and TENS. However, special precautions apply to the neonate and infant.

Pre-term and full-term neonates

Stimulation of any sort, including stimuli felt as pleasant in infants and older children, should be administered cautiously to the neonate, especially the premature neonate. In a pre-term infant, simple stroking of the skin may cause an intense physiological response. Hence, bathing by immersion in warm water rather than sponge bathing is recommended for pre-term and full-term neonates (Als et al, 1986).

Cutaneous stimulation such as stroking above or below the site of pain is recommended for older children and adults for pain relief, but it does not appear to be helpful to neonates. For example, stroking the premature neonate's leg above the site of a heel lance may dramatically increase heart rate and other responses to pain. Research shows that the greatest percentage change in heart rate occurs during the first 10 seconds after application of stimuli such as touch and/or heel lance (Beaver, 1987). Hence, in the neonate, a convenient and quick method of assessing the effect of any stimulation, whether it is painful or intended to decrease pain, may be to observe immediate changes in heart rate.

Toddlers and older children

Special considerations in the use of certain cutaneous stimulation techniques for toddlers and older children are:

- *Cold and ice* applications are usually readily accepted by children, whereas adults are often reluctant to use them. Simply handing the injured child an ice cube can be distracting, and helping the child to rub it above or below the injury or contralaterally may also relieve pain. Children with headaches or undergoing orthodontic adjustments are often receptive to trying ice-cube massage to the web of the hand.

  A cold pack made from a disposable plastic glove may be especially useful with children since the fingers of the glove will cover small areas or get into narrow spaces between tiny body parts. The glove may be filled with ice chips and water, or placed in the freezer after filling with two-thirds water and one-third alcohol (alcohol keeps it from freezing into a hard mass). Further, if the cold pack must be sterile, sterile gloves may be used.

  A recommended site for cutaneous stimulation, especially when the site of pain is not accessible, is between pain and the brain. A common method of increasing fluid intake in young children, e.g. postoperatively, is the ice pop. Interestingly, this also serves the purpose of placing cold between pain and the brain.

  Alternating applications of heat and cold is one of the most effective methods of pain relief with cutaneous stimulation. The child may be given both heat and cold packs, with instructions to alternate them at his/her own discretion. This may also distract the child and give a sense of control.

- *TENS* reportedly is helpful to many children, although not to all, who have chronic non-malignant pain (Beyer and Leven, 1987; Epstein and Harris, 1978). It may relieve some types of procedural pain, such as IV insertion, burn graft donor site pain, and prolonged pain from bone metastasis (Eland, 1988c).

Distraction

Children seem to be especially talented in the use of distraction, especially physical activity, to make pain more bearable. Therefore over-use of this technique must be avoided. Fatigue may occur easily, and pain persists in the presence of distraction, sometimes requiring analgesics in addition to distraction. For example, energetic distraction such as play is frequently followed by fatigue, irritability, and an increased awareness of pain, and analgesics are often indicated at that time.

Those distraction techniques discussed in Chapter 6 that are especially appropriate for pre-school and older children for brief painful procedures are listening (and if appropriate, participating in) to recorded music or stories, anything funny, and pictures, particularly pop-up books. For children of all ages, maintaining normal sensory input is helpful in coping with on-going pain. However, stimulation of all sorts must be used with caution in the very young.

Pre-term infants. An infant at this age is easily overwhelmed by what is considered ordinary sensory stimuli. To decrease stress and promote self-regulation in the pre-term infant, certain stimuli should be avoided or minimized, e.g. unnecessary touching, stroking, or taking out of the incubator. The pre-term infant should be placed away from noises such as telephones, radios, areas of heavy activity and traffic, and bright lights. Feeding may need to take place in a shielded incubator or quiet corner of the room with the infant swaddled and often should not be accompanied by talking to or looking at the infant. Care must be taken not to offer too many types of stimuli at the same time. Appropriate stimuli for the pre-term infant include listening to soothing instrumental music and opportunities to grasp a finger roll or to suck (Als et al, 1986).

Pre-school and older children. Pre-school and older children often produce or initiate distraction to deal with pain. For painful procedures such as lumbar punctures, children 3 years of age and older may benefit from something as ordinary as squeezing someone's finger, clenching their fists, or engaging in an interesting conversation (McGrath and de Veber, 1986; Ross and Ross, 1984).

Out of 63 children between the ages of 6 and 19 years observed during bone marrow aspiration, 18 were bothered very little by the procedures. Fourteen were able to give significant clues about how they handled the procedure. Explanations included deliberate use of the following before and during the procedure: muscle contraction, e.g. clenching the fist or gripping the side of the table; screaming *prior* to pain, i.e. the needle injection; conversation, especially humourous and lively; and fantasy (Hilgard and LeBaron, 1984).

For painful procedures, a pop-up book may be especially suitable for the toddler. It has the advantage of providing multiple new and novel stimuli that are helpful in recapturing the child's attention whenever he/she focuses on the painful procedure. The child may stop looking at the book at times and observe the procedure or make some remark about it, but attention is fairly easily returned with a new pop-up. Being able to name the pictures in the book may also give the child a sense of achievement. The effectiveness of this distraction usually increases with practice or with experience using it in repeated painful procedures. Children report that the pop-up surprises seem to help the procedure go more quickly (Kuttner, 1986).

For children from 3 years of age through to adolescence, listening to music or a story is highly effective during a variety of brief painful procedures (Eland, 1988b). Naturally, allowing a child to select the story or music helps increase the effectiveness.

To use humour, keep in mind that a child's sense of humour differs from an adult's. For example, television cartoons are usually much funnier to school-age children than to adults.

Maintaining normal sensory input. For children confined to bed, especially in a hospital, avoiding boredom can be a challenge. Putting up mirrors so the child can see around the room and outside the room may help. Whenever possible, move the bed to the hallway, playroom, or outside. Provide physical exercise for the extremities with games such as throwing (with hands or feet) bean bags or wadded paper into the wastebasket. A daily project might be decorating the bed as a spaceship or with pictures drawn daily or with cards received in the mail. For many adolescents, a telephone is a necessary lifeline to the rest of the world.

Relaxation

Relaxation primarily reduces distress rather than pain, and it is not usually an appropriate substitute for pain-relief measures such as the administration of analgesics. However, it is a helpful coping mechanism for children and adults. Those relaxation strategies discussed in Chapter 6 that are useful for children 3 or 4 years of age and older include the deep breath/tense, exhale/relax, yawn exercise; humour; and progressive relaxation. It is especially helpful to tape record the recollection of the pleasant memories.

The presence of the parent, especially the child's mother, is helpful in reducing distress associated with pain in almost all age groups. As soon as the child is able to recognize the parent, probably in early infancy, encourage the parent to stay with the child during painful procedures or on-going pain, allowing the parent to touch, stroke, and hold the child whenever possible. From infancy up to age 4 years, the parent's holding of the child during painful procedures such as intramuscular injections or lumbar punctures, has been shown to result in less distress (Brown, 1984; Hallstrom, 1968).

Pre-term infants. Certain interventions appear to reduce stress and promote self-regulation in these infants during or between painful or other stressful events. Bedding and clothing may consist of a water mattress, sheepskin, and rolls of cloth to provide boundaries similar to those in the womb. When painful procedures are performed, an effort can be made to avoid interrupting deep sleep and to sequence activities to allow time in between. During the procedure the infant can be shielded from light and placed in as comfortable a position as is possible, such as supported in the prone or side-lying positions (not lying on the back). The infant can be swaddled, allowed to suck, and provided with something to grasp (see additional suggestions in Als et al, 1986). Dummies are offered to infants and toddlers to help reduce stress of on-going pain.

Toddlers and older children. Blowing bubbles is an especially effective technique, providing both relaxation and distraction. Most children are familiar with this activity. The child can count the bubbles as they float around the room, burst them, blow them around, or simply watch what happens to them. Or, blowing alone may be helpful. The child can be instructed to take a deep breath and slowly blow away anything that bothers him/her, such as hurt or scarey feelings. Ideally this is taught prior to a painful event (Kuttner, 1986).

Bubble-blowing may evolve into a form of slow rhythmic breathing without the bubbles. During a painful procedure, particularly one where the child must be very still or a sterile field is required, blowing bubbles may not be possible, but the technique can then be done without the bubbles. The young child may not be able to be distracted or to relax during the actual painful procedure, but the bubbles or slow breathing may reduce anxiety prior to the procedure.

Imagery

Imagery techniques designed to relieve pain are discussed in Chapter 6. Those that may be adapted for toddlers and older children include conversational imagery, breathing out pain, and an individualized imagery technique.

Examples of possible conversational imagery with the older child are suggestions to imagine medication travelling through the body to the pain or imagine blowing out the hurt with each exhalation. For a headache, the child can be instructed to gently blow air, e.g. enough to cause thin paper to flutter, and imagine the headache getting smaller and smaller each time he/she blows out.

Retelling or playing a tape recording of the child's favourite story during a painful procedure can be particularly effective. Prior to a painful event, if possible, find out what story is the child's favourite, or ask if he/she has a favourite outing such as going to the zoo. If the story or outing is unfamiliar to you, ask the child to tell you about it. During pain, the child can become involved in this, closing his eyes and pretending to be there in the imagination. The nurse can help the child become actively involved in this imagery by asking questions about what is seen, where he/she goes, and suggesting different possibilities in the story. The favourite story technique seems to be effective in reducing distress during painful procedures for children as young as 3 years of age, because it appears to provide distraction and relaxation, and may also produce dissociation from the pain (it does not, however, significantly reduce pain).

Chronic pain

Children suffer from almost all the various forms of chronic pain that occur in adults, e.g. recurrent acute pain as in migraine and chronic non-malignant pain as in musculoskeletal problems. (See Chapter 2 for classifications of chronic pain.) Of course, prolonged cancer pain occurs from infancy through to adulthood, but some types of chronic pain are more common with children, e.g. recurrent abdominal pain. However, chronic pain in children, except for cancer pain, has received very little attention. Although there are numerous multidisciplinary pain clinics for adults, very few exist for children.

Cancer pain in children is treated according to the same principles involved in treating adults. A considerable amount of literature addresses relief of cancer pain in children, particularly procedural pain, e.g. bone marrow aspirations. Pharmacological approaches are similar to those recommended for adults, and have been discussed earlier in this chapter.

Examples of chronic non-cancer pain in children include that resulting from cystic fibrosis, haemophilia, burns, headaches, recurrent abdominal pain, reflex sympathetic dystrophy, juvenile arthritis (JA, juvenile rheumatoid arthritis, juvenile chronic polyarthritis), and sickle cell disease. Some of the approaches suggested in Chapter 7 are helpful. For example, the number and severity of chronic migraine and non-migrainous headaches may be reduced in adolescents by teaching them relaxation techniques (Larsson et al, 1987).

Recurrent abdominal pain is one of the most common types of chronic non-malignant pain in children. Recently a simple approach proved effective in 52 children aged 5–15 years of age. Fewer attacks of recurrent abdominal pain occurred after only 6 weeks on a simple regimen of two corn fibre biscuits per day (McGrath and Feldman, 1986).

Sickle cell crisis, on the other hand, must usually be relieved with IV narcotics (for specific guidelines see annotated reference Cole, Sprinkle, Smith and Buchanan, 1986). IV PCA may be especially appropriate. Unfortunately, lack of knowledge of pharmacology and exaggerated fears of addiction have interfered with pain relief and research in this area (Schechter, Berrien and Katz, 1988).

When pain is prolonged in the child, achievement of age-related developmental tasks may be hampered. For example, pain may adversely affect motor development in the infant, play in the toddler, and peer relationships in the adolescent. Special efforts are required to decrease the intensity of the pain and teach the child coping mechanisms such as relaxation and distraction. For example, a comprehensive programme has been used for management of chronic non-malignant pain in children from pre-school age through to adolescence. Increased adherence to rehabilitation programmes has been successfully achieved with techniques such as guided imagery, relaxation, and modification of environmental factors that influence pain behaviours (Varni, Jay, Masek and Thompson, 1986). An increase in non-pain behaviours and the ability to avoid crying during a procedure probably also increase the child's self-esteem.

Adolescents may tend to report more pain than do school-age children (Beales, Kean and Lennox-Holt, 1983). This may be especially true when pain is chronic and not the result of a visible injury. Past experience with chronic pain may contribute to increased expression of pain because chronic pain may affect the child's life in ways that increase the child's awareness of the meaning of pain, e.g. decreased activity of juvenile arthritis.

When a child of any age is very expressive in response to prolonged or recurrent pain, there is sometimes a temptation to ignore the child's behavioural responses in an effort to decrease the intensity or frequency of the behaviour. Such an approach can easily lead to one of the historical problems in managing pain in adults— trying to minimize expression of pain without trying to relieve pain. This results from the health-care system holding the health-care team responsible for controlling a patient's expression of pain without being held responsible for relieving the pain (see Chapter 1).

In both children and adults with pain it is essential to remember the following about the relationship between behavioural expression and presence of pain:

- Lack of expression of pain does not necessarily mean lack of pain.
- Minimizing behavioural response to pain by ignoring the behaviour does not relieve the pain. Adults may be more comfortable if the child stops crying or clinging, but simply ignoring this behaviour is not an appropriate way to change it.
- If behavioural responses to pain are used by the child to gain attention or some other reward, the desired and appropriate rewards should be given to the child in situations other than pain.
- The best way to minimize behavioural response to pain is to relieve the pain or help the child learn ways of making the pain more tolerable.

The child's responses to pain must be met with appropriate attention and concern along with suggestions and efforts to relieve the pain or make it more bearable. When a child has pain, no matter how he/she expresses or responds to the pain, that child deserves our respect.

RESOURCES FOR CHILDREN, PARENTS, AND NURSES

The Oucher. Several studies (e.g. Beyer and Aradine, 1988) support the content and construct validity of this tool for self-reporting of pain intensity in white children aged 3–12 years. Although research on its use with non-white children has not been completed, the tool may be offered to these youngsters. A small picture of this much larger poster-like scale is shown in Fig. 8.4 (actual size is approximately 11 inches wide and 16 inches tall). The two scales, of numerical and photographic faces, facilitate use of the Oucher by children of varied ages and abilities. Those who can count to 100 may use the

Fig 8.4 The Oucher, copyright 1983 by the University of Virginia. Reprinted with permission.

numerical scale, while those who cannot may use the six faces. Since this tool is copyrighted, the reader must order it. Parents may find it helpful in the home care of children with pain; alternatively, the tool might be posted in several places in a facility caring for children, e.g. treatment rooms where painful procedures are performed. For a copy of the Oucher scale, user's manual, and technical report, send $9.95 to Judith E. Beyer, RN, PhD, Associate Professor, University of Colorado Health Sciences Center, School of Nursing, Campus Box C288, 4200 East Ninth Ave, Denver, CO 80262.

SELECTED ANNOTATED REFERENCES THAT CITE RESEARCH OR GIVE CLINICAL SUPPORT

Als, H.: Toward a synactive theory of development: promise for the assessment and support of infant individuality. *Infant Mental Health J.*, MDBO 3: 229–243, Winter 1982. A theoretical model to understand and assess the individual pre-term infant, 24–27 weeks postconception, is presented. The focus is on the dynamic, continuous interplay of various subsystems: autonomic, motor, state organizational, attentional-interactive, and self-regulatory. Specific interventions are suggested for accomplishing the goal of decreasing the stress accompanying manipulation of the infant and enhancing stabilization. Suggestions include introducing stimuli to the baby during a transition state and avoiding introduction of stimuli when the baby is soundly asleep or quietly alert, helping the infant into a flexed position, providing a soft, graspable roll for both hands, facing the baby away from a direct light source, avoiding the supine position, avoiding eye contact with certain infants during feeding, and being alert to cues that too much input is being provided. Such cues include the infant yawning, averting his gaze, sneezing, or hiccoughing. Tables of stress reactions and of self-regulatory behaviours are included.

Anand, K.J.S., and Hickey, P.R.: Pain and its effects in the human neonate and fetus. *N. Engl. J. Med.* **317**:1321–1329, Nov 19, 1987. This review of the literature includes 201 references to pain in the human fetus and neonate. Based on the findings of numerous studies, the authors state some of the following conclusions in an attempt to help correct widespread misconceptions about the fetus or neonate not feeling pain. Cutaneous sensory receptors have spread to all cutaneous and mucous surfaces by the 20th week of gestation, and the density of nociceptive nerve endings in the skin of newborns is similar to or greater than that in adult skin. Also, by 20 weeks the fetal neocortex has a full complement of

neurons, and several tests suggest functional maturity. Lack of myelination does not support the argument that neonates are not capable of pain perception. Even in the peripheral nerves of adults, nociceptive impulses are carried through unmyelinated fibres. Incomplete myelination merely implies a slower conduction velocity in the nerves, which is offset completely in the neonate by the shorter distances traveled by the impulses. The authors conclude, "Thus, human newborns do have the anatomical and functional components required for the perception of painful stimuli" (p. 1323). Regarding memory of pain, they point out that even adults cannot remember pain, only the experiences associated with pain. Further, memory and learning depend on brain plasticity, which is known to be highest during the late prenatal and neonatal periods.

Studies of neonates undergoing painful procedures reveal changes in cardiovascular variables, transcutaneous partial pressure of oxygen, and palmar sweating. Local anaesthesia for circumcision prevents changes in heart rate, blood pressure, and decreases in transcutaneous partial pressure of oxygen, but use of a pacifier during heel stick does not alter the preterm neonate's cardiovascular or respiratory responses to pain. Detailed hormonal studies in pre-term and full-term neonates undergoing surgery with minimal anaesthesia document marked metabolic stress responses that can be inhibited by potent anaesthetics such as halothane and fentanyl. In fact, preliminary evidence suggests that neonates having light anaesthesia during major cardiac surgery have increased postoperative morbidity and mortality. Evidence for increased sensitivity to pain with decreased age includes several studies of the cry response to painful procedures in neonates and older infants (3–12 months). The authors conclude that the evidence shows that "marked nociceptive activity clearly constitutes a physiologic and perhaps even a psychological form of stress in premature or full-term neonates" (p. 1326).

Anand, K.J.S., Sippell, W.G., and Aynsley-Green, A.: Randomized trial of fentanyl anaesthesia in preterm babies undergoing surgery: effects on the stress response. *Lancet* **1**:62–66, Jan 10, 1987. In a study of pre-term infants undergoing ligation of patent ductus arteriosus (PDA) and anaesthetized with nitrous oxide and d-tubocurarine, 8 with fentanyl (10 μg/kg IV) added and 8 without fentanyl, major hormonal responses to surgery were significantly greater in the non-fentanyl than in the fentanyl group. Some responses remained greater in the non-fentanyl group on the third postoperative day. Compared with the fentanyl group, the non-fentanyl group members were more likely to require an increase in ventilatory support after surgery and to have circulatory or metabolic complications. Two in the non-fentanyl group developed intraventricular haemorrhages during or soon after surgery. The authors conclude that the substantial stress response to surgery under anaesthesia with nitrous oxide and curare can be prevented by the addition of fentanyl and that this may improve postoperative outcome. They also conclude that the degree of analgesia in paralysed and ventilated infants can be assessed reliably only by measurement of the biochemical and endocrine markers of stress. The authors cite studies showing that surgical stress responses last longer in pre-term than in full-term babies and are greater in magnitude than those of adult patients. Further analysis of 40 published reports showed that 77% of newborn babies undergoing surgical ligation of PDA received either muscle relaxants alone or with nitrous oxide given intermittently.

Beasley, S.W., and Tibballs, J.: Efficacy and safety of continuous morphine infusion for postoperative analgesia in the paediatric surgical ward. *Aust. N.Z. J. Surg.* 57:233–237, Apr 1987. Continuous infusion of morphine following major surgery in 121 non-ventilated children resulted in few side effects with adequate pain relief as rated by the patient, if able, and the parents and nurses. The article includes the protocol for morphine infusion. A therapeutic range of 10–40 µg/kg/hr was used, usually starting at 20–25 µg/kg/hr. The age range was from less than 1 year (13 infants, 4 weighing less than 5kg) to 14 years. Only 26 of the 121 patients had complications attributed to morphine, the most frequent problem being vomiting (27 patients). Respiratory depression did not occur in any patient. The authors recommend continuous morphine infusion as a routine method of analgesia for children following major surgery.

Beaver, P.K.: Premature infants' response to touch and pain: can nurses make a difference? *Neonatal Network,* 6:13–17, Dec 1987. Intraventricular haemorrhage (IVH) is a major cause of death among premature infants. Decreasing crying and hypoxic episodes may decrease the incidence of IVH. Thus, painful stimuli may be life threatening if they result in crying in these neonates. This study of 8 premature infants exposed to touch only, heel lance only, and heel lance plus stroking on the medial side of the same leg, revealed that the latter situation caused the greatest increase in heart rate and blood pressure and decrease in transcutaneous oxygenation. The greatest percentage of change from baseline for both heart rate and blood pressure occurred during the first 10 seconds after the stimuli. The author suggests that to reduce the magnitude of the premature's response to stimulation, stimulation might be done as quickly as possible and the infant should be allowed to recover before being exposed to the next set of stimuli.

Bell, S.G., and Ellis, L.J.: Use of fentanyl for sedation of mechanically ventilated neonates. *Neonatal Network,*

6:27–31, Oct 1987. This article combines a good review of the literature with the authors' clinical experience. It is fairly common practice to use low to moderate doses (2–4 µg/kg) for sedation of the mechanically ventilated infant who is agitated and/or in pain. Neonates' responses to noxious stimuli include agitation, cyanosis, bradycardia, hypoxia, and hypercarbia. Advantages of fentanyl for neonates are a faster onset and shorter duration than morphine. Given IV it has an almost immediate onset with peak respiratory depression occurring in 5–10 minutes. These authors have successfully used fentanyl for sedation and pain relief in both ventilated and nonventilated infants, e.g. for postoperative pain or one-time doses for painful procedures such as insertion of a chest tube. For sedation they recommend fentanyl 2–4 µg/kg given IV over a minimum of 2 minutes (preferably over 15 minutes to avoid respiratory muscle rigidity), with frequency determined on an individual basis. Because fentanyl binds to tissues, the infant must be observed for rebound fentanyl plasma levels. As with all narcotics, there is a risk of seizure activity. Fentanyl should be avoided in patients who are hypotensive or have impaired hepatic function. During the initial administration of fentanyl to the ventilated infant, a respiratory therapist probably should be present to evaluate the need for changing ventilatory settings. When fentanyl is discontinued after prolonged use, the infants should be observed for signs of withdrawal syndrome.

Beyer, J.E., and Aradine, C.R.: Patterns of pediatric pain intensity: a methodological investigation of a self-report scale. *Clin. J. Pain,* 3:130–141, 1987. This study of 95 hospitalized children 3–12 years old supported the construct validity of a self-report scale called the Oucher, copyrighted in 1983 by The University of Virginia. (Construct validity is the degree to which an instrument measures the concept, e.g. pain under investigation.) For more information on the Oucher, see p. and Fig. 8.4.

Billmire, D.A., Neale, H.W., and Gregory, R.O.: Use of IV fentanyl in the outpatient treatment of pediatric facial trauma. *J. Trauma* 25:1079–1080, Nov 1985. For repair of facial lacerations in 2000 children between the ages of 12 months and 12 years, a dose of 2–3 mg/kg body weight was administered slowly intravenously to provide sedation and analgesia. The rapid onset and short duration (30–40 minutes) of fentanyl make it advantageous for use in brief painful procedures where rapid recovery is desired. The IV dose was administered over 3–5 minutes since more rapid administration might result in paralysis of the respiratory muscles or apnoea. Peak respiratory depression from fentanyl may not occur for 5–15 minutes. Only 3 apnoeic episodes occurred and all were successfully reversed with naloxone.

Interestingly, the authors report that children aged 18–36 months usually required the full calculated dose while older children usually required less than the calculated dose. Facial pruritis was a minor problem. Few difficulties were encountered with nausea and vomiting, and there were no episodes of delirium or muscular rigidity. Local anaesthesia was used after fentanyl became effective. An additional benefit of using fentanyl was that the children were less fearful when they returned for suture removal.

Brown, S.R.: An anxiety reduction technique during lumbar punctures in infants and toddlers. *J. Assn Pediatr. Oncol. Nurs.* **1**:24–25, Summer 1984. In 8 children between the ages of 1 and 4 years, a total of 25 lumbar punctures were performed with the mother holding the child upright in her arms with a pillow at the child's abdomen to help arch the back. The children exhibited minimal crying and movement, and the parents were pleased to be able to offer comfort.

Burne, R., and Hunt, A.: Use of opiates in terminally ill children. *Palliative Med.* **1**:27–30, 1987. A review of the records of 21 children, ranging in age from infancy to 14 years, who had received morphine or diamorphine during terminal care, revealed that the highest 4-hourly doses were in the young age group, 1–4 years. The doses included the equivalent of 360mg of morphine PO 4 hourly in one child and 240mg 4 hourly in another. High doses also occurred in the age group 5–9 years, with one child receiving 150mg 4 hourly and another receiving 90 mg 4 hourly. These doses were determined by titration according to the individual's response. Respiratory depression was not seen in any child. Routine administration of laxatives, but not antiemetics, is likely to be necessary in children receiving strong opiates.

Cole, T.B., Sprinkle, R.H., Smith, S.J., and Buchanan, G.R.: Intravenous narcotic therapy for children with severe sickle cell crisis pain. *Am. J. Dis. Child* **140**:1255–1259, 1986. The records of 38 children and adolescents (age range not specified) with 98 episodes of sickle cell vaso-occlusive crisis were reviewed, in which 76 episodes were treated with a continuous IV narcotic infusion. The authors used a protocol consisting of bolus IV injection of 0.15mg/kg morphine or 1.0mg/kg meperidine upon arrival at the hospital, followed by narcotic continuous infusion at a dose rate of 0.07–0.10 mg/kg/hr morphine or 0.5–0.7 mg/kg/hr meperidine, with bolus injections as needed, titrated upward by increments of about 25% 3 hourly until satisfactory pain relief was achieved (usually based on ratings by patient or the parents). Patient comfort was usually achieved in a little over 3 hours after initiating the protocol. Narcotic infusions usually continued for about 72 hours, and then some were stopped abruptly and others tapered with doses of oral acetaminophen with codeine. Seizures did not occur with meperidine, as had been reported by others, but the authors specify that they did not use phenothiazines as did the others because phenothiazines lower seizure threshold and do not enhance analgesia. Side effects of narcotic therapy were frequent, especially lethargy, but were not serious. No addictive behaviour was observed in any patients.

Dilworth, N.M., and MacKellar, A.: Pain relief for the pediatric surgical patient. *J. Pediatr. Surg.* **22**:264–266, Mar 1987. In 144 patients ranging in age from 6 months to 15 years who had received 155 variable-rate IV narcotic infusions, respiratory rate dropped below the set minimum in only one patient. Reduction of drug dosage was sufficient and naloxone was not required. Restriction of movement troubled the 1–2-year-old children and sometimes led to early termination of the IV. In an additional 242 infusions in children, only one patient suffered respiratory depression and required a small dose of naloxone. Contrary to the fears of medical and nursing staff, respiratory depression was very infrequent, promptly recognized, and easily corrected. The authors discuss other methods of postoperative pain relief and stress the importance of including this in pediatric surgical textbooks.

Dothage, J.A., Arndt, C., and Miser, A.W.: Use of continuous intravenous morphine infusion for pain control in an infant with terminal malignancy. *J. Assn. Pediatr. Oncol. Nurs.* **3**:22–24, 1986. In a 10-month-old, 8kg infant with prolonged cancer pain, the dose of IV morphine required to relieve pain seemed to be successfully titrated by using two independent observers (the mother and the nurse) who rated pain on a visual analog scale using behaviour that predictably varied with tumour size and analgesic administration. Types of behaviour that indicated pain and that improved with increased narcotic dose were holding the painful area, failure to move the painful limb, decrease in general activity, poor sleep, poor food intake, fretfulness, and crying. Physiological parameters, which have been shown to change in newborns in response to acute pain, were not reliable. At the time of his death the continuous IV infusion dose of morphine had remained at 0.25mg/hr for 2 days. At this dose the mother could hold him without his crying out in pain, and he seemed to sleep comfortably, ate small amounts, and occasionally smiled at his parents.

Eland, J.M.: Children's pain: developmentally appropriate efforts to improve identification of source, intensity and relevant intervening variables. In Felton, G., and Albert, M., eds: *Nursing research: a monograph for non-nurse researchers*, pp 64–79, U of Iowa Press, Iowa City, 1983. This publication cites research data regarding the least painful injection site as being the ventrogluteal muscle. The vastus lateralis is more painful, and the rectus is the most painful of the three. (See also Eland, 1988a.)

Forlini, J., Morin, D.M., and Treacy, S.: Painless peds procedures. *Am. J. Nurs.* **87**:321–323, Mar 1987. The authors report on the use of the ultra–short-acting anaesthetic ketamine for brief procedural pain in children as young as 7 months. Appropriate procedures include lumbar puncture, intrathecal chemotherapy, bone marrow aspiration, removal of an indwelling central catheter, laryngoscopy, burn debridement, circumcision, and dental work. Usually it is given IV, and loss of consciousness occurs in about 30 seconds and lasts approximately 10 minutes.

Haslam, D.R.: Age and the perception of pain. *Psychon. Sci.* **15**: 86–87, 1969. This is one of the few studies that addresses the issue of pain perception in relation to age in children. Using increasing pressure to the tibia to cause pain, the pain thresholds of 115 well school children aged 5–18 years were measured. The results indicated that pain threshold increases between the ages of 5 and 18, indicating that the perception of pain begins to decline at a very early age. In other words, between the ages of 5 and 18, the younger the child, the lower the pain threshold and the more pain is felt. (These findings are in direct opposition to the common belief that younger children feel less pain than older children and adults.)

Johnston, C.C., and Strada, M.E.: Acute pain response in infants: a multidimensional description. *Pain,* **24**:373–382, 1986. Responses of 14 infants, ages 2 and 4 months, undergoing routine immunization were observed. There was wide variability between infants, but facial expression was consistent. The facial expression consisted of brows lowered and drawn together, bulging forehead with vertical furrows between the brows, a broadened nasal root, eyes tightly closed, and an angular, squarish mouth. The pattern of response was characterized by several phases: an initial drop in heart rate and a long, high-pitched cry followed by a period of apnoea, rigid torso and limbs, and a facial expression of pain. This was followed by a sharp increase in heart rate, lower-pitched but dysphonated cries, less body rigidity, and a facial expression of pain, and finally a continued elevation in heart rate, lower-pitched and more rhythmic cries with a rising-falling pattern, and a return to normal body posture.

Katz, E.R., Kellerman, J. and Siegel, S.E.: Behavioural distress in children with cancer undergoing medical procedures: developmental considerations. *J. Consult Clin. Psychol.* **48**:356–365, 1980. An observational behaviour rating scale was used to measure anxiety responses to bone marrow aspirations in 115 children with cancer, ages 8 months to 17 years and 9 months. A significant relationship was found between age and both quantity and type of anxious behaviour, with younger children tending to respond with a greater variety of anxious behaviours over a longer period of

time than older children. With advancing age the children responded with more withdrawal and muscle tension. These data clearly show that children do not "get used to" painful procedures.

Katz, E.R., et al: Beta-endorphin immunoreactivity and acute behavioural distress in children with leukemia. *J. Nerv. Ment. Dis.* **170**:72–77, 1982. Beta-endorphin levels were measured in 75 children with leukaemia, ages 8 months to 18 years 4 months, undergoing routine lumbar puncture. Behavioural measures of distress included objective behaviour, nurse ratings of anxiety, and self-reports of pain and fear. Results of the study support the hypothesis that pain and stress produce increased endorphin levels. In the children over 4 years of age, endorphin decreased with age, suggesting greater distress and pain in the younger children. Inconsistent results were obtained for children younger than 4 years of age, possibly because of antineoplastic chemotherapeutic variables. Interestingly, girls were found to have lower endorphin levels than boys, suggesting that boys may be biologically more adept at minimizing pain and stress because of their enhanced ability to produce endorphin. Alternatively, girls may have less need for endorphin because of better expressive abilities and less internal stress. All of these findings, of course, must be considered preliminary. Further research is needed.

Krishnan, A., Tolhurst-Cleaver, C.L., and Kay, B.: Controlled comparison of nalbuphine and morphine for post-tonsillectomy pain. *Anaesthesia* **12**:1178–1181, 1985. Pain relief following tonsillectomy helps prevent crying and straining that might precipitate bleeding. Morphine 0.2 mg/kg IM, nalbuphine 0.3mg/kg IM, and placebo were compared following tonsillectomy in 60 children aged between 4 and 12 years. One of the drugs was administered 5 minutes before the conclusion of surgery. Pain, restlessness, and side effects were assessed 1 and 2 hours later. (It is not clear how pain was assessed.) No significant differences were found between the two narcotics. Drowsiness occurred but other side effects were uncommon. Nalbuphine may offer advantages compared with morphine in regard to safety. Choice of dose with nalbuphine is less critical than it is with morphine since nalbuphine has a proven maximal respiratory depressant effect.

Lynn, A.M., Opheim, K.E., and Tyler, D.C.: Morphine infusion after pediatric cardiac surgery. *Crit. Care Med.* **12**:863–866, 1984. After cardiac surgery, 44 children, aged 14 months to 17 years, received a continuous IV infusion of morphine ranging from 10–50mg/kg/hr, with the majority on 10–30mg/kg/hr.

Lynn, A.M., and Slattery, J.T.: Morphine pharmacokinetics in early infancy. *Anesthesiology* **66**:136–139, 1987. Pharmacokinetic studies of morphine in 10 infants showed longer elimination half-lives in those 1–4 days of age than in older infants

17–65 days of age, mean 6.8 hours and 3.9 hours, respectively. Clearance in the young ones was less than half that found in the older infants. The combination of lower clearance and longer elimination half-life in the newborns may explain the prolonged duration of action of morphine in very young infants. However, in infants older than 1 month of age, morphine clearance reaches or surpasses the adult level, and they are not more sensitive to respiratory depressant effects of morphine than are adults.

Miser, A.W., Chayt, K.J., Sandlund, J.T., Cohen, P.S., Dothage, J.A. and Miser, J.S.: Narcotic withdrawal syndrome in young adults after the therapeutic use of opiates. *Am. J. Dis. Child* **140**:603–604, June 1986. Five young adults, including one 14- and one 15-year-old, developed narcotic withdrawal 6–48 hours after abrupt discontinuation of narcotic therapy that had been administered for 6–21 days. The symptoms included agitation, irritability, muscular jerks, abdominal pain, diarrhoea, burning sensations, "gooseflesh", and itching. Four of the patients, including the two adolescents, were successfully weaned without recurrence of withdrawal symptoms. The fifth patient was continued on methadone because of continuing pain. Important points include the fact that physical dependence on narcotics refers to an altered physiological state produced by prolonged or repeated exposure to a drug that results in withdrawal syndrome when the drug is abruptly discontinued. It is not addiction, defined as a behavioural pattern of drug use and overwhelming involvement with use of a drug. Further, cancer patients may frequently become physically dependent but rarely become addicted to narcotics. Families need to be assured that physical dependency is not synonymous with addiction. The aetiology of physical dependence and the withdrawal symptoms that follow abrupt discontinuation of narcotics are not fully understood. However, continuous morphine infusion may more rapidly lead to physical dependence than an intermittent narcotic schedule. Several methods may be used to manage withdrawal symptoms. The authors chose to use oral methadone, a long-acting narcotic, given in a tapering schedule over approximately 5 days.*

Nover, R.A.: Pain and the burned child. *J. Am. Acad. Child Psychiatry*, **12**:499–505, July 1973. This is one of the early studies of children's reactions to pain. A case study of a 5-year-old boy with a 3% second and third degree burn on the leg and buttocks, but no sense of pain in the area due to a spinal cord anomaly, revealed this child reacted far less to the burn than other children who felt the sensation of pain. The child showed very little regressive tendency and no hostile behaviour toward the staff. Consequently the author says that negative feelings of the staff toward the child were absent. (Apparently it was common for staff to react to burned children with judgments of "good and bad", failing to understand that a child's hostile behaviour and lack of cooperation were due to pain.)

Owens, M.E., and Todt, E.H.: Pain in infancy: neonatal reaction to heel lance. *Pain,* **20**:77–86, 1984. Responses in 20 2-day-old newborns to heel lance showed that crying and increased heart rate occurred consistently. Heart rate increased to an average of 179 beats per minute, a rise of 49 beats per minute, with this increase lasting an average of 3.5 minutes until a return to baseline.

Rogers, B.M., Webb, C.J., Stergios, D., and Newman, B.M.: Patient-controlled analgesia in pediatric surgery. *J. Pediatr. Surg.* **23**:259—262, Mar 1988. PCA (patient controlled analgesia) using IV boluses of morphine without continuous infusion, was evaluated in 15 children between 11 and 18 years old undergoing major abdominal or thoracic surgery. All were mentally alert, had no history of narcotic abuse, and were able to understand the instructions. Several different approaches to pain rating were used, and apparently satisfactory pain relief was obtained in all patients. Compared with 15 patients receiving the usual IM analgesia postoperatively, the 15 children on IV PCA self-administered about twice as much narcotic during the first 24 hours, but the dose was still well within the recommended therapeutic range. This finding is also typical of adult patients on IV PCA. No significant respiratory depression occurred. By the third day, the PCA patients were administering less narcotic than the comparison group receiving IM narcotic. (Authors' note: There was no evidence of narcotic abuse postoperatively in the group using IV PCA.) Only two patients did not like IV PCA, and both experienced burning at the site of infusion of morphine, which the researchers thought was due to rapid infusion of a relatively large bolus dose, i.e. greater than 2.5mg. They conclude that the most satisfactory degree of analgesia is achieved with smaller doses of morphine at shorter lockout intervals. They suggest a loading dose of morphine 2–4 mg (0.05–0.10 mg/kg) and bolus doses of 1–2mg (0.025–0.05mg/kg) with a lockout interval of 10–15 minutes. (Authors' note: This study was done before most PCA pumps had the capacity for continuous infusion in addition to boluses. Based on the researchers' recommendations, a combination of continuous infusion with boluses as needed would

---

*This reinforces the merit of an intermittent schedule of oral narcotics when this is possible. When IV narcotics are necessary, the health-care team should be alert to withdrawal syndrome and institute appropriate treatment. The higher likelihood of withdrawal syndrome with IV narcotics should not prohibit their use, since withdrawal can be successfully handled in several ways.

probably be better than bolus alone.)

The advantages of PCA IV were that the child had control of analgesia and did not have to wait for nurses to bring doses. The children apparently had no difficulty understanding how to use PCA IV boluses. The researchers recommend PCA for patients 10 years of age or older and are now exploring the possibility of allowing responsible parents to use PCA IV to provide postoperative analgesia for younger children.

Ross, D.M., and Ross, S.A.: Childhood pain: the school-aged child's viewpoint. *Pain,* **20**:179–191, 1984. Semi-structured interviews of 994 children, age 5–12 years, revealed great diversity in children's preference for the timing of information about pain. The trend was for a preference toward having a longer rather than a shorter period between receiving information and the actual event. Parents in particular need to be aware of their child's preference. Only 213 children reported use of self-initiated strategies for coping with pain, with distraction and physical activity, such as fist clenching, being the more frequent.

Stang, H.J., Gunnar, M.R., Snellman, L., Condon, L.M., and Kestenbaum, R.: Local anaesthesia for neonatal circumcision: effects on distress and cortisol response. *J.A.M.A.* **259**:1507–1511, Mar 11, 1988. Although there is no absolute medical indication for routine circumcision of the newborn, it continues to be done in the United States and typically in the absence of anaesthesia. Oddly, it is the only elective surgical procedure routinely performed without anaesthesia. In a controlled, double-blind study of healthy male newborns, 60 subjects were randomly assigned to three groups for circumcision with lidocaine, saline, or no injection. The results revealed that dorsal penile nerve block was safe, easy, and effective in reducing behavioural distress and modifying the adrenocortical stress response. However, there was still discomfort and stress associated with circumcision. During the circumcision, babies in the lidocaine group cried 23% of the time, while babies in the saline and control groups cried 68% and 71% of the time, respectively, the latter two figures showing striking increases in the percentage of time spent crying compared with crying during the injection period and the precircumcision nursery observation period. Overall, the lidocaine injection attenuated the adrenocortical response to circumcision, as compared with the response in the saline and no-injection groups. Further, in the majority of instances, observers were able to correctly distinguish between infants who had received saline and those who had received lidocaine.

The process of injecting the lidocaine did not increase stress reactions and did not offset the beneficial effects of anaesthesia. In fact, during the injection period (strapped on the restraint board 5 minutes before circumcision), the babies in the lidocaine and saline groups did not cry more than did the babies in the no-injection group. Thus the restraint itself caused as much crying as the injection. Several research studies are cited as evidence that the absence of crying following circumcision is the result of coping mechanisms, not the result of lack of postoperative pain. The authors state that if circumcisions are to be performed, they should be done as humanely as possible.

Stewart, C.F., and Hampton, E.M.: Effect of maturation on drug disposition in pediatric patients. *Clin. Pharm.,* **6**:548–564, July 1987. Age-related changes in biotransformation (the chemical alterations that a substance undergoes in the body) are extremely complex. It is almost impossible to predict the effect of maturation on a biotransformation process based solely on the postnatal age of an infant. For most drugs, biotransformation is decreased in the neonate, increased from 1 to 5 years of age, and decreased after puberty, eventually reaching adult values. Maturational changes from infancy to adolescence have a more striking effect on drug response than do changes associated with aging. Still, biological maturation has a poorly understood effect on drug disposition. Children remain "therapeutic orphans", and many drugs marketed in the United States for adults have not been studied in children and thus carry the warning on the drug insert that safe drug usage has not been established for certain young age groups.

Wong, D.L., and Baker, C.M.: Pain in children: comparison of assessment scales. *Pediatr. Nurs.,* **14**:9–17, Jan-Feb 1988. The validity, reliability, and preference of 6 pain assessment scales (simple descriptive, numeric of 0–10, faces, water glasses, chips, and colours) were investigated in 150 hospitalized children aged 3–18 years. With all scales, validity increased with advancing age. Reliability increased from the 3–7 year to the 8–12 year group, but decreased for most scales in the 13–18 year age group, suggesting the possibility that the younger children remembered pain more vividly than did older children. The most preferred scale overall was the faces scale. Of the 116 events the children reported as painful, the most commonly reported were those involving needles, e.g. injections and venepuncture.

Wong, D.L., and Whaley, L.F.: *Clinical handbook of pediatric nursing,* ed 2, The C.V. Mosby Co, St. Louis, 1986. This book is a practical guide to many aspects of caring for the child and family. Specific information that is particularly helpful in caring for children with pain includes both general and age-specific guidelines for preparing children for procedures (pp 363 to 366), play activities for specific procedures (p 368), and suggestions for assessing and relieving pain in children (pp 372 to 378).

BRITISH LITERATURE ON PAIN

Burn, R. and Hunt, A.: Use of opiates in terminally ill children. *Palliative Med.* 1(1):27–30, 1987.

Chambers, E.J., Oakhill, A., Cornish, J.M. and Cumick, S.: Terminal care at home for children with cancer. *B.M.J.* **298**:937–940, 1989.

Chapman, J. and Goodhall, J.: Symptom control in ill and dying children. *J. Maternal and Child Health*, 5:144–154, 1980.

Goldman, A. and Bowman, A.: The role of oral, controlled-release morphine in pain relief in children with cancer. *Palliative Med.* 4(4):279–285, 1990.

Hunt, A.M.: Open house, *Nurs. Times*, 1986.

Hunt, A.M.: A survey of signs, symptoms, and symptom control in 30 terminally ill children. *Developmental Med. and Child Neurology* 32:341–346, 1990.

Mann, R.A., Freeman, A., and Clark, E.: Children with cancer. In Walsh, TD (ed), *Symptom Control*, Blackwell Scientific Publications, Oxford, 1985.

REFERENCES AND SELECTED READINGS

Als, H., Lawhon, G., Brown, E., Gibes, R., Duffy, F.H., et al: Individualized behavioural and environmental care for the very low birth weight preterm infant at high risk for bronchopulmonary dysplasia: neonatal intensive care unit and developmental outcome. *Pediatrics* **78**:1123–1132, Dec 1986.

Als, H., Lester, B.M., Tronick, E.Z., and Brazelton, T.B.: Toward a research instrument for the assessment of preterm infants' behaviour (APIB). In Fitzgerald, H, Lester, BM, and Yogman, MW, eds: *Theory and research in behavioral pediatrics* 1:3563, Plenum Press, New York, 1982.

Anand, K.J.S., and Aynsley-Green, A.: Metabolic and endocrine effects of surgical ligation of patent ductus arteriosus in the human preterm neonate: are there implications for further improvement of postoperative outcome? *Mod. Probl. Paediatr.* **23**:143–157, 1985.

Anand, K.J.S., Brown, M.J., Causon, R.C., Christofides, N.D., Bloom, S.R., and Aynsley-Green, A.: Can the human neonate mount an endocrine and metabolic response to surgery? *J. Pediatr. Surg.* **20**:41–48, Feb 1985.

Anand, K.J.S., et al: Studies on the hormonal regulation of fuel metabolism in the human newborn infant undergoing anesthesia and surgery. *Horm. Res.* 22:115–128, 1985.

Anand, K.J.S. and McGrath, P.J.: *Neonatal pain and distress.* Elsevier Science Publishers, Inc., Amsterdam, 1989.

Anand, K.J.S., Sippell, W.G., and Aynsley-Green, A.: Randomized trial of fentanyl anaesthesia in preterm neonates undergoing surgery: effects on the stress response. *Lancet* 1:243–248, 1987.

Aradine, C.R., Beyer, J.E., and Tompkins, J.M.: Children's pain perception before and after analgesia: a study of instrument construct validity and related issues. *J. Pediatr. Nurs.* 3:11–23, Feb 1988.

Axton, S.E., and Fugate, T.: A protocol for pediatric IV Meds. *Am. J. Nurs.* **87**:943–945, July 1987.

Baker, C.M., and Wong, D.L.: Q.U.E.S.T.: a process of pain assessment in children. *Orthopaed. Nurs.* **6**:11–20, Jan-Feb 1987.

Beales, J.G., Kean, J.H., and Lennox-Holt, P.J.: The child's perception of the disease and the experience of pain in juvenile chronic arthritis. *J. Rheumatol.* **10**:61–65, 1983.

Benitz, W.E., and Tatro, D.S.: The pediatric drug handbook. Year Book Medical Publishers, Chicago, 1981.

Beyer, J.E.: *The Oucher: a user's manual and technical report.* Judson Press, Evanston, Ill, 1984.

Beyer, J.E., and Aradine, C.R.: Content validity of an instrument to measure young children's perceptions of the intensity of their pain. *J. Pediatr. Nurs.* 1:386–394, Dec 1986.

Beyer, J.E., and Aradine, C.R.: Convergent and discriminant validity of a self-report measure of pain intensity for children. *Child Health Care* **16**:274–282, Spring 1988.

Beyer, J.E., Ashley, L.C., Russell, G.A., and DeGood, D.E.: Pediatric pain after cardiac surgery: pharmacologic management. *Dimens Crit. Care Nurs.* 3:326–334, Nov-Dec 1984.

Beyer, J.E., and Byers, M.L.: Knowledge of pediatric pain: the state of the art. *Child Health Care* **13**:150–159, Spring 1985.

Beyer, J.E., DeGood, D.E., Ashley, L.C., and Russell, G.A.: Patterns of postoperative analgesic use with adults and children following cardiac surgery. *Pain* **17**:71–81, 1983.

Beyer, J.E., and Knapp, T.R.: Methodological issues in the measurement of children's pain. Child Health Care 14:233–241, Spring 1986.

Beyer, J.E., and Levin, C.R.: Issues and advances in pain control in children. *Nurs. Clin. North Am.* **22**:661–676, Sept 1987.

Bhatt-Mehta, V., and Rosen, D.: Management of actue pain in chdilren. *Clin. Pharm.*, **10**:667–685, Sept 1991.

Bradshaw, C., and Zeanah, P.D.: Pediatric nurses' assessments of pain in children. *J. Pediatr. Nurs.* 1:314–322, Oct 1986.

Broadman, L.M., et al: Post-circumcision analgesia—a prospective evaluation of subcutaneous ring block of the penis. *Anesthesiology* **67**:399–402, Sept 1987.

Brown, L.: Physiologic responses to cutaneous pain in neonates. *Neonatal Network* **6**:18–22, Dec 1987.

Clarke, S., and Radford, M.: Topical anaesthesia for venepuncture. *Arch. Dis. in Childhood* **61**:1132–1134, 1986.

Collins, L.: Pain sensitivity and ratings of childhood experience. *Percept Mot Skills* 21:349–350, 1965.

Cowlay, C.K. and Bogs, R.A.: Fatal outcome with use of rectal morphine for postoperative pain control in an infant. *B.M.J.* **304**:766–767, Mar, 1992.

Craig, K.D., McMahon, R.J., Morison, J.D., and Zaskow, C.: Developmental changes in infant pain expression during immunization injections. *Soc. Sci. Med.* 19:1131–1137, 1984.

Davidson, J.A.H., and Boom, S.J.: Warming lignocaine to reduce pain associated with injection. *B.M.J.* **305**:617–618, 1992.

Duncan, A.: The postoperative period. *Clin. Anesthesiol.* **3**:619–632, July 1985.

Eland, J.M.: The child who is hurting. *Semin. Oncol. Nurs.* 1:116–122, May 1985a.

Eland, J.M.: Pain in children. In Hockenberry, M., and Coody, D., eds: *Pediatric hematology-oncology: perspectives in care*, pp 394–406. The CV Mosby Co. St Louis, 1986.

Eland, J.M.: Pediatrics. In *Pain. Nursing now* series, pp 108–118, Springhouse Corp. Springhouse, Pa, 1985b.

Eland, J.M.: Persistence in pediatric pain research: one nurse researcher's efforts, *Recent Adv. Nurs.* 1988a.

Eland, J.M.: Personal communication, University of Iowa, Iowa City, Iowa, 1988b.

Eland, J.M.: Pharmacologic management of acute and chronic pediatric pain. *Issues Comp. Pediatr. Nurs.* 11:93–111, 1988c.

Eland, J.M. and Anderson, J.E.: The experience of pain in children. In Jacox, A, ed: *Pain: a sourcebook for nurses and other health professionals*, pp 453–473, Little, Brown & Co, Boston, 1977.

Epstein, M.H., and Harris, J., Jr: Children with chronic pain: can they be helped? *Pediatr. Nurs.* 4:42–44, 1978.

Favaloro, R.: Adolescent development and implications for pain management. *Pediatr. Nurs.* 14:27–29, Jan–Feb 1988.

Feychting, H.: Premedication and psychological preparation. *Clin. Anaesthesiol.* 3:505–514, July 1985.

Fisher, D.M., Robinson, S., Brett, C.M., Perin, G., and Gregory, G.A.: Comparison of enflurane, halothane, and isoflurane for diagnostic procedures in children with malignancies. *Anesthesiology* 3:647–650, Dec 1985.

Flower, R.J., Moncada, S., and Vane, J.R.: Drug therapy of inflammation. In Gilman, A.G., Goodman, L.S., Rall, T.W., and Mural, F., eds: Goodman and Gilman's *The pharmacological basis of therapeutics*, ed 7, pp 674–715, Macmillan Publishing Co, Inc., New York, 1985.

Fowler-Kerry, S., and Lander, J.R.: Management of injection pain in children. *Pain* 30:169–175, 1987.

Gaffney, A., and Dunne, E.A.: Developmental aspects of children's definitions of pain. *Pain* 26:105–117, 1986.

Gunnar, M., Fisch, R., and Malone, S.: The effects of pacifying stimulus on behavioral and adrenocortical responses to circumcision. *J. Am. Acad. Child Adolesc. Psychiatry* **23**:34–38, 1984.

Hallstrom, B.: Contact comfort: its application to immunization injections. *Nurs. Res.* 17:130, 1968.

Hatch, D.J., and Sumner, E.: Neonatal anaesthesia. *Clin Anaesthesiol* 3:633–655, July 1985.

Hawley, D.D.: Postoperative pain in children: misconceptions, descriptions and interventions. *Pediatr. Nurs.* 10:20–23, Jan–Feb 1984.

Hester, N.O.: The preoperational child's reaction to immunizations. *Nurs. Res.* **28**:250–254, 1979.

Hester, N.O., and Barcus, C.S.: Assessment and management of pain in children. Pediatrics: *Nurs. Update* 1:2–7, 1986.

Hickey, P., et al: Blunting of stress responses in the pulmonary circulation of infants by fentanyl. *Anesthesiol. Analg.* **64**:11371142, 1985.

Hilgard, J.R., and LeBaron, S.: *Hypnotherapy of pain in children with cancer*. William Kaufmann, Inc., Los Altos, Cal, 1984.

Hockenberry, M.J., and Balogna-Vaughan, S.: Preparation for intrusive procedures using noninvasive techniques in children with cancer: state of the art vs. new trends. *Cancer Nurs.* 8:97–102, Apr 1985.

Hopkins, C.S., Buckley, C.J., and Bush, G.H.: Pain-free injections in infants. *Anaesthesia* **43**:198–201, 1988.

Hurley, A., and Whelan, E.G.: Cognitive development and children's perception of pain. *Pediatr. Nurs.* 14:21–24, Jan–Feb 1988.

Hurwitz, E.S., Barrett, M.J., Bergman, D., Gunn, W.J., Pinsky, P., et al: Public Health Service study of Reye's syndrome and medications: report of the main study. *J.A.M.A.* **257**:1905–1911, Apr 10, 1987.

Jaffe, J.H., and Martin, W.R.: Opioid analgesics and antagonists. In Gilman, A.G., Goodman, L.S., Rall, T.W., and Mural, F., eds: Goodman and Gilman's *The pharmacological basis of therapeutics*, ed 7, pp 491–531, Macmillan Publishing Co., New York, 1985.

Jay, S.M., Ozolins, M., Elliott, C., and Caldwell, S.: Assessment of children's distress during painful medical procedures. *J. Health Psychol.* **2**:133–147, 1983.

Jeans, M.E.: The measurement of pain in children. In Melzack, R., ed: *Pain measurement and assessment*, pp 183–189, Raven Press, New York, 1983.

Kaiko, R.F.: Age and morphine analgesia in cancer patients with postoperative pain, *Clin Pharmacol. Ther.* **28**:823–826, Dec 1980.

Kavanagh, C.: A new approach to dressing change in the severely burned child and its effect on burn-related psychopathology. *Heart Lung* **12**:612–619, Nov 1983.

Koehntop, D., et al: Pharmacokinetics of fentanyl in neonates. *Anesthesiol. Analg.* **65**:227–232, 1986.

Koren, G., et al: Pediatric fentanyl dosing based on pharmacokinetics during cardiac surgery. *Anesthesiol. Analg.* **63**:577–582, 1984.

Kuttner, L.: Favorite stories: a hypnotic pain-reduction technique for children in acute pain. *Am. J. Clin. Hypn.* **30**:289–295, Apr 1988.

Lacouture, P.G., Gaundreault, P., and Lovejoy, F.H.: Chronic pain of childhood: a pharmacologic approach. *Pediatr. Clin. North Am.* **31**:1133–1151, 1984.

Lamontagne, L.L., Mason, K.R., and Hepworth, J.T.: Effects of relaxation on anxiety in children: implications for coping with stress. *Nurs. Res.* **34**:289–292, Sept–Oct 1985.

Langer, J.C., Shandling, B., and Rosenberg, M.: Intraoperative bupivacaine during outpatient hernia repair in children: a randomized double blind trial. *J. Pediatr. Surg.* **22**:267–270, Mar 1987.

Larsson, B., Daleflod, B., Hakansson, L., and Melin, L.: Therapist-assisted versus self-help relaxation treatment of chronic headaches in adolescents: a school-based intervention. *J. Child Psychol. Psychiatry* **28**:127–136, Jan 1987.

Levy, D.M.: Observations of attitudes and behavior in the child-health center. *J. Public Health* **41**:182–190, 1951.

Levy, D.M.: The infant's earliest memory of inoculation: a contribution to public health procedures. *J. Genet. Psychol.* **96**:3–46, 1960.

Liebeskind, J.C., and Melzack, R.: The international pain foundation: meeting a need for education in pain management. *Pain* **30**:1–2, 1987.

Loadman, W.E., Arnold, K., Volmer, R., Petrella, R., and Cooper, L.Z.: Reducing the symptoms of infant colic by introduction of a vibration/sound based intervention. *Pediatr. Res.* **21**:182A, 1987.

Lutz, W.J.: Helping hospitalized children and their parents cope with painful procedures. *J. Pediatr. Nurs.* **1**:24–32, Feb 1986.

Marshall, R.E., Stratton, W.C., Moore, J.A., et al: Circumcision. I. Effects on newborn behavior, *Infant Behav. Dev.* **3**:1–14, 1980.

Martin, B.B.: Where are all the children. *Am. J. Hospice Care* **2**:6–7, Mar-Apr 1985.

Martin, R.G.: Drug disposition in the neonate. *Neonatal Network* **4**:14–19, Feb 1986.

Martyn, J.A.J.: Ketamine pharmacology and therapeutics. *J. Burn Care Rehabil.* **8**:146–148, Mar-Apr 1987.

Matheus, B.A.: Quick dissolve. *Nursing* **17**:66, Sept 1987.

Mather, L., and Mackie, J.: The incidence of postoperative pain in children. *Pain* **15**:271–282, 1983.

Maunuksela, E.L., Olkkola, K.T., and Korpela, R.: Intravenous indomethacin as postoperative analgesic in children: acute effects on blood pressure, heart rate, body temperature and bleeding. *Ann. Clin. Res.* **19**:359–363, 1987.

Maunuksela, E.L., Rajantie, J., and Silmes, M.A.: Flunitrazepam-fentanyl-induced sedation and analgesia for bone marrow aspiration and needle biopsy in children. *Acta Anaesthesiol. Scand.* **30**:409–411, 1986.

McCaffery, M.: IV morphine for children. **Am. J. Nurs. 84**:11–53, Sept 1984.

McGrath, P.A., and de Veber, L.L.: The management of acute pain evoked by medical procedures in children with cancer. *J. Pain Sympt. Manag.* **1**:145–150, Summer 1986.

McGrath, P.A., de Veber, L.L., and Hearn, M.T.: Multidimensional pain assessment in children. In Fields, H.L., Dubner, R., and Cervero, F., eds: *Advances in pain research and therapy*, vol 9, pp 387–393, Raven Press, New York, 1985.

McGrath, P.J., Johnson, G., Goodman, J.T., Schillinger, J., Dunn, J., and Chapman, J.: The CHEOPS: a behavioral scale to measure postoperative pain in children. In Fields, H.L., Dubner, R., and Cervero, F., eds: *Advances in pain research and therapy*, vol 9, pp 395–402, Raven Press, New York, 1985.

McGrath, P.J., Cunningham, S.J., Goodman, J.T., and Unruh, A.: The clinical measurement of pain in children: a review, *Clin. J. Pain* **1**:221–227, 1985.

McGrath, P.J., and Feldman, W.: Clinical approach to recurrent abdominal pain in children. *Devel. Behav. Pediatr.* **7**:56–63, 1986.

McGrath, P.J., and Unruh, A.M.: *Pain in children and adolescents.* Elsevier Science Publishing Co, Inc, New York, 1987.

Mischel, H.N., Fuhr, R., and McDonald, M.A.: Children's dental pain: the effects of cognitive coping training in a clinical setting. *Clin. J. Pain* **1**:235–242, 1985.

Miser, A.W., McCalla, J., Dothage, J.A., Wesley, M., and Miser, J.S.: Pain as a presenting symptom in children and young adults with newly diagnosed malignancy. *Pain* **29**:85–90, 1987.

Miser, A.W., Dothage, J.A., and Miser, J.S.: Continuous intravenous fentanyl for pain control in children and young adults with cancer. *Clin. J. Pain* **3**:152–157, 1987.

Molsberry, D.: Young children's subjective quantifications of pain following surgery. Unpublished master's thesis, University of Iowa, 1979.

Orlowski, J.P., Gillis, J., and Kilham, H.A.: A catch in the reye. *Pediatrics* **80**:638–642, Nov 1987.

Owens, M.E.: Pain in infancy: conceptual and methodological issues. *Pain* **20**:213–230, Nov 1984.

Pagliaro, L.A., and Pagliaro, A.M.: Age-dependent drug selection and response. In Pagliaro, L.A., and Pagliaro, A.M., eds: *Pharmacologic aspects of nursing*, pp 130-139. The CV Mosby Co., St. Louis, 1986.

Penticuff, J.H.: Neonatal nursing ethics: toward a consensus. *Neonatal Network* **5**:7–16, June 1987.

Perin, G., and Frase, D.: Development of a program using general anesthesia for invasive procedures in a pediatric outpatient setting. *J. Assn. Pediatr. Oncol. Nurs.* 3:8–10, 1985.

Perry, S., and Heidrich, G.: Management of pain during debridement: a survey of US burn units. *Pain* 13:267–280, 1982.

Piaget, J.: *The child's concept of physical causality.* Routledge & Kegan-Paul, London, 1930.

Poland, R.L., Roberts, R.J., Gutierrez-Mazorra, J.F., and Fonkalsrud, E.W.: Neonatal anesthesia. *Pediatrics* 80:446, Sept 1987.

Purcell-Jones, G., Dormon, F., and Sumner, E.: Paediatric anesthetists' perceptions of neonatal and infant pain. *Pain* 33:181–187, May 1988.

Quinton, D., and Rutter, M.: Early hospitalization and later disturbances of behaviour. *Devel. Med. Child Neurol.*, 18:447–459, 1976.

Rana, S.R.: Pain—a subject ignored. *Pediatrics* 79:309, 1987.

Rawlings, D.J., Miller, P.A., and Engel, R.R.: The effect of circumcision on transcutaneous PO_2 in term infants. *Am. J. Dis. Child* 134:676–678, 1980.

Ross, D.M., and Ross, S.A.: *Childhood pain*, Urban & Schwarzenberg, Inc., Baltimore, 1988.

Ross, D.M., and Ross, S.A.: Pain instruction with third- and fourth-grade children: a pilot study. *J. Pediatr. Psychol.* 10:55–63, 1985.

Rowe, P.C., ed: *The Harriet Lane handbook: a manual for pediatric house officers,* ed 11, Year Book Medical Publishers, Inc., Chicago, 1987.

Savedra, M.: Coping with pain: strategies of severely burned children. *MCN* 5:197–203, Fall 1976.

Savedra, M., Gibbons, P., Tesler, M., Ward, J., and Wegner, C.: How do children describe pain?: a tentative assessment, *Pain* 14:95–104, 1982.

Scanlon, J.: Barbarism, *Perinatal Press* 9:103–104, 1985.

Schechter, N.L., and Allen, D.: Physicians' attitudes toward pain in children. *J. Devel. Behav. Pediatr.* 7:350–354, 1986.

Schechter, N.L., Allen, D.A., and Hanson, K.: The status of pediatric pain control: a comparison of hospital analgesic usage in children and adults, *Pediatrics* 77:11–15, 1986.

Schechter, N.L., Berrien, F.B., and Katz, S.M.: The use of patient-controlled analgesia in adolescents with sickle cell pain crisis: a preliminary report. *J. Pain Sympt. Manag.* 3:109–113, Spring 1988.

Schultz, N.V.: How children perceive pain. *Nurs. Outlook* 19:670–673, Oct 1971.

Sentivany, S.: Personal communication, Children's Hospital at Stanford, Palo Alto, Calif, 1988.

Smith, M.S., and Womack, W.M.: Stress management techniques in childhood and adolescence: relaxation training, meditation, hypnosis, and biofeedback: appropriate clinical applications, *Clin Pediatr* 26:581–585, Nov 1987.

Stevens, B., Hunsberger, M., and Browne, G.: Pain in children: theoretical, research, and practice dilemmas. *J. Pediatr. Nurs.* 2:154–166, June 1987.

Steward, D.J.: Paediatric diseases which may cause anaesthetic problems: prematurity. In Gomez, Q.J., Egay, L.M., and de al Cruz-Odi, M.F., eds: *Anaesthesia—safety for all,* pp 189–193, Excerpta Medica, New York, 1984.

Swafford, L.I., and Allan, D.: Pain relief in the pediatric patient. *Med. Clin. North Am.* 52:131–136, Jan 1968.

Tichy, A.M., Braam, C.M., Meyer, T.A., and Rattan, N.S: Stressors in pediatric intensive care units. *Pediatr. Nurs.* 14:40–42, Jan-Feb 1988.

Tree-Trakarn, T., Pirayavaraporn, S., and Lertakyamanee, J.: Topical analgesia for relief of post-circumcision pain. *Anesthesiology* 67:395–399, Sept 1987.

Ubell, E.: Should infants have surgery without anesthesia? *Parade Magazine,* p 17, Apr 12, 1987.

Varni, J.W., Jay, S.M., Masek, B.J., and Thompson, K.L.: Cognitive-behavioral assessment and management of pediatric pain. In Holzman, A.D., and Turk, D.C., eds: Pain management: a handbook of psychological treatment approaches, pp 168–192, Pergamon Press, New York, 1986.

Varni, J.W., Katz, E.R., and Dash, J.: Behavioral and neurochemical aspects of pediatric pain. In Russo, D.C., and Varni, J.W., eds: *Behavioral pediatrics: research and practice,* pp 177–224, Plenum Press, New York, 1982.

Walsh, V.R.: Making medication tasteless. *Nursing* 17:66, Sept 1987.

Wandless, J.G.: A comparison of nalbuphine with morphine for post-orchidopexy pain. *Eur. J. Anaesthesiol* 4:127–132, Mar 1987.

Westfall, L.K., and Pavlis, R.W.: Why the elderly are so vulnerable to drug reactions. *RN* 50:39–42, 1987.

Wetchler, B.V.: The role of anesthesia in outpatient surgery. *Today's OR Nurse* 4:18–23, 62, Sept 1982.

Whaley, L., and Wong, D.: *Essentials of pediatric nursing,* ed 3, The CV Mosby Co, St. Louis, 1989.

Wiley, F.: Personal communication, University of California Medical Center, Los Angeles, Calif, May 1988.

Woffard, L.G.: Pain in children with cancer: an assessment. *J. Assn. Pediatr. Oncol. Nurs.* 2:34–37, Spring 1985.

Yaster, M.: Analgesia and anesthesia in neonates. *J. Pediatr.* 111: 394–395, Sept 1987.

9

Pain in the Elderly

Special Considerations

Tremendous advances have been made in the scientific understanding and clinical management of pain. However, the special needs of and considerations applying to the elderly with pain is a neglected area. In the 1991 United Kingdom Census of the Population, there were found to be 10,595,495 elderly people. This included 6,959,395 women over 60 years of age and 3,636,100 men over 65 years (OPCS, 1991). The Government Actuaries Office predicts the number of elderly will be 12,095,000 by the year 2011 including 7,685,000 women over 60 years of age and 4,410,000 men over 65 years. This illustrates the increasing number of elderly people in the UK.

Despite the continuing growth of this segment of our population, research examining the effects of age on various pain control modalities is scarce. As a result, strategies for effective pain control in this population are at present based mostly on clinical experience and application of pain-control methods shown to be useful with younger adults. There is a need for research in all areas of pain control for the elderly; too many questions remain unanswered.

■ The authors would like to thank Susan C. Schafer, RNC, MS, Clinical Research Nurse, Pain Research Clinic, National Institutes of Health, Bethesda, Maryland, and Madelyn Miscally, RN, MSN, Geriatric Clinical Specialist, Bowman Gray School of Medicine, Winston-Salem, North Carolina for their review of this chapter, helpful comments and suggestions, and for supplying many of the patient examples.

PURPOSE AND LIMITATIONS OF THIS CHAPTER

The purpose of this manual is to present specific, clinical pain-control strategies for the nurse in any health-care setting. In this chapter, however, there are many gaps because the answers are simply not yet known. Our frustration as we prepared this chapter was the realization that although the elderly comprise the fastest growing segment of our population, the least amount of research on pain control exists in this age group. Thus we present this chapter with the hope that it will serve as a catalyst to stimulate thinking and generate exploration.

The primary purpose of this chapter is to address the areas of greatest need in the care of the elderly with pain:

- Raising questions about our lack of knowledge.
- Correcting misconceptions.
- Preventing the perpetuation of misinformation that may ultimately interfere with effective assessment and treatment of pain in the elderly population.

An initial step is to acknowledge that older patients may have different responses and needs from younger ones concerning assessment and interventions for pain control. It is beyond the scope of this chapter to present a thorough exploration of all the important aspects of gerontology.

Similar to the explosion of literature on pain control in children over the last several years, research in the elderly undoubtedly will continue to evolve. The authors look forward to developing this chapter further as more information on pain and the elderly becomes available.

For now, however, it is important for us to be particularly vigilant in applying scientific skills that include avoiding generalizations about elderly patients, being sceptical of assumptions that lack a research base, and continually reminding ourselves that each person, regardless of age, reacts individually to any treatment modality.

MISCONCEPTIONS ABOUT PAIN IN THE ELDERLY

Many of the misconceptions previously discussed in Chapter 2 on assessment and Chapter 7 on chronic non-malignant pain apply to the older person with pain, and the reader is encouraged to review these. Following are misconceptions that are specific to the elderly. In addition, several misconceptions are restated from Chapter 7 because of their relevance to the older person with pain. Refer to this chapter and the annotated references (pp. 218) for more detailed discussion.

Misconception: Pain is a natural outcome of growing old.

Correction: Pain is in fact not an inevitable part of aging, and its presence necessitates assessment, diagnosis, and treatment similar to the case with pain in any age group (Butler and Gastel, 1980; Harkins et al, 1984). This assumption can no longer be tolerated. Harkins et al (in press) suggest that this erroneous assumption may even be responsible for the lack of research on pain in the elderly.

The illogical nature of this misconception is best illustrated by the 101-year-old male participant in a study on aging as described by Butler and Gastel (1980). When he stated that his left leg hurt, the doctor suggested that it was to be expected at age 101. The man then asked him to explain why his right leg, which was also 101 years old, did not hurt a bit.

Although pain is not an inevitable result of aging, the elderly are at greater risk from many disorders that may result in pain, e.g. arthritic disorders, cardio-vascular diseases, osteoporosis, and cancer (Rowe and Besdine, 1982). The incidence of less common painful disorders such as postherpetic neuralgia and trigeminal neuralgia also are increased in elderly populations (Butler and Gastel, 1979). Further, injuries such as falls and hip fractures are more common in the elderly population and may result in chronic pain (Rubenstein and Robbins, 1984).

Is the lack of interest in pain in the elderly a reflection of our fear of aging? Butler and Gastel (1980) eloquently remind us that this neglect cannot continue. The elderly are "our future selves" (p.297) and the quality of our own lives as we grow older may in fact depend on the extent of our efforts at understanding pain in the older generation.

Misconception: Pain perception, or sensitivity, decreases with age.

Correction: This assumption is unsafe. In addition to the fact that conflicting data exist, this generalization results in our missing important indications of pain. The consequences are needless suffering and undertreatment of both pain and the underlying causes.

Results of experimental studies on pain perception in the elderly fail to conclusively report age-related differences in pain perception (Clark and Mehl, 1971; Harkins et al, 1986; Harkins et al, (in press); Harkins and Chapman, 1976).

Instances of atypical presentations of clinical pain include silent myocardial infarctions and the absence of abdominal pain in the elderly with peptic ulcer disease (Clinch et al, 1984; MacDonald, 1984). However, these reports of pain absence cannot be generalized to all disorders that may result in pain, or to all elderly people who may experience myocardial infarcts or ulcers. Further, if an elderly person has atypical absence of pain, this cannot be generalized to mean that pain will be absent in other conditions as well.

Failure to report pain must not be interpreted as absence of pain. The elderly may not report pain readily; however, this does not necessarily mean that they feel it any less. Further research is needed to understand all components of the pain experience in this segment of the population.

Misconception: The potential side effects of narcotics make them too dangerous to use to relieve pain in the elderly.

Correction: Narcotics may be used safely in the elderly if the person's response to medication is followed and evaluated closely and the pharmacokinetics in this population are recognized (Portenoy, 1987). Although the elderly may be more sensitive to narcotics, this does not justify withholding narcotics and failing to treat the pain. The potentially dangerous side effects of narcotics can be readily monitored with careful and frequent assessments of the individual's response to the narcotic, and usually avoided by adjustment of dose and interval between doses. If necessary, the most life-threatening side effect, respiratory depression, can be reversed by the antidote naloxone.

Misconception: If the elderly patient appears to be occupied, sleeps, or can be otherwise distracted from pain, then he/she does not have much pain.

Correction: The older patient need not act like he is in pain to be in pain. Lack of pain expression does not mean lack of pain (Chapter 1). The older person may have experienced pain for a long time and for many different reasons may minimize the expression of pain.

The elderly patient may not believe it is acceptable to show pain, so he/she may have a variety of ways to keep him/herself occupied or distracted from the pain. Assumptions about the presence or absence of pain cannot be solely based on a person's behaviour.

Misconception: If the older person is depressed, especially if there is no known cause for the pain, then depression is causing the pain. Pain is a symptom of depression and would subside if the depression were effectively treated.

Correction: It is normal to be depressed because of chronic pain. Chronic pain may cause depression. Some types of depression are present prior to the onset of pain but are not likely to be the cause of pain. However, a pre-existing depression does affect the person's ability to cope with the pain.

When the symptoms of chronic pain are compared with those of depression, the similarities between the two make it easy to see how they can become confused and how a patient can be mistakenly identified as being "only depressed" (see Table 7.1, Features of Chronic Pain and Depression, p. 205).

It is dangerous to assume that treatment of the depression is all that is needed to alleviate the pain. With this assumption, we run the risk of omitting a thorough pain assessment, not treating the pain, and ultimately allowing suffering to continue (refer to annotated references in Chapter 7: Ahles et al, 1987; Bouckoms et al, 1985; Hendler, 1984; Krishnan et al, 1985, Parts I and II; Pilowsky et al, 1985).

Misconception: Narcotics are totally inappropriate for all patients with chronic non-malignant pain.

Correction: There is little evidence to support this view. However, this belief has been held for many years. This bias is compounded by the additional suggestion that side effects from narcotics are more pronounced in the elderly, and therefore they should be used only for severe acute episodes of pain.

Several studies have shown that prolonged narcotic therapy for selected patients with chronic non-malignant pain can be a safe and humane alternative to no treatment. Portenoy and Foley (1986) reported on 38 patients, 25–82 years of age, in which 19 patients were maintained on narcotics for 4 or more years. Most researchers suggest that prolonged narcotic therapy for chronic non-malignant pain be considered after other reasonable attempts to control pain have been unsuccessful and only in patients without a history of drug abuse (see annotated references in Chapter 7: Crook and Tunks, 1985; Portenoy and Foley, 1986).

ASSESSMENT OF PAIN

At the present time, pain assessment tools specifically tailored for the elderly are lacking, as is research examining the special considerations when questioning this population about pain. The many unanswered questions and lack of information on specific strategies make this section particularly difficult to present to the reader. For the present, we must recognize our lack of knowledge, but never stop asking questions that promote our exploration of this area.

Factors that influence assessment

Following are factors to consider concerning the assessment process in the elderly. Those elderly people who are active and have minimal memory and cognitive problems may not require any adjustments in the assessment process already discussed in Chapter 2. However, for others, these problems will present special needs and may influence the patient's report of pain. Although these factors are by no means an all-inclusive list, they are proposed to define our lack of knowledge and to stimulate thought in this area.

Communication Problems

Some elderly people may have hearing or vision problems that complicate their ability to report their pain experience or apply pain-control strategies. In some cases, we may not be aware of these problems and may have to determine them through the use of open-ended questions and observations. For example, requests to "Describe what the pain feels like", or "Read me the prescription label on your bottle of pills" may alert the nurse to these problems.

For those patients in whom self-reporting about pain is not clear or possible, the nurse may need to rely on reports from family or caregivers. Observations of changes in level of functioning may be an indication of pain, e.g. a change in gait or guarding of a part of the body. Asking the family what they notice about the patient's level of activity during the day may be helpful. Are there any changes in the way the individual moves or any decrease or increase in activity?

Patient Example

A couple in their mid 70s living at home receive regular visits from the district nurse. The husband is unable to articulate thoughts and feelings because of a stroke. Although the wife has periods of mild memory loss, she still functions well with household activities. The wife reports that her husband has headaches and asks if there is any medication she can give him. Because of the wife's mild cognitive impairment, the nurse tries to confirm the accuracy of her pain report. She asks the wife how she knows about her husband's pain. The wife describes her husband's grimaces and rubbing his head and face. The nurse observes this behaviour during her visit, and together they plan strategies to control the husband's headaches (Kelly, 1988).

The older patient with confusion or dementia in addition to pain presents a particularly complex situation. Some patients with dementia may be able to tell you that they hurt; however, they may be unable to describe the pain. Detailed questions may result in their becoming frustrated.

Patient Example

Mrs P., 84 years old with severe memory deficit, repeatedly tells the district nurse that she has pain and points to her upper abdominal area. She asks over and over "Why do I have pain?" The nurse tries to ask detailed questions about the pain; however, Mrs P. is not able to answer them and instead becomes frustrated and anxious. Although the patient has a history of ulcerative disease, the nurse decides that a further examination is needed. The wisdom of further investigation is supported when Mrs P. is admitted to the hospital, and diagnostic tests reveal gallstones (Kelly, 1988).

There are no easy, straightforward answers to assessment in the demented or confused patient. We may attempt to use what we already know about pain assessment, but we must understand that in these complex situations, it may fail to help us. To date no definitive information exists as to the most effective approaches for controlling pain and relieving suffering in the demented or confused patient (Harkins et al, in press).

Although it is beyond the scope of this chapter to discuss assessment of dementia and confusion, attention to these factors is vital to individualized nursing care and certainly impacts on effective pain control measures. Many screening tools, e.g. the Short Portable Mental Status Questionnaire and the Mini-Mental Status, are available, and nurses interested in pursuing this further are referred to other sources (Foreman, 1986; Freund, 1987; Linderborn, 1988; Travis, 1988; Williams et al, 1988).

Many questions and considerations remain about assessment of the confused or demented elderly person in pain. These include:

- Are there common types of pain behaviour that might alert us? Do they differ from those of the non-demented elderly in pain?
- How might the current tools for dementia and confusion be adapted to include assessment strategies for pain?
- How does unrelieved pain contribute to confusion?
- What role does polypharmacy, which may involve both prescription drugs and over-the-counter medications, play in confusion or dementia?
- Can patients who are confused and need restraints still verbalize and remember their pain experience? Research has shown that some restrained elderly people are capable of vividly describing their pain (Strumpf and Evans, 1988).
- Does behaviour change after administration of an analgesic? In a situation where self-reporting of pain is unclear and family observations are not possible, a trial dose of analgesics monitored using an assessment sheet may be worthwhile.

Inadvertent denial of pain

Some older patients may not ordinarily use the word "pain". Therefore they may deny pain when asked about it. Use other terms such as discomfort, aches, soreness, hurt, or pressure, to obtain more complete information.

Other patients may expect and accept pain as a natural result of aging. They may have been told that there is nothing that can be done to relieve it. They may believe that because of their age, health-care providers ignore their statements about pain. As a result, they may simply stop talking about their pain (Gioiella and Bevil, 1985).

Explain to the patient that pain is not a normal consequence of growing older, and that you will work with him/her and other health-care team members to achieve control of the pain. Assure the patient that you want to know about the pain, and that you will not abandon him/her.

The "passive recipient" role of health-care consumers in earlier generations continues today. Patients of all ages, but especially doctors, may assume that physicians and nurses know when they hurt. Stress the importance of reporting the fact that they feel pain.

Deliberate Cover-up

Patients who grew up in an era when hospitals were only for the dying may deny pain even when asked. They may fear that the consequences of admitting pain may lead to diagnostic procedures, hospitalizations, and additional expense. It is important to discuss the risks involved and the options that are available.

A multidimensional approach to pain assessment in the elderly

For those elderly people who cannot communicate verbally about their pain, observations must be made of non-verbal behaviour. Guidelines are lacking for behaviour that clearly indicates pain. For the patient who cannot communicate, it is important to understand that relying solely on behavioural responses has serious limitations. For instance, older people may sleep in spite of severe pain or may distract themselves with music or television. Even when the patient can communicate, verbal statements are not always correctly interpreted.

Therefore the task of pain assessment is not always straightforward. The importance of a multidimensional approach and considering all aspects of a patient's situation is clearly illustrated in the following example.

Patient Example

A 70-year-old man, cognitively alert, presented to the hospital with statements of severe stomach pain. He lived alone. His demented wife had recently been placed in a nursing home because he was unable to care for her. After a complete examination, no cause was found for the stomach pain. At this point he was given food, and the pain stopped. In this instance, the patient perceived hunger as pain, but he never articulated that he was hungry (Petrucci, 1988). Perhaps he did not know that his hunger caused the pain, or he may have thought that he clearly communicated the nature of his stomach pain.

The concepts contributing to a multidimensional approach are summarized in the box on p. 274. They are addressed further in the initial pain-assessment tool.

Assessment tools

The initial pain-assessment tool and the pain assessment sheet discussed in Chapter 2 are tools that promote identification of specific needs and implementation of pain-control measures, followed by the continuous process of evaluation or assessment of the safety and effectiveness of these measures.

Although we suggest the use of these tools in the elderly, it remains to be seen whether they are appropriate ones to use in this special population. The authors look forward to expanding and revising this section as more research and clinical data become available.

Following is a brief summary of these tools (the reader is referred to Chapter 2 for a complete discussion and examples).

Initial pain-assessment tool

Sections of the initial pain-assessment tool that merit special considerations for the elderly include:

I. Location. Because the elderly patient may have multiple areas of pain, it is important he/she marks on the figures or traces on his/her body all areas that hurt. It may be helpful for the patient to prioritize the pains by asking which pain is bothering him/her the most right at the moment?

Multidimensional Approach to Pain Assessment in the Elderly

- Initiate discussions about pain. Do not assume that the presence of pain will automatically be reported. Emphasize to the family and patient that the health-care team does not always know when the patient is hurt. If the patient is unable to tell you about the pain felt, help the family articulate any behaviour that they observe that might be an expression of pain.
- Obtain a self-report. In the patient who is confused or unable to communicate, this may be impossible. However, do not automatically assume that it is not possible in the confused patient.
- Identify the presence of pathology or occurrence of procedures that are known to cause pain in others.
- Notice vocalizations that may indicate pain. These might include grunting or groaning. Look for changes in vocalizing pattern, e.g. the individual who was talkative then becomes quiet.
- Observe facial expressions. Those associated with pain may include a wrinkled forehead, tightly closed or widely opened eyes, tightly closed or widely opened mouth, or any distorted expression. Of course, older people will vary widely in their facial expressions of pain. The family may be helpful in identifying these expressions.
- Observe body movements. For example, moving head from side to side, rocking, pulling legs into abdomen, slight increase in hand/finger movements, inability to keep hands still, or increase in pacing behaviour.
- Ask about any changes in daily activities, gait and behaviour. For example, sudden increase in activity, guarding of a part of the body, increase in rest periods, irritability, decrease in social interactions, and sudden cessation of common routines. A sudden onset of confusion may indicate pain, although it may also be related to other underlying conditions such as infection, malnutrition, or electrolyte imbalance.
- Consider a trial dose of analgesic and observe the response. This may be particularly helpful when the question arises whether the behaviour is due to pain, anxiety, or confusion.

II. Intensity. The patient is asked to use a numerical scale, e.g. 0–10 (0 = no pain, 10 = worst pain). If the individual has difficulty with this concept, use phrases, e.g. no pain, a little pain, a lot of pain, too much pain, to rate the intensity of the pain. As there may be multiple sites of pain, be sure the patient specifies which pain rating applies to which pain.

Patient Example

A 72-year-old woman in an outpatient research setting with pain from shingles had been rating her pain at 5 on a 0 to 10 scale (0 = no pain, 10 = worst pain) for the past 2 weeks. Suddenly the pain rating changed to 9. The nurse was puzzled by this sudden change and asked the patient if this rating was due to the shingles pain. The patient stated that this was an entirely new pain that bothered her more now than the shingles pain (Schafer, 1988).

III. Quality. What words would the patient use to describe his pain? Reporting pain may be unacceptable in the older person's culture. The older person may combine a sense of humour with his description of pain. For example, one 70-year-old man chuckled when he described the pain in his left arm as "a bunch of jangling, rusty tin cans."

IV. Onset, duration, variation, and rhythms. Ask about these qualities in terms of the individual's daily activities. "How is your pain upon waking in the morning?" "What happens to the pain during your daily walk?"

V. Manner of expressing pain. Learning the patient's expression of pain is particularly important if the patient is unable to communicate or is unable to hear. Family members who are familiar with the patient's expression of pain may be able to tell you what clues they look for. If the patient is able to

CONTINUOUS-ASSESSMENT SHEET FOR PAIN

Age: 92 years

Patient **Mrs W**   Date **5/11**

*Pain rating scale used **Behaviours indicating pain: continuous grunting, eyes tightly closed, legs pulled in toward abdomen, picks at bed covers.**

Purpose: To evaluate the safety and effectiveness of the analgesic(s).

Analgesic(s) prescribed:

Time	*Possible* ~~Pain rating~~ **behaviors**	Analgesic	R	P	BP	Level of arousal	*Possible* ~~Other†~~ **comfort behaviors**	Plan and comments

Figure 9.1 Example of how the assessment sheet from p. 38 may be adapted for the non-communicating elderly person.

communicate, facial expressions or body posture should be used only as clues, not as sole indicators.

VI. What relieves the pain? Explore remedies commonly used years ago, e.g. menthol or plasters.

VII. What causes or increases the pain? Ask about these in terms of the older person's daily activities.

VIII. Effects of the pain. Ask "If you had a 50% reduction in pain daily, what would you be doing?"

Pain assessment sheet

The pain assessment sheet provides a quick and easy tool to evaluate the safety and effectiveness of analgesics and other pain-control measures. The assessment sheet may be adapted for use with the non-communicating elderly person. Ask the family or someone who knows the patient well to help you list types of behaviour that might indicate pain and those that indicate comfort. Figure 9.1 shows an example of how the assessment sheet may be modified for a noncommunicating elderly person.

Daily diary

The daily diary (Appendix) may be kept by the patient or family and may be especially helpful in gathering data when the pain picture is confusing and the elderly person is at home. Although every hour does not need to be recorded, it is important to note when medication is taken, or when the level of activity alters a previous pain rating. The Patient/Family Teaching Point for use of Daily Diary (Appendix) may be duplicated for patients and family members.

PAIN-CONTROL INTERVENTIONS

Chapters 4–6 discuss in detail pharmacological and non-pharmacological pain-control measures. Therefore the purpose of this section is to build on this information and present an overview of research, clinical strategies, and unanswered questions concerning effective pharmacological and non-invasive pain-control methods for the elderly.

275

Pharmacological interventions

This section addresses the following issues:

- Physiological changes as a result of aging and the resulting pharmacological implications as they apply to analgesics.
- Key concepts of analgesic therapy.
- Non-narcotic analgesics.
- Narcotic analgesics.
- Adjuvant analgesics.

Physiological changes influencing drug therapy

"...Ageing is a unique and individual process that occurs at different rates in different individuals" (Pagliaro and Pagliaro, 1983, p. 1). Knowledge of how this process affects the distribution, metabolism, and elimination of drugs provides a framework for understanding altered pharmacological responses to analgesics in the elderly. With more research, our knowledge of the most effective ways to monitor and adjust analgesic therapy will be refined.

Distribution of Drugs

Factors that affect the distribution of drugs are altered by increasing age and include the following (Ouslander, 1981; Pagliaro and Pagliaro, 1986; Reidenberg, 1982; Schmucker, 1984; Westfall and Pavlis, 1987):

- Changes in body composition. An increase in the proportion of body fat may cause delayed onset and accumulation with repeated dosing of drugs that are fat soluble, e.g. diazepam. Heart, kidney, and muscle mass decrease with age. As a result, a usual adult dose may need to be decreased to avoid toxic drug levels in the blood and tissue.
- Serum proteins. Many drugs bind to plasma proteins, leaving a portion of each drug circulating unbound or free for pharmacological activity. Although the normal aging process probably does not reduce serum proteins, malnutrition and chronic disease, observed more often in this population, may contribute (Lamy, 1983; Mitchell and Lipschitz, 1982). Decreased circulating proteins potentially result in greater drug effect from higher concentrations of unbound drug, with a greater risk of toxic effect. Non-narcotic analgesics that are protein bound and likely to be associated with

greater pharmacological effect include: ibuprofen, naproxen, indomethacin and piroxicam (Flower, Moncada and Vane, 1985).

Metabolism of Drugs

The liver is the major site of drug metabolism. However, the effect of aging on hepatic metabolism is complex, difficult to predict, and has not been well studied in humans (Greenblatt et al, 1982; Ouslander, 1981). It appears that the capacity of the liver to metabolize drugs may not be uniformly affected by aging and that most drugs are normally metabolized in the older population (Ouslander, 1981; Pagliaro and Pagliaro, 1986). Although it cannot be generalized to all other drugs, the rate of some forms of hepatic metabolism may be decreased in specific drugs, e.g., paracetamol (Pagliaro and Pagliaro, 1986). The practical application of this finding may be to allow for the longer period of metabolism of the drug dose by anticipating the need for a longer interval between doses.

Excretion of Drugs

As a result of age, both structural and functional changes occur in the kidney. These include a decrease in renal mass, renal blood flow, glomerular filtration rate, and tubular secretion. Dehydration and heart failure occur rather frequently in ill elderly patients and may further reduce renal function (Lonergan, 1988; Ouslander, 1981; Pagliaro and Pagliaro, 1983). Consequently, drugs or the active metabolites of drugs that are eliminated by the kidney may remain in the body longer, resulting in prolonged therapeutic and/or toxic effects.

The clinical importance of poor kidney function is apparent with the narcotic pethidine. An active metabolite of pethidine, nor-pethidine may accumulate with repeated doses, causing central nervous system excitation (Kaiko, 1983). This appears to be more likely to occur in patients with compromised renal function (American Pain Society, 1987).

Research documenting renal metabolism of drugs in the elderly is just beginning; it is suggested that there will be increasing evidence of the importance of the kidney in the elimination of opiates and other drugs (Hanks and Aherne, 1985; Lonergan, 1988).

Clearance of Drugs

Kaiko and associates (1982) report that morphine clearance from the plasma decreases with age. As a result, morphine may remain in the body longer and at higher concentrations, suggesting that its effects could be greater and last longer in the elderly as opposed to younger patients. Therefore in clinical situations, this finding alerts us to the fact that individual patients' responses need to be assessed for adjustments that may include lower doses of narcotic given less frequently.

Drug Receptors

It has been suggested that a decreased number of drug receptors or decreased responsiveness of these receptors in the elderly may account for increased sensitivity to drug effects (Pagliaro and Pagliaro, 1986). However, there is little data to suggest that aging is accompanied by a decrease in number or effectiveness of drug receptors (Schmucker, 1984).

> **KEY POINT:** In attempting to explain the effect of aging on the pharmacokinetics of drug therapy for pain, it is clear that this is an underdeveloped area of research.

The impact of the above potential physiological changes is not totally clear, and the difficulty in predicting individual responses remains. The following principles, e.g. titrating to effect by adjusting drug dose and interval according to individual response, remain vital strategies for effective pain control in all ages.

Key concepts in analgesic therapy

The following three concepts have already been discussed at length in Chapter 4. The reader is encouraged to refer to Chapter 4 for detailed guidelines and patient examples. The concepts are summarized briefly here as a reminder of their importance, and any variations specific to the elderly are noted:

1. Use a Preventive Approach

Use a preventive approach and stay on top of the pain. A preventive approach means that the analgesic is given or taken before pain occurs or before it increases, that is:

- Regularly — this schedule is appropriate if the pain occurs consistently and predictably throughout a 24-hour period.

  For some elderly patients a 4-hourly or 6-hourly schedule of pain medication may be easily forgotten or confused. It may be helpful in this situation to arrange the medication around specific activities throughout the day, as long as they occur consistently, or to prescribe slow-release preparations as often as possible.

Patient Example

Mr S. is taking ibuprofen 400mg for rib and back pain from metastatic prostate cancer. After a careful assessment, the district nurse notes that he takes it irregularly and only when the pain becomes unbearable. The nurse encourages Mr S. to try a new regime for a trial of 3–4 days: take ibuprofen 400mg after each meal. By linking the pain pill regime with specific activities he does every day, Mr S. is able to readily remember when to take the pain medicine. After a trial of 2 days, he is amazed at the difference in his comfort level, and he continues with this regime.

- PRN (as needed, requires nursing assessment and evaluation), for pain that cannot be predicted. However, it should be used preventively, as soon as pain begins and before it gets out of control. An analgesic prescribed "PRN for pain" may be implemented on a regular basis for on-going pain (Chapter 4).

2. Dosage Adjustment to Effect

Adjust and individualize the analgesic for each patient. This involves tailoring analgesics by adjusting the following:

- Dose. Although it has been found that the elderly may be more sensitive to narcotics (Kaiko et al, 1982), this finding cannot be generalized to rule out the use of narcotics or to mean that all elderly patients need lower doses of analgesics. If greater sensitivity is noted in an older person, analgesics must be monitored and adjusted more vigilantly.

  At first, it was suggested that age should be the main criterion for choosing an initial analgesic dose (Bellville et al, 1971); however, current research suggests that age influences frequency of dosing more than dosage (Kaiko et al, 1982).

The only safe and effective way to administer an analgesic is to monitor the individual's response to the drug. For some elderly patients, it may be appropriate to administer a relatively low starting dose of medication (Portenoy, 1987). It is important that this dose is then immediately adjusted up or down depending on the patient's response. Interestingly, height, weight, and body surface are not accurate guides for narcotic dose requirements in the elderly (Bellville et al, 1971).

Use an assessment sheet and look at patient responses, in the following order:

a. Respiratory function.

b. Pain rating, descriptive phrase, or non-verbal behaviour.

c. Based on the above, determine what should be done with the number of milligrams of analgesic the patient is receiving. *The last thing you look at are milligrams being given; look at effect first.*

- Interval between doses. Older patients may experience a longer duration of action of narcotics (Kaiko, 1980; Kaiko et al, 1982). Therefore increasing age should prompt close monitoring of the frequency of narcotic administration. For example, in the elderly, sustained-release morphine may last longer than 12 hours, in some instances up to 24 hours.

  Again the key here is monitoring each patient individually; the assessment sheet may be a particularly helpful tool for this.

- Route. Adjust the route of drug administration according to the individual patient's needs, remembering that even severe pain may be controlled with oral narcotics. These needs might include such considerations as convenience, side effects, and onset of analgesia. The present discussion is limited to potential problems with the IM and continuous subcutaneous infusion route in the elderly. Refer to Chapter 4 for detailed discussion of other routes of administration, remembering that the oral route is preferred. When this is not possible other routes such as PR, SC, IM, IV and epidural should be considered.

  Absorption of IM injections and continuous subcutaneous infusions are important factors when determining appropriate routes of administration for the elderly. Drug absorption is highly variable and likely to be diminished for a number of reasons. As a result, the drug may not be readily absorbed and there may be delayed onset of action (Lukacsko, 1987). Following are factors that interfere with absorption:

Degenerated muscle from inactivity, poor nutrition, or dehydration.

Absorption of IM narcotics may be poor, especially in the immediate postoperative period (Austin et al, 1980). In the elderly, especially in this postoperative period, peripheral circulation may be diminished. Circulatory problems may then result, and insufficient plasma concentration of drugs may be particularly significant.

Variability in absorption poses a specific danger in the postoperative period when an IM dose is repeated. For instance, as a result of poor absorption, the first IM dose may not provide pain relief for the elderly person. The dose may be repeated. As circulation improves, the initial dose may be absorbed just as the second dose is taking effect. The result may be an elderly patient who is in pain just before the second dose, and afterward is more likely to be sedated or have respiratory depression.

- Choice of drug. The choice of analgesic may to a great degree be influenced by its potential adverse effects. The following considerations that influence drug selection in the elderly are discussed in the section on narcotic analgesics:

  — Hazards of pethidine.

  — Problems with agonists/antagonists.

  — Problems with narcotics with long duration.

  Other factors may influence an elderly patient's willingness to accept the health-care team's choice of analgesic.

3. Patient Controlled Analgesia (PCA)

In its broadest sense, the key concept of PCA may be defined as the patient's self-administration of all forms of pain control by methods that consider safety as well as the patient's ability and willingness to exercise control. The elderly person who feels the pain is the individual who must have, to the maximum extent possible, control over all measures to relieve it.

Some elderly patients may be unable or unwilling to exercise control. They may look to the doctor or nurse for direction concerning all aspects of health care.

Other elderly people may have changes in mental status and be unable to determine or direct pain relief. In this case, the patient's indications of pain are carefully monitored and the form and/or the amount of pain control is adjusted according to the individual patient.

Non-narcotic analgesics (NSAIDs)

The following principles of non-narcotic therapy have been discussed at length in Chapter 4: indications, disadvantages, mechanism underlying effects of NSAIDs, adverse side effects, promising uses, and guidelines for their effective use along with patient teaching tools that may be readily adapted for use with the elderly patient.

It is beyond the scope of this chapter to discuss the long-term use of anti-inflammatory medications for the chronic treatment of highly inflammatory conditions such as rheumatoid arthritis. The interested reader is referred to other sources for this information (Baskin and Goldfarb, 1983; Gall, 1982; Lamy, 1986; Morgan and Furst, 1986; Polisson, 1987; Schlegel and Paulus, 1986).

Reminders of the important aspects of using non-narcotics as analgesics include:

- Non-narcotic analgesics are often undervalued as effective pain-relieving medications. For example, two aspirin or paracetamol (500mg) relieve as much pain as codeine 30mg orally.
- Combining a non-narcotic with a narcotic is a simple yet frequently overlooked strategy. It provides a safe and logical method of pain control.
- When NSAIDs are used for brief episodes of pain, the incidence or severity of side effects may not bear comparison with those seen with long-term treatment. For example, when indomethacin is given rectally over 3 days for postoperative pain, side effects are likely to pose less of a problem than when indomethacin is given orally over several months.

In the elderly patient, there may be a concern about increasing side effects if a narcotic dose is increased. Adding an NSAID to the narcotic instead of increasing a narcotic dose may result in increased analgesia without increasing side effects (Weingart et al, 1985).

Dosage of Non-narcotic Analgesics

One study of 17 healthy men and women from 65 to 78 years of age found that age had minimal effect on the absorption, distribution, metabolism, and excretion of ibuprofen. Therefore Albert et al (1984) suggest that the dosage of ibuprofen does not need to be adjusted for age.

Side Effects of Non-narcotic Analgesics

Cognitive dysfunction, i.e. memory loss, inability to concentrate, confusion, and personality change, was noted in eight patients over 65 years of age who took naproxen or ibuprofen over a period of 1 year. These symptoms cleared in all of the patients within 2 weeks after stopping the NSAID (Goodwin and Regan, 1982). Particularly noteworthy is the fact that none of the patients volunteered information about side effects. Instead, knowledge of adverse symptoms came from family members' remarks or as a result of direct questioning of the patient. One of the patients was relieved to learn that the distraction and memory loss she experienced were a result of the naproxen. She assumed she was "becoming senile" and that her family would have to put her in a nursing home.

Impaired renal function is another common side effect of NSAIDs in the elderly (Polisson, 1987; Schlegel and Paulus, 1986). Patients at increased risk of this side effect include those with (Schlegel and Paulus, 1986):

- Reduced cardiac output associated with congestive heart failure.
- Hepatic disease with cirrhosis and ascites.
- Diuretic-induced volume depletion.
- Atherosclerotic cardiovascular disease who are receiving concurrent diuretic therapy.

Upon initiation of NSAIDs, especially for chronic use, monitoring of renal function, electrolytes, and mental status is important. Following are important nursing-care guidelines for using nonnarcotics as analgesics in the elderly:

- Discuss the possible side effects of NSAIDs with the patient and family.
- Initiate questions about symptoms of cognitive dysfunction or mood alterations.

Narcotic Analgesics (Opioids)

The following principles of narcotic therapy have been discussed in detail in Chapter 4: mode of action, reasons for under-treatment, equianalgesic doses, selection of appropriate narcotics, selection of appropriate route of administration, and side effects, in addition to numerous patient examples and patient/family teaching tools.

Following are reminders of important aspects of narcotic analgesics that are particularly pertinent to the elderly:

1. Hazards of Pethidine

Although pethidine is a frequently prescribed IM narcotic, several characteristics of this drug make it an undesirable choice:

- Tissue irritation with the potential for severe muscle tissue fibrosis with frequent injections (Jaffe and Martin, 1985). This problem may be compounded in the elderly patient with decreased muscle mass.
- Possible neuropsychiatric effects, such as disorientation, bizarre feelings, and hallucinations. These occur frequently with parenteral pethidine (Miller and Jick, 1978).
- Toxicity, due to the accumulation of an active metabolite, nor-pethidine, which is a central nervous system stimulant (Kaiko et al, 1983; Szeto et al, 1977). Because decreased renal function increases the likelihood of this side effect, elderly patients may be particularly vulnerable (Portenoy, 1987).

2. Problems with Agonists/Antagonists (or partial agonists)

Because all drugs in this group, for example nalbuphine, pentazocine, and buprenorphine, have a limit to the amount of respiratory depression they cause, it may be particularly tempting to prescribe this group of drugs for the elderly. However, pentazocine may cause psychotomimetic effects such as confusion and hallucinations (American Pain Society, 1987). Respiratory depression with buprenorphine is rare and this is the only case when such narcotic-induced respiratory depression is not readily reversed with naloxone.

However, if the narcotic antagonist property of nalbuphine and pentazocine is not understood, the following difficulties may occur in relation to "pure" narcotic agonists such as codeine and morphine:

- They may precipitate withdrawal in someone who has been taking a "pure" narcotic for a week or more.
- They may reverse analgesia of "pure" narcotics if an agonist/antagonist is given at the same time or alternately.

3. Problems with Narcotics with Long Half-Lives

The half-life of a narcotic refers to the time it takes for the drug to fall to half its initial plasma concentration. Methadone has a long half-life, and therefore the plasma levels of this drug slowly rise over many days after initiating a dosing schedule. As a result, the risk of delayed toxicity is much greater than with drugs of shorter half-life such as morphine or diamorphine. In the elderly population where sensitivity to narcotics may be increased, the use of methadone must be approached with caution and particularly vigilant monitoring of the patient's response. If this drug is used, refer to Chapter 4 for suggestions on dosing.

4. Side Effects of Particular Concern: Confusion and Constipation

In some patients, polypharmacy (simultaneous administration of many medications, both prescription and over-the-counter), multiple medical problems, and age-related physiological changes with pharmacological impact may present a complex inter-relationship contributing to many side effects, especially confusion and constipation. Frequently, narcotic analgesics are automatically blamed. While cognitive impairment in the elderly patient may be drug-induced (Larson et al, 1987), investigation into its cause should not be limited to narcotics.

Constipation may be of particular concern to some elderly patients. Many have probably established their own patterns for treating it. New suggestions for handling this side effect may not be followed. Therefore if possible, it is important to augment whatever strategies the patient currently uses. Refer to appendix for patient/family teaching point and p. 111 for suggested regimes.

It is important to tell patients that constipation is an expected side effect of narcotics and some adjuvant analgesic medications and that it can be prevented.

Patient Example

Mrs T., 60 years old, began a course of amitriptyline for foot and abdominal pain from diabetic neuropathy. She stopped the drug on her own because of constipation. She was never told to expect it or how to prevent it. When she learned that this was an expected side effect and how to prevent it, she resumed the amitriptyline (Schafer, 1988).

Adjuvant analgesics

The following principles of adjuvant analgesic therapy have been discussed at length in Chapter 4: appropriate uses; disadvantages; so-called potentiators; adjuvant analgesics for sleep disturbances, anxiety, depression, shock-like pain, sedation, and muscle spasms.

Following are reminders of important aspects of using adjuvant analgesics:

- Adjuvant analgesics are not a substitute for adequate doses of narcotics or non-narcotic analgesics. Adjuvant analgesics should be used in combination with narcotics/non-narcotic analgesics for specific pain syndromes.
- The choice of an adjuvant analgesic is appropriate when there is: (1) a component to the pain that narcotics alone cannot address, e.g. depression, sleeplessness, or anxiety, and (2) a pain syndrome that may not respond to narcotics, e.g. phantom limb pain, post-herpetic neuralgia, or causalgia.

Precautions and Side Effects

Adjuvant analgesics must be used with caution in the elderly. Sedation, confusion, and constipation may be compounded by the sedative and anticholinergic effects of many of the adjuvant medications (Portenoy, 1987). Low starting doses, in some cases one half to two thirds that of doses normally used, are suggested for these medications (Cunha, 1986; Peabody et al, 1986; Portenoy, 1987). Any increase in dosage should be gradual.

If an elderly patient taking a narcotic and adjuvant analgesic reports unacceptable side effects, decrease or discontinue the adjuvant medication first. After evaluating the patient's response, it may then be necessary to change the narcotic (Portenoy, 1987).

Postural hypotension (a severe drop in blood pressure when changing from a lying to a standing position) is one of the most common and serious cardiovascular complications of the tricyclic

medications (Peabody et al, 1986). This complication may directly affect the elderly person's mobility by potentially resulting in injury from falls.

In the elderly patient, there is a tendency to use the benzodiazepines to sedate the agitated patient or better control behaviour (Meyer, 1982). This is particularly true for the anxious patient with uncontrolled pain. The long half-life of many of these drugs makes them a poor choice in the elderly patient. Although increased sensitivity of the elderly to this group of drugs needs further exploration, the following question alerts us to potential problems: "Do the benzodiazepines have an effect in producing accidental injury in the elderly?" (Meyer, 1982, p. 1021).

Non-invasive interventions

Cutaneous stimulation (Chapter 5), distraction (Chapter 6, pp. 161–168), relaxation (Chapter 6, pp. 168–180), and imagery (Chapter 6, pp. 180–190) have previously been discussed, and the reader is referred to the corresponding chapters for detailed discussions, annotated references, and patient/family teaching points.

Rather than review the previously discussed concepts, this section presents special considerations in using selected techniques for the elderly patient.

Cutaneous stimulation: use of cold and topical preparations

Cold may be very effective for conditions that are traditionally treated with heat, e.g. low back pain and arthritis. However, elderly persons may be particularly reluctant to try the local application of cold. They may associate cold weather or dampness with increased pain; therefore it is helpful to clarify that the application of cold to a small body area does not necessarily produce the same results as cold damp weather. For an added sense of warmth and comfort while cold is being applied, suggest the use of a heating pad on other parts of the body.

A topically applied substance containing menthol, for example, is a type of external analgesic that may be particularly appealing to an elderly person. Menthol-containing preparations may have been a popular home remedy for this generation. In our present age of frequent medication use and a highly technical approach to health care, elderly patients may assume that menthol is an inappropriate and unscientific pain-control measure, especially for use in the hospital setting. Initiating conversation about menthol products and encouraging the patient to use what has worked for him/her before may foster a sense of control and open-mindedness that can be applied to other pain-control strategies.

Distraction: listening to music, life review, and the use of pets

Listening to music can provide powerful distraction from pain (Glynn, 1986; Herth, 1978). Selection of music according to the preference of the patient is crucial to its effectiveness. For some elderly, this may mean selecting music from a different era.

Patients with a hearing aid may find it difficult to use a headset. If there is a problem using the two together, it may be helpful to use the speech and hearing department of a hospital as a resource. It is also important to note that problems with hearing aids are often the result of dead batteries, simple to correct, yet frequently overlooked.

Life review may be used as a means of distraction for the elderly person experiencing pain (Dietsche, 1979; Murray et al, 1980; Ryden, 1981). A tendency of the elderly to self-reflect and reminisce may be viewed as part of cognitive loss or onset of senility. However, Butler (1963) discovered the significance of these activities, recognized them to be a normal process, and named them Life review.

Life review is defined as "a naturally occurring, universal mental process characterized by looking back over the life lived and recalling either pleasurable memories or unresolved conflicts which can be surveyed and integrated" (Murray et al, 1980, p. 284). While talking with an elderly patient, you may note recurrent themes that are frequently talked about. When using life review as a distraction technique for pain, ask the patient to tell you more about that particular event or period of time. To initiate reflecting or reminiscing behaviour, ask the patient to look back over his/her life and tell you what stands out in his/her mind (Ryden, 1981).

Patient Example

Mrs L., 79 years old with pancreatic cancer, was admitted to the hospital for severe abdominal pain, nausea, and vomiting. During one of her daily visits, the geriatric clinical nurse specialist found her lying in bed with her eyes tightly closed. Mrs L. stated that she could not talk right now because the pain was so bad. After Mrs L. received additional pain medication, the nurse asked if she could sit with the patient. Mrs L. began to talk about her life. She talked about her childhood and an early marriage to an abusive husband. She talked of raising her own children in addition to some of her brothers and sisters. She stated that she was proud of her accomplishments even though there had been some bad times. The nurse reinforced the fact that she certainly made the best of many difficult situations. Mrs L. then said that her pain was much better and that she was tired and needed to rest. She thanked the nurse for staying and said that it really helped to talk (Miscally, 1988).

Many homes for the elderly have pets such as cats or dogs. The unconditional love from a pet can be a soothing distraction, especially for those whose lives have always included animals.

Relaxation/imagery

The term relaxation may be unacceptable to the elderly patient. It may be more appropriate to encourage the patient to tell you what brings them "peace of mind or comfort".

Other patients may respond to specific techniques by being encouraged to release any contractions in their muscles. One study of 20 adults aged 56–89 years examined the effects of a jaw relaxation technique (dropping the lower jaw, relaxing the tongue, and using coordinated breathing) on the postoperative comfort level of patients with fractured hips. The use of this technique increased the level of the patients' postoperative comfort (Ceccio, 1984).

Griffin (1986) reports on the successful use of imagery in her health care of the elderly practice. One of her techniques, the use of an "inner advisor", is explained to patients as a way to "help you get in touch with YOU again" (p. 806).

Patient Example

Mrs J., a 67-year-old widow, developed abdominal pain 3 months after her husband died. She identified a ball of fire aiming rays at her stomach causing the pain. Weekly sessions with the nurse enabled her to stand up to this ball of fire and talk to it. Over a 2-month period, it shrank and finally disappeared. Although the pain was gone 1 year later, Mrs J. continued to use a variation of this technique to increase her energy and help her sleep soundly (Griffin, 1986).

THE FUTURE

Much remains to be done about pain in the elderly. Beginning attempts are necessarily frustrating because we:

- Identify what we do not know.
- Tentatively apply to the elderly what we know about effective pain-control measures used for younger patients.
- Attempt to formulate questions that are sensitive to the needs of the elderly.

In the years to come, it is our hope that the following quote will be no longer applicable: "...Pain is most poorly managed in those most defenceless against it—the young and the elderly" (Liebeskind and Melzack, 1987, p. 66).

SELECTED ANNOTATED REFERENCES THAT CITE RESEARCH OR GIVE CLINICAL SUPPORT

Albert, K.S., Gillespie, W.R., Wagner, J.G., et al: Effects of age on the clinical pharmacokinetics of ibuprofen. *Am. J. Med.* **77**:47–50, July 13, 1984. The pharmacokinetics of one dose of 400, 800, and 1200mg of ibuprofen (Motrin), respectively, were studied after administration to 17 healthy men and women aged 65–78 years. The findings were then compared with those in a similar study in young males aged 22–35 years. According to the results, advanced age has minimal influence on the absorption, distribution, metabolism, and excretion of ibuprofen. Therefore the authors suggest that the dosage does not need to be adjusted for elderly patients.

Bellville, J.W., Forrest, W.H., Miller, E., and Brown, B.W.: Influence of age on pain relief from analgesics. *J.A.M.A.* **217**:1835–1841, Sept 27, 1971. This is a particularly meaningful study because in it were used well-controlled conditions to determine the correlation between age and analgesia. Seven hundred and twelve patients received 10mg of morphine IM or 20mg of pentazocine IM or both for acute postoperative pain and were studied for correlations between the degree of pain relief and patient characteristics such as age, height, weight, body surface, operative site, and variations among hospitals. Age proved to be the most important variable in that the older age group reported more pain relief following IM administration of an analgesic. No difference was found between the incidence of side effects reported by patients aged 58 and older and those reported by patients younger than 58. No correlation was found between the sedation score and age. The authors suggest therefore that their findings concerning age cannot be explained purely on the basis of altered drug absorption and distribution, otherwise they would have expected to be able to correlate age with the sedative side effects. The authors state that it is more important to adjust dosage of a narcotic in relation to a patient's age than in relation to height, weight, or other patient characteristics.

Faherty, B.S., and Grier, M.R.: Analgesic medication for elderly people post-surgery. *Nurs. Res.* **33**:369–372, 1984. One hundred and forty-two patients from 25 to 107 years old following abdominal surgery were studied to determine if elderly patients receive less analgesic medication than younger patients, and, if so, how the physician's prescriptions and the nurse's administration contribute to this finding. The data from this study indicate that older postsurgical patients have less analgesic medication prescribed and administered. The smaller amounts of analgesic medication given to elderly patients may have been influenced by the smaller amounts prescribed for this age group. However, nurses also administered a smaller percentage of the smaller amount prescribed for the elderly patients. Of the 83 patients who were aged 55 years or older, 50 (60.2%) received less than 50% of the dose prescribed.

Harkins, S.W., Kwentus, J., and Price, D.D.: Pain and the elderly. In Benedetti, C., Chapman, C.R., and Morrica, G., eds: *Advances in pain research and therapy*, vol 7, pp. 103–121, Raven Press, New York, 1984. A review article examines age differences in pain perception under conditions staged in the laboratory and as a result of pathology. The authors conclude that any changes in pain sensitivity and perception related to age are difficult to document and may in fact be of little significance. Acute and chronic pain are reviewed with comments about the sensitivity of the elderly to narcotics and non-steroidal anti-inflammatory medications. Depression and chronic pain, pain and dementia, and social environment and pain are briefly discussed.

Harkins, S.W., Price, D.D., and Martelli, M.: Effects of age on pain perception: thermonociception. *J. Gerontol.* **41**:58–63, 1986. Forty-four young (20–36 years), middle-aged (45–60 years), and elderly (65–80 years) volunteers received noxious heat stimuli to several areas on the forearm. The participants used visual analogue scales to rate the intensity and unpleasantness of the heat stimuli. The researchers found minimal differences with age between how strong the pain felt and the unpleasantness of the pain. There were more similarities in pain perception than differences among age groups.

Kaiko, R.F.: Age and morphine analgesia in cancer patients with postoperative pain. *Clin. Pharmacol. Ther.* **28**:823–826, 1980. The responses of 947 postoperative cancer patients receiving 8 and 16mg doses of IM morphine were studied. Age was the significant factor associated with duration of analgesia, i.e. the older patient had a longer duration of analgesia than the younger patient. Seventy-one percent of patients aged 70–89 years continued to experience pain relief 4 hours after morphine IM. However, only 28% of patients aged 18–29 years felt pain relief after 4 hours. The results of this study suggest that age is a significant factor for anticipating the duration of morphine analgesia and therefore the frequency of administration.

Kaiko, R.F., Wallenstein, S.L., Rogers, A., et al: Narcotics in the elderly. *Med. Clin. North Am.* **66**:1079–1089, 1982. A report of three studies designed to further develop the observations of Bellville and colleagues (discussed above). Seven hundred and fifteen patients who received 8mg and 16mg doses of morphine were studied to determine the following factors: the significance of age relative to dose and demographic and pain variables, age and peak vs. duration of morphine analgesia, and age and morphine plasma levels. Of the variables examined, age, race, sex, pretreatment intensity, character, and site of pain, the difference in age was associated with the greatest difference in analgesia. The patients who were particularly old responded to morphine as though they had received three to four times the dose given to young adult patients. Age-related increase in analgesia is primarily a function of an increase in duration rather than an increase in peak analgesic effect. These studies in combination with previous ones suggest that morphine clearance decreases with age. The authors' data suggest that age should be used as the criterion for choosing initial dosing frequency. The authors stress that pain should be managed by adjustment of dose and dosing frequency according to individual patients' responses.

Nolan, L., and O'Malley, K.: Prescribing for the elderly. Part I. Sensitivity of the elderly to adverse drug reactions. *J. Am. Geriatr. Soc.* **36**:142–149, 1988. The article reviews the in-patient and outpatient studies which report the relationship of adverse drug reactions to increasing patient age. While the incidence of adverse drug reactions may be greater in the elderly, there is no evidence to conclusively link these reactions to the biological effects of aging. It is suggested that polypharmacy is more consistently associated with adverse drug reactions, and that severe illness, multiple pathology, and its associated high level of prescribing are more important than age.

Portenoy, R.K., and Kanner, R.M.: Patterns of analgesic prescription and consumption in a university-affiliated community hospital. *Arch. Intern. Med.* **145**:439–441, 1985. The records of 208 medical and 103 surgical patients were reviewed. The type of analgesic and psychotropic medications, dosage, and dosing intervals were noted. The older patients in this study were prescribed for and took fewer narcotics. Two-thirds of the patients were more than 60 years old, yet only half of the analgesics prescribed went to this group. More than 50% of the 18- to 40-year-old patients took an analgesic, in contrast to only 19% of those older than 80. Only 20% of the members of the older group who took an analgesic used a narcotic, compared with 88% of the younger group members. The authors suggest that the age-related differences in both prescribing patterns and consumption of analgesics may be a result of concern about increased risk of side effects in older patients. However, they state that there is inadequate information on this. The data also suggest additional findings concerning treatment of cancer pain, polypharmacy, and prescribing of psychotropics.

Roy, R., and Thomas, M.: Elderly persons with and without pain: a comparative study. *Clin. J. Pain* **3**:102–106, 1987. Two hundred and five people, aged 60–89, who were ambulatory and capable of participating in a variety of activities were surveyed to assess prevalence of pain problems in the healthy elderly and how they compared with elderly without pain. Seventy per cent of the people studied reported some kind of problem with pain, and yet disability due to pain was almost non-existent. There were no signs of depression in this group, and all group members were part of an organization that promoted community involvement and organized social activities. Under these circumstances, pain and disability during the older years can be virtually eliminated.

REFERENCES AND SELECTED READINGS

Amadio, P., Cummings, D.M., and Amadio, P.B.: Pain in the elderly: management techniques. *Pain Manag.* **1**:33–41, 1987.

American Pain Society: Principles of analgesic use in the treatment of acute pain and chronic cancer pain: a concise guide to medical practice. The Society, Washington, DC, 1987.

Austin, K.L., Stapleton, J.V., and Mather, L.E.: Multiple intramuscular injections: a major source of variability in analgesic response to meperidine. *Pain* **8**:47–62, 1980.

Avorn, J.: Drugs and the elderly. *Harvard Medical School*

Health Letter 9:3–4, June 1984.

Baskin, S.I., and Goldfarb, A.H.: Age-associated changes of non-narcotic analgesics. In Goldfarb, P.B., and Robers, J., eds: *CRC Handbook on pharmacology of aging*, pp. 113–125, CRC Press, Florida, 1983.

Butler, R.N: The life review: an interpretation of reminiscence in the aged. *Psychiatry* 26:65–76, 1963.

Butler, R.N., and Gastel, B.: Care of the aged: perspectives on pain and discomfort. In Ng, L.K., and Bonica, J., eds: *Pain, discomfort and humanitarian care*, pp. 297–311, Elsevier, North Holland, 1980.

Ceccio, C.M.: Postoperative pain relief through relaxation in elderly patients with fractured hips. *Orthoped. Nurs.* 3:11–19, 1984.

Clark, W.C., and Mehl, L.: Thermal pain, *J. Abnorm. Psychol.* 78: 202–212, 1971.

Clinch, D., Banerjee, A.K., and Ostick, G.: Absence of abdominal pain in elderly patients with peptic ulcer disease. *Age Ageing* 13:120–123, 1984.

Cunha, U.V.: Antidepressants: their use in nonpsychiatric disorders of aging. *Geriatrics* 41:63–72, 1986.

Dietsche, L.M.: Facilitating the life review through group reminiscence. *J. Gerontol. Nurs.* 5:43–46, 1979.

Eland, J.M.: Pain management and comfort. *J. Gerontol. Nurs.* 14:10–15, 1988.

Engelking, C.: Comfort issues in geriatric oncology. In Frank-Stromberg, M., and Welch-McCaffery, D., eds: *Semin. Oncol. Nurs.* 4:198–207, Aug 1988.

Fakouri, C., and Jones, P.: Relaxation rx: the slow stroke back rub. *J. Gerontol. Nurs.* 13:32–35, 1987.

Ferrell, B.A., and Ferrell, B.R.: Assessment of chronic pain in the elderly. *Geriatr. Med. Today.* (in press)

Flower, R.J., Moncada, S., and Vane, J.R.: Drug therapy of inflammation. In Gilman, A.G., et al, eds: Goodman and Gilman's *The pharmacological basis of therapeutics*, pp. 674–715, ed 7, Macmillan Publishing, New York, 1985.

Foreman, M.D.: Acute confusional states in hospitalized elderly: a research dilemma. *Nurs. Res.* 35:34–38, 1986.

Freund, G.: Drug and alcohol-induced dementia. In Wood, W.G., and Strong, R., eds: Geriatric clinical pharmacology, pp. 95–105, Raven Press, New York, 1987.

Gall, E.P.: Analgesic and anti-inflammatory agents. In Conrad, K.A., and Bressler, R., eds: *Drug therapy for the elderly*, The CV Mosby Co, St Louis, 1982.

Gioiella, E.C., and Bevil, C.W.: Nursing care of the aging client, pp. 291-310, Appleton-Century-Crofts, Norwalk, Conn, 1985.

Glynn, N.J.: The therapy of music. *J. Gerontol. Nurs.* 12:6–10, 1986.

Goodwin, J.S., and Regan, M.: Cognitive dysfunction associated with naprosyn and ibuprofen in the elderly. *Arthritis Rheumatism* 25:1013–1015, 1982.

Government Actuaries Department 1993: Personal Communication.

Greenblatt, D.J., Sellers, E.M., and Shader, R.I.: Drug disposition in old age, *N. Engl. J. Med.* 306:1081–1088, May 6, 1982.

Griffin, M.: In the mind's eye. *Am. J. Nurs.* 86:804–806, 1986.

Hanks, G.W., and Aherne, G.W.: Morphine metabolism: does the renal hypothesis hold water? *Lancet* 1:221–222, Jan 26, 1985.

Harkins, S.W., and Chapman, C.R.: Detection and decision factors in pain perception in young and elderly men. *Pain* 2:253–264, 1976.

Harkins, S.W., Kwentus, J., and Price, D.D.: Pain and suffering in the elderly. In Bonica, J., ed: *Clinical management of pain.* Lea and Febiger, Philadelphia.

Herth, K.: The therapeutic use of music. *Supervisor Nurs.* 9:22–23, 1978.

Jaffe, J.J., and Martin, W.R.: Opioid analgesics and antagonists. In Gilman, A.G., Goodman, L.S., Rall, T.W., and Murad, F., eds: *The pharmacological basis of therapeutics*, pp 532–581, ed 7. Macmillan Publishing, New York, 1985.

Johnson, J.: Drug treatment for sleep disturbances: does it really work? *J. Gerontol. Nurs.* 11:9–12, 1985.

Kaiko, R.F., Foley, K.M., Grabinski, P.Y., et al: Central nervous system excitatory effects of meperidine in cancer patients. *Ann. Neurol.* 13:180–185, 1983.

Kelly, N.: Personal communication, 1988. This patient example was given to us by Nancy Kelly, RN, MSN, Geriatric Intake and Assessment Nurse, East Boston Neighborhood Health Center, Boston, Mass. We are appreciative of her willingness to share this example.

Kwentus, J.A., Harkins, S.W., Lignon, N., and Silverman, J.J.: Current concepts of geriatric pain and its treatment. Geriatrics 40: 48–57, 1985.

Lamy, P.P.: The elderly, undernutrition, and pharmacokinetics. *J. Am. Geriatr. Soc.* 31:560–562, Sept 1983.

Lamy, P.P.: Pain management, drugs and the elderly. *Am. Health Care Assoc. J.* 10:32–36, July 1984.

Lamy, P.P.: Adverse drug reactions and the elderly: an update. In Ham, R.J., ed: *Geriatric medicine annual* 1986, pp. 128–154. Medical Economics Books, Oradell, NJ, 1986.

Larson, E.B., Kukull, W.A., Buchner, D., and Reifler, B.V.: Adverse drug reactions associated with global cognitive impairment in elderly persons. *Ann. Intern. Med.* 107:169–173, 1987.

Liebeskind, J.C., and Melzack, R.: The international pain foundation: meeting a need for education in pain management. *Pain* 30:1–2, 1987.

Linderborn, K.M.: The need to assess dementia. *J. Gerontol. Nurs.* 14:35–39, 1988.

Lonergan, E.T.: Aging and the kidney: adjusting treatment to physiological change. *Geriatrics* 43:27–33, 1988.

Lukacsko, P.: A guide to the parenteral management of moderate to severe pain. *Hosp. Pharm.* 22:361–412, Apr 1987.

MacDonald, J.B.: Presentation of acute myocardial

infarction in the elderly. *Age Ageing* **13**:196–200, 1984.

Mather, L.E., Tucker, G.T., Pflug, A.E., et al: Meperidine kinetics in man. *Clin Pharmacol Ther* **17**:21–30, 1975.

McCaffery, M.: Narcotic analgesia for the elderly. *Am. J. Nurs.* **85**:296–297, 1985.

Meyer, B.R.: Benzodiazepines in the elderly. *Med. Clin. North Am.* **66**:1017–1035, 1982.

Miller, R.R., and Jick, H.: Clinical effects of meperidine in hospitalized medical patients. *J. Clin. Pharmacol.* **18**:180–189, 1978.

Miscally, M.: Personal communication, 1988. This example was given to us by Madelyn Miscally, RN, MSN, Geriatric Clinical Nurse Specialist, Bowman Gray School of Medicine, Winston-Salem, NC. Ms. Miscally was also a reviewer and consultant for this chapter. We are very appreciative of her willingness to share her expertise on care of the elderly.

Mitchell, C.O., and Lipschitz, D.A.: Detection of protein-calorie malnutrition in the elderly. *Am. J. Clin. Nutr.* **35**:398–406, 1982.

Morgan, J., and Furst, D.E.: Implications of drug therapy in the elderly. *Clin. Rheumat. Dis.* **12**:227–243, 1986.

Murray, R., Huelskoetter, M., and O'Driscoll, D.: *The nursing process in later maturity*, pp. 284–293. Prentice-Hall, Englewood Cliffs, NJ, 1980.

Office of Population Census and Surveys, Population Estimates Unit O.P.C.S. Crown Copyright, 1991.

Ouslander, J.G.: Drug therapy in the elderly. *Ann. Intern. Med.* **95**:711–722, 198.1

Pagliaro, L.A., and Pagliaro, A.M.: Introduction. In Pagliaro, L.A., and Pagliaro, A.M., eds: *Pharmacological aspects of aging*, pp. 1–6, The CV Mosby Co, St Louis, 1983.

Pagliaro, L.A., and Pagliaro, A.M.: Age-dependent drug selection and response. In Pagliaro, L.A., and Pagliaro, A.M., eds: *Pharmacological aspects of nursing*, pp. 130–139, The CV Mosby Co, St Louis, 1986.

Peabody, C.A., Whiteford, H.A., and Hollister, L.E.: Antidepressants and the elderly. *J. Am. Geriatr. Soc.* **34**:869–874, 1986.

Petrucci, K.: Personal communication, 1988. This patient example was given to us by Kerry Petrucci, RN, MSN, Nurse Gerontologist, Clinical Center Nursing, National Institutes of Health, Bethesda, Md. We appreciate her willingness to share this example.

Polisson, R.P.: Selecting a NSAID for elderly patients. *Hosp. Ther.* **12**:17–32, 1987.

Portenoy, R.K.: Postherpetic neuralgia: a workable treatment plan. *Geriatrics* **41**:34–48, 1986.

Portenoy, R.K.: Optimal pain control in elderly cancer patients. *Geriatrics* **42**:33–44, 1987.

Portenoy, R.K., and Foley, K.M.: Chronic use of opioid analgesics in non-malignant pain: report of 38 cases. *Pain* **25**:171–176, May 1986.

Reidenberg, M.M.: Drugs in the elderly. *Med. Clin. North Am.* **66**:1073–1078, 1982.

Rowe, J.W., and Bresdine, R.W., eds: *Health and disease in old age*, Little, Brown & Co, Boston, 1982.

Rubenstein, L.Z., and Robbins, A.S.: Falls in the elderly: a clinical perspective. *Geriatrics* **39**:67–78, 1984.

Ryden, M.B.: Nursing intervention in support of reminiscence. *J. Gerontol. Nurs.* **7**:461–463, 1981.

Schafer, S.C.: Personal communication, 1988. This patient example was given to us by Susan Schafer, RNC, MS, Clinical Research Nurse, Pain Research Clinic, National Institutes of Health, Bethesda, Md. Ms. Schafer was also a reviewer and consultant for this chapter. We are very appreciative of her willingness to share her expertise on pain in the elderly.

Schlegel, S.I., and Paulus, H.E.: Non-steroidal and analgesic therapy in the elderly. *Clin Rheumat Dis* **12**:245–273, 1986.

Schmucker, D.L.: Drug disposition in the elderly: a review of the critical factors. *J. Am. Geriatr. Soc.* **32**:144–149, 1984.

Strumpf, N.E., and Evans, L.K.: Physical restraint of the hospitalized elderly: perceptions of patients and nurses. *Nurs. Res.* **37**: 132–137, 1988.

Sturgis, E.T., Dolce, J.J., and Dickerson, P.C.: Pain management in the elderly. In Carstensen, L., and Edelstein, B.A., eds: *Handbook of clinical gerontology*, pp. 190–203, Pergamon Press, New York, 1987.

Szeto, H., Inturrisi, C., Houde, R., et al: Accumulation of normeperidine, an active metabolite of meperidine, in patients with renal failure or cancer. *Ann. Intern. Med.* **86**:738–741, 1977.

Thomas, M.R., and Roy, R.: Age and pain: a comparative study of the "younger and older" elderly. *Pain Manag.* **1**:174–179, July–Aug 1988.

Thorsteinsson, G.: Chronic pain: use of TENS in the elderly. *Geriatrics* **42**:75–82, 1987.

Todd, B.: Narcotic analgesia for chronic pain. *Geriatr. Nurs.* **7**:53–55, Jan–Feb 1986.

Travis, S.S.: Observer-rated functional assessments for institutionalized elders. *Nurs. Res.* **37**:138–143, 1988.

Triozzi, P.L., Goldstein, D., and Lazlo, J.: Supportive care of the patient with cancer. In Cohen, H.J., ed: *Clin. Geriatr. Med.* **3**:505–516, Aug 1987.

Weingart, W.A., Sorkness, C.A., and Earhart, R.H.: Analgesia with oral narcotics and added ibuprofen in cancer patients. *Clin. Pharm.* **4**:53–58, Jan-Feb 1985.

Westfall, L.K., and Pavlis, R.W.: Why the elderly are so vulnerable to drug reactions. *RN* **50**:39–42, 1987.

Whall, A.: Psychotropic medications and side effects in the elderly. *J. Gerontol. Nurs.* 10:35, 1984.

Williams, M.A., Ward, S.E., and Campbell, E.B.: Confusion: testing versus observation. *J. Gerontol. Nurs.* **14**:25–30, 1988.

Appendix
Patient/Family Teaching Points

Photocopy these and use them with your patients and their families

List of Patient/Family Teaching Points in alphabetical order:

DAILY DIARY

NAME: _____   DATE: _____

Time	Pain-rating scale	Medication type & amount taken	Other pain-relief measures tried or anything that influences your pain	Major activity being done: lying sitting standing/walking
12 MIDNIGHT				
1 AM				
2				
3				
4				
5				
6				
7				
8				
9				
10				
11				
12 NOON				
1				
2				
3				
4				
5				
6				
7				
8				
9				
10				
11				

COMMENTS _____

_____

Use of Daily Diary

TO: _____ (patient's name)   DATE: _____

Filling out a daily diary will help us understand how pain affects your daily activities. With this information, we can work together toward the best possible control of your pain. An explanation of the columns in the diary follows. **Pain rating.** Use whatever pain rating you and the health-care team have decided is easiest for you to use. The scale you are to use is:

_____

Medication. Fill in the name of the medication and the amount you take at the time noted in the far left column.

Other pain-relief measures. Fill in any measures that you might use to get good control of the pain. This might include your favourite hobby, listening to music, or use of heat or cold over the painful area.

Major activity being done. It is important for us to know how well you sleep and if walking or other activities have an effect on your pain.

Have your record available when you see the nurse or doctor next. **Remember:** You are the only one who can tell us what your pain is like. The more you tell us about your pain, the more information we have to plan with you ways to make the pain better.

Additional comments: _____

_____

_____

_____

If you have any questions or problems with this record, contact:

Name: _____   Phone: _____

■ May be duplicated for use in clinical practice. From McCaffery, M., Beebe, A., and Latham , J. (ed.): *Pain: Clinical Manual for Nursing Practice*, Mosby, an imprint of Times Mirror International Publishers Ltd, London, 1994.

Preventive Approach with Pain Medication

TO: _____ (patient's name)   DATE: _____

Your Pain Medication(s):

- _____
- _____
- _____

Important Points about Pain Medication

- If you are in hospital, you may have to ask the nurse for pain medication. Do not assume that it is included with your other tablets and do not assume that the nurse knows when you hurt; you must tell her.

- Ask the doctor or nurse how your pain medication is prescribed for you.

- Your pain medication may be prescribed to be given or taken regularly at certain hours. However, if it is not, ask for it, and let the nurse know when the pain *first starts.*

- If you are at home, take the medication when you first notice the pain.

- Do not wait until the pain is bad before you call for or take the pain medication. Trying to "wait a little longer" only allows the pain to get worse and means that it will take longer to control it and you may need higher doses of medication if it becomes severe.

- You may be holding off because you are worried about getting "hooked" on the medication. Remember you are taking the medication for a medical reason: pain relief. When the pain stops, the overwhelming majority of people stop taking the medication.

- Tell the nurse or doctor if the medicine does not help the pain so they can adjust it until you are comfortable.

Additional comments: _____

_____

_____

If you have any questions about the above, contact:

Name: _____ Phone: _____

Instructions for Using Non-Narcotic Analgesics at Home

TO: _____ (patient's name)   DATE: _____

Facts about your pain reliever and how to take it. This non-narcotic medicine is sometimes called a non-steroidal anti-inflammatory drug (NSAID) or an aspirin-like drug. It is commonly used for arthritis but also may be used to relieve many other types of pain. Pain relief is usually felt within 2 hours or less after taking it. In addition to relieving pain, it reduces inflammation and fever. This medicine does not, however, cure the cause of your pain. To relieve your discomfort or pain, you are taking the following non-narcotic medicine:

Name of medicine: _____   (other names): _____

Dose: _____   (number of tablets per dos:): _____

How often: _____

The method indicated below is the appropriate approach for relief of your pain:

_____   For on-going pain, it is usually recommended that you take this on a regular daily basis, every day, without missing a dose. This helps keep your pain under control.

_____   For occasional or unpredictable pain, you may be instructed to begin taking this at the onset of pain, and then take it on a regular basis, without missing a dose, until the pain goes away.

Take this medicine with food or at least a full glass of milk to avoid stomach upset. If this does not prevent stomach upset or indigestion, you may try an antacid. If stomach upset continues, notify your nurse or doctor. *Do not take it with alcohol* because stomach irritation can occur.

Never take this on an empty stomach. Even if it does not upset your stomach, it can still damage the stomach. If you take two or more doses as prescribed and the medicine does not relieve your pain, notify your nurse or doctor. It may be necessary to increase the dose or change to another medicine.

Do not take any additional medicine known as a non-narcotic or nonsteroidal anti-inflammatory drug (NSAID) except for paracetamol, unless it is recommended by a doctor who knows what you are taking now. Taking more than one non-narcotic pain reliever can dramatically increase side effects and/or cause serious organ damage that you would not necessarily notice initially.

Watch for non-prescription products with "hidden aspirin". Many cold remedies and other over-the-counter medicines contain aspirin. The addition of aspirin could increase your risk of side effects. If you are already taking aspirin, this additional aspirin could raise your dose to a dangerous level.

If you have any side effects from your medicine that you cannot control by trying the suggestions on this form, stop taking the medicine and notify your nurse or doctor. Some of the side effects that may occur with some of the NSAIDs are stomach upset or indigestion; dizziness; headache; blurred vision; ringing in the ears or hearing loss; swelling in legs, ankles, or neck; skin rash; shortness of breath; black bowel movements; diarrhoea or constipation; unusual bleeding; onset of or increase in symptoms of asthma; depression; or confusion. Elderly patients should be especially alert to possible memory loss, inability to concentrate, or personality change

Contra-indications: Before you take this medicine, notify your nurse or doctor if you are pregnant; breast-feeding; taking anticoagulant, antidiabetic, or anticonvulsant drugs; have bleeding problems; heart disease; kidney problems; stomach ulcers; or allergy or sensitivity to aspirin. Also, notify your nurse or doctor if any of these occur while you are taking this medicine.

Additional comments: _____

_____

If you have any questions or problems with the above, contact:

Name: _____   Phone: _____

■ May be duplicated for use in clinical practice. From McCaffery, M., Beebe, A., and Latham, J. (ed.): *Pain: Clinical Manual for Nursing Practice*, Mosby, an imprint of Times Mirror International Publishers Ltd, London, 1994.

Common Side Effects of Narcotics

.TO: _____ (patient's name)   DATE: _____

Possible Side Effects Resulting from Narcotics
Constipation, drowsiness, and nausea are all possible effects of taking regular doses of narcotic medication for pain. Something can usually be done about each of these.

Constipation Caused by Narcotics: Important Points to Remember
- If you are taking pain medication regularly, you will become constipated.
- However, constipation is something that can be prevented; or if it occurs, it can be treated.
- It is unacceptable to be told that your pain medication cannot be increased because of constipation. Constipation can be prevented or controlled by careful assessment of your habits, and by adjustments in your constipation medication and food and liquids.
- The usual methods you use to stay regular probably will not work well enough alone. Several approaches will be required and may be intensified as needed. We will try to incorporate your preferences for bowel care as far as is possible.
- The usual goal is a bowel movement at least every 2–3 days.
- While medication to relieve and prevent constipation is important, combining this with non-medicine methods can be even more effective. These include the following suggestions:

1. Eat foods that help you have regular bowel movements. These include:

_____

_____

2. Drink as much water or other fluid as possible. Aim for _____ glasses each day of these fluids:

_____

_____

3. Exercise daily—such as walking. If you are in bed, exercises are important too. Your daily exercise routine will include:

_____

_____

4. The urge to go to the bathroom is a natural message. Ignoring it can lead to constipation or make it worse.
5. Take your time while having a bowel movement; hurrying can be as bad as delaying the urge to go.
6. Do not strain or make a lot of effort to have a movement.
   - If more than 2 days pass without a bowel movement, notify your nurse or doctor immediately so that he/she can help you correct this problem.

Your daily medications for constipation are:

_____

_____

continued

Common Side Effects of Narcotics (cont'd.)

As long as you take narcotics, you must continue these measures to keep constipation under control. Do not stop any of these approaches simply because you have a bowel movement. You need to continue them in order to keep from being constipated.

Additional comments:

Nausea and Vomiting Caused by Narcotics: Important Points to Remember
• Some people become nauseated and vomit after first starting on pain medication.
• If this happens to you, let your nurse or doctor know so that you can begin on an anti-nausea medication (anti-emetic).
• Nausea and vomiting should stop after several days. The dose of anti-nausea medication can then be decreased or stopped. However, some people need to continue on this medication as long as they are on narcotics.
• Sometimes there are causes of nausea other than the pain medication. Your doctor may look at other medications that you are taking or other things going on in your body.

Your medications for nausea are:

Additional comments:

Drowsiness Caused by Narcotics: Important Points to Remember
• Some people feel drowsy after first starting on pain medication.
• This drowsiness usually goes away after several days.
• You may have had no sleep because of the pain. When your body finally gets some relief, it is natural that you will probably sleep a lot at first because of total exhaustion.
• If sitting or lying in bed quietly, many people on pain medication find that they "catnap" throughout the day. This is normal and should not be seen as a bad effect. However, discuss this with your nurse or doctor if the drowsiness interferes with your ability to concentrate, talk with friends, or do the things that are important to you. They will work with you to try to correct this problem.
• If you are taking medications to control nausea, they may make you drowsy. Drowsiness from these medications will go away when you stop taking them.
• Other causes of drowsiness (other than the narcotic) may be explored by your doctor.
Additional comments:
If you have any questions or concerns about the above, contact:

Name: Phone:

(Nurse's signature)

Antidepressant Medications to Help with Pain Control

TO: _____ (patient's name)   DATE: _____

You are taking a medication called an antidepressant. Although this drug at higher doses may help depression, you are taking it at lower doses for other reasons. These are:
- Relief of pain.
- Relief of sleep problems.
- Relief of anxiety.

This drug can be very effective along with your pain medication. However, you may not notice the effects for 7–14 days. Do not give up and stop taking it! With regular doses you will feel a difference, but it does take time.

One effect that you may notice right away is a really good night's sleep after one or two doses. Another effect that you may experience is a dry mouth.

Let your doctor or nurse know if you experience an excessively dry mouth, inability to urinate, extreme drowsiness, or dizziness when standing. These are possible side effects which need attention if they occur.

Additional comments: _____

_____

_____

_____

_____

_____

If you have any questions or problems with the above information, contact:

Name: _____   Contact: _____

Massage of Body, Hands, or Feet

TO: _____ (patient's name)   DATE: _____

Almost everybody likes to receive a massage. You and the person who will be giving the massage, referred to as the massager, may consider the following tips on making it as beneficial as it can be.

1. *What area is best?* Most people think of the traditional back rub that includes the area from the lower back to the shoulders. Arms and legs can be added. However, if these areas are inconvenient, try massage of both hands or both feet.

2. *When should it be done?* You may enjoy it most when you're tired, when your pain increases, when you get anxious, or just before you go to sleep. If possible, you may want to set aside a specific time each day for a massage, perhaps the same time every day. This will give you something to look forward to.

3. *How long should it last?* This depends a lot on how much time is available to you and your massager. You'll have a better idea of what seems best for you after you've had a massage. Note the time massage begins and then note how long it takes for you to feel the benefits. Some people benefit from only a few minutes of massage. You may want to establish an exact period of time so you can enjoy the massage without wondering how long it will last or if you should give the massager permission to stop.

4. *Bare hands or lotion?* Do what feels best. If your skin is dry, you may want a moisturizing lotion. Warm the lotion in a microwave oven or by placing the bottle in a sink of hot water. Or, you may want to try powder. Either keeps the movement slippery, preventing uncomfortable friction on the skin or pulling tiny hairs.

5. *What position?* Both you and your massager should be in relaxed positions.

6. *How is the rubbing done?* Massage over the trunk and extremities is usually done with the palms of both hands, conforming to the body contours and using long strokes with firm enough pressure not to be ticklish. For massage of the feet or hands the massager usually uses the fingers of both hands. The entire foot or hand is massaged, including separate massage for each toe or finger. Initially, you need to tell your massager what feels good to you. Regardless of the type or area of massage, the movements should almost always be continuous, even, and rhythmical.

7. *Should you talk during a massage?* Probably not. Let your massager know this so neither of you will feel obligated to talk. Just concentrate on how good the massage feels.

As a reminder, you may wish to complete the following:

Date: _____ Massager: _____

Area to be massaged: _____ Warm lotion, oil, or powder? _____

Time of day: _____ Length of time for massage: _____

Special considerations: _____

From: _____ Contact: _____

■ May be duplicated for use in clinical practice. From McCaffery, M., Beebe, A., and Latham, J. (ed.): *Pain: Clinical Manual for Nursing Practice*, Mosby, an imprint of Times Mirror International Publishers Ltd, London, 1994.

Pain Relief with Heat? Cold? Both?

TO: _____ (patient's name) DATE: _____

You've probably used heat and cold before for relief of discomfort. Maybe you used a heating pad for a backache or a cold pack for a black eye. You may have been taught to use cold on a new injury for the first 24–48 hours to reduce bleeding and swelling, and then switch to heat. But cold relieves pain too, long after the initial injury. Sometimes heat and cold can be used interchangeably. But did you know that sometimes cold relieves pain better than heat? Even for arthritis!

If you're thinking about using *either heat or cold*, consider the following:

1. *Is either one contra-indicated?* In general, heat is contra-indicated the first 12–24 hours after an injury or if there is swelling or bleeding. Cold is usually contra-indicated if it increases pain. Otherwise there are not many common conditions for which cold is contra-indicated. If you have questions, talk with your nurse or doctor.

2. *Use what has worked for you before,* or simply follow your hunches. You can always change to the other. What works for one person or one type of pain will not necessarily work for another person or another type of pain. Heat and cold work differently for different people and different pains.

3. *Intensity.* Heat or cold should be applied at a comfortable level of intensity, not too hot or cold. It should not be painful or uncomfortable. Containers of heat or cold can be wrapped to make them less hot or cold. Moist cloth makes them feel hotter or colder.

4. *Precautions with heating.* To prevent burns it is safer not to lie on heating devices. Also, use a towel or cloth to soak up sweat beads (moisture) that could increase the temperature, and remove jewellery or other metal objects that come in contact with the heat.

5. *Length of time.* Heat or cold is usually applied for 20–30 minutes. It can be left on longer. The minimum effective time is about 5–10 minutes.

6. For better pain relief that lasts longer after the removal of heat or cold, try applying it for a longer period of time, e.g.up to 1 hour. But remember, heat and cold numb the skin to some extent and you won't be as sensitive to the heat or cold. Continuing with heat or applying fresh cold packs must be done carefully to avoid temperatures so cold or hot that skin damage occurs.

7. Site. Heat or cold is usually applied to the site of pain, but if you can't get to the pain site or if it is too tender to touch, heat or cold may be applied in other areas such as:
   • Around the pain site.
   • Between pain and the brain.
   • Beyond the pain, i.e. pain is between the brain and the heat or cold.
   • Opposite side of body corresponding to the pain site (contralaterally).
   • Acupuncture or trigger points. (Your nurse may be able to give you a diagram of these or help you find them.)
   To find the most effective site, experiment with different sites for about 5 minutes each.

8. Many people are reluctant to try cold, but remember:
   • A cold pack, not ice, will be applied.
   • The cold pack can be wrapped sufficiently to prevent an uncomfortable degree of cold. It can be wrapped so well that the first sensation is merely cool, not cold. Then unwrap gradually over a period of minutes, but avoid skin irritation, e.g. redness.
   • If cold causes generalized chilling, be sure to wrap yourself well, e.g. sweater or electric blanket, or cuddle up with a heating pad.

continued

Pain Relief with Heat? Cold? Both? (cont'd.)

• Changes in the weather, e.g. cold weather, and dampness often increase pain, but increased pain does not necessarily occur with the local application of cold, i.e. application of cold to a small area.

• Research shows that cold may be very effective for conditions that are traditionally treated with heat, e.g. low back pain, arthritis.

• If cold relieves the pain, cold probably will work better than heat because

It relieves pain faster.

It relieves more pain.

Pain relief lasts longer after cold is removed.

9. If pain is severe or if you desire more relief:
   • Interrupt the application. Heat may be taken on and off, or heat and cold may be alternated. Intervals as frequent as 5 seconds or as long as several minutes may be used. Experiment to find your own rhythm.
   • Increase the intensity of heat or cold, but be careful not to cause pain or tissue damage.

10. If you have a muscle or joint injury and if you experience pain relief following use of heat or cold (most likely with cold), be careful not to perform any activities that would cause further injury. However, with proper supervision, therapeutic exercises are commonly recommended following heat or cold.

11. Heat and especially cold decrease skin sensitivity after removal. Be cautious to avoid injuries to the skin after use, since the skin is less able to feel pain and act as a warning signal of impending damage.

12. Topical analgesic/anaesthetic preparations may be applied to the skin along with cold, but not with heat since burns can result.

13. Water or moisture with heating is often recommended but must be used cautiously because of the increased risk of burns. (Burns are caused by a high rate of heat transmission to the skin, and water is an excellent conductor of heat.) Dry towelling, a poor conductor of heat, may be used over skin to reduce intensity of heat and risk of burn.

14. Whenever possible, use heat or cold before pain occurs or becomes severe.

15. Discontinue use if increased pain or skin irritation occurs.

16. If cold causes chilling or shivering, discontinue.

As a reminder to yourself or those assisting you, fill in the following blanks.

Type of heat or cold: _____

Keep it from being too hot or too cold by: _____

Body site for application: _____

When should it be applied? _____

How long? _____

Precautions: _____

continued

Pain Relief with Heat? Cold? Both? (cont'd.)

Keep a record of what happened, e.g. when you used it, how well it relieved pain, and any changes you made in how you used it. (For results, you may use a pain-rating scale of 0 = no pain to 10 = worst pain, recording pain rating before and after use of heat or cold.)

Date	Time	Results	Any Changes?

Instead of the above, you may ask your nurse for the "Daily Diary" form.*

From: _____   Contact: _____

*"Daily Diary" form is on p. 288.

■ May be duplicated for use in clinical practice. From McCaffery, M., Beebe, A., and Latham, J. (ed.): *Pain: Clinical Manual for Nursing Practice*, Mosby, an imprint of Times Mirror International Publishers Ltd, London, 1994.

Ice Application or Massage for Pain Relief

TO: _____ (patient's name)   DATE: _____

Using ice to relieve pain may sound questionable at best. It doesn't feel good at the time. In fact, it often hurts briefly.
So why should you try ice for pain relief? Because:

- Ice may work better and longer than other methods of stimulating the skin.
- Pain relief usually lasts for I hour or longer after ice is used. It almost always relieves pain for longer than heat or cold.
- Research has shown that in some conditions pain relief from ice is equal to or better than relief from acupuncture or TENS (transcutaneous electrical nerve stimulation, a relatively expensive, new technique that uses electrodes on the skin to transmit mild electrical impulses).
- Acupuncture and TENS sometimes hurt too.
- The sensations from the ice may over-ride other sensations. The discomfort of the ice may be better than feeling the discomfort of the other pain.

If use of ice is intolerable or ineffective the first time, consider trying it again. It may take several attempts before you find a way to tolerate the cold or before ice produces pain relief.
Two easy and inexpensive ways to apply ice are:
1. Immerse the painful part, e.g. hand, in water with melting ice.
2. With ice cubes or very cold water in cups that can be thrown away, e.g. paper or plastic cups.
Technique of ice massage:

- Ice should be in contact with the skin. Do not cover the ice with anything waterproof. The melting of the ice as it comes in contact with the skin is a safety factor that prevents tissue damage.
- Use a cloth to wipe up melting ice.
- Gently rub the ice on the skin, using circular or back-and-forth motions. Avoid pressure, especially over boney prominences.

How does ice feel? Ice application or massage is uncomfortable. Within 5 to 10 minutes, the sequence of sensations usually felt is: cold; burning; occasional itching; aching; and numbness. Sometimes the feeling of cold proceeds directly to numbness.

What is the normal skin reaction? Usual changes in skin appearance begin with redness. This may proceed to blanching (white or pale), but at this point icing should not be allowed to proceed much longer.

When should icing be stopped? Discontinue ice after 10 minutes of constant application or if any of the following occur:

- Sensation is intolerable.
- Muscle chilling.
- Shivering.
- Numbness.
- "Hunting reaction", alternating blanching and dilatation of vessels (occurs several minutes after blanching). This is called an end-point; further icing may injure the skin.

Avoid injuries after use. The skin is at least partially numb and is unable to send a warning signal of impending damage. Also, underlying muscles may be relieved of pain and care should be taken not to perform physical activities that would injure the muscles. Therapeutic exercises under supervision are, however, frequently recommended.
Apply a hand lotion after ice massage to prevent skin dryness.

From: _____ Contact _____

■ May be duplicated for use in clinical practice. From McCaffery, M., Beebe, A., and Latham , J. (ed.): *Pain: Clinical Manual for Nursing Practice*, Mosby, an imprint of Times Mirror International Publishers Ltd, London, 1994.

Distraction for Brief Pain with Slow Rhythmic Breathing

TO: _____ (patient's name)   DATE: _____

1. Keep your **eyes open and focus** steadily on one stationary spot or object. If you wish to close your eyes, picture the air going in and out of your lungs.

2. To begin, **take a slow deep breath.**

3. Then **breathe slowly**, at whatever depth is comfortable for you. Breathe in slowly, breathe out slowly, at about 6–9 breaths per minute. Do not hold your breath and do not breathe too deeply, but do take a deep breath whenever you feel the need.

4. **Breathe in a slow rhythm.** Concentrate on your breathing, thinking of the air going in and out of your lungs. Establish your rhythm by counting or saying phrases silently to yourself. Example of counting: "In, 2, 3, out, 2, 3." Example of phrases: When you breathe in, say to yourself "Breathe in slowly." When you breathe out, say to yourself "Breathe out slowly."

5. **End with a slow, deep breath.**

6. If this is **not effective, try adding** one or more of the following: rhythmic massage of a body area; inhalation through nose and exhalation through lips; abdominal or chest breathing; raising and lowering finger with inhalation and exhalation.

Additional points: This technique does not require much physical or mental exertion and is fairly relaxing. It may be used for up to 10 or 15 minutes, or off and on for about an hour.

From: _____   Contact: _____

Distraction for Brief Pain by Describing a Series of Pictures

TO: _____ (patient's name)   DATE: _____

1. **Obtain pictures** that interest you.
   • Types of pictures. There are many possibilities, such as pictures from magazines; photographs of friends, family, or a holiday; or books with pictures of a specific subject such as aeroplanes or historic events. You may want pictures on the same subject or different subjects. Avoid any pictures that you find disturbing or that remind you of your discomfort.
   • Number of pictures. The number of pictures you need will depend on several factors, such as how long your discomfort will last, how much detail you describe, and how fast you talk.

2. You may need **assistance.** If you do not have much time or energy, you may consider asking a friend to obtain the pictures for you, e.g. cut out magazine pictures. You may also want someone to hold the pictures up for you to see as you describe them and help you with your descriptions by asking you for some of the details discussed below.

3. **Look at the pictures and describe** them in any manner that interests you. Usually it is best to continue looking at the pictures while you describe them (as opposed to looking at the picture briefly, hiding it, and then trying to remember the details of the picture). Ways of describing or talking about the pictures include the following—to help you keep your attention focused on the pictures, you may want a friend to have this list and ask you about these items:
   • Pretend you are in the picture. What would you do?
   • Count the number of items in the picture.
   • Name each item in the picture.
   • Name the colours.
   • What is happening in the picture? Make up a story about the picture.
   As soon as you are no longer interested in the picture, put it away and look at another picture. Proceed from one picture to another as rapidly as you wish. If the picture reminds you of something you would like to describe or discuss, try doing so. What the picture reminds you of may be more distracting than the actual picture.

4. If this is **not effective enough, try adding or changing** one or more of the following: massage an area of your body while you are describing the pictures; try different pictures or different questions; reverse the procedure and ask questions of the person who is assisting you; include at random some surprise pictures that may be difficult to describe but have novel value, e.g. simple cartoons or scantily clad figures; if the discomfort increases, try changing the pictures more rapidly; if you feel self-conscious talking aloud, try describing the pictures to yourself silently.

Additional points: If you enjoy talking, you may find this technique useful in a number of situations. You may be able to use it for a few minutes during a very painful procedure, and use a variation of it for an hour or so with a visitor to help you with on-going mild to moderate pain.
This technique may be an ideal way to involve someone who has extra time and wants to help you with your pain. A friend or carer may gather pictures in his/her spare time and give them to you prior to a painful event, or the person might be there to show you the pictures and ask questions.

From: _____ Contact: _____

Handling Boring or Strange Days

TO: _____ (patient's name) DATE: _____

Do you have this problem? Are most of your days boring or full of strange sights and sounds? Are you doing very little of what you did before this illness and pain? This may be causing you more trouble than you realize. Boring or strange days may make you more and more aware of your pain, and you may find it becoming more difficult to tolerate. You may feel bored, tense, angry, frustrated, lonely, or sad. Getting back to a more normal daily life may help.

The *goal* is to plan your whole day, from getting up to going to bed, so that it includes specific activities that are somewhat like your more normal, healthy days. Try the following suggestions:

1. Think about the details of **what you used to do every day**. You might want to try making a list. What did you do almost every day? Which were most important? Most enjoyable? Little things like catching 10 minutes of morning news on the radio may be just as important as the big items such as working 8 hours. What were the special treats?

2. Which things could you still do with **just a little effort?** Examples that might apply to you: wear cologne, drink a second cup of coffee and read the morning newspaper, listen to the radio station you used to hear on the way to work, telephone a friend, get a copy of your favourite magazine, watch favourite TV programmes, get a plant to water and feed.

3. Can you do some **small part of important, but currently impossible activities?** Examples that might apply to you: if you used to enjoy dressing carefully for the day, put on some personal and attractive clothing item or accessory each morning; if you enjoyed the conversation with peers at morning breaks or lunch, ask one of them to include you by telephone each day; if you enjoyed your work and if someone is taking over your work responsibilities, offer to assist (within your limits) by telephone each day, perhaps at a specified time; if you enjoyed a bedtime ritual with your child or anyone else, talk with the person by phone before retiring.

4. Be especially alert to the possibility of including something related to each of the following since they tend to have many benefits, such as the relaxing qualities of some types of music:
   • **Music** with headset (headset blocks out other sounds and avoids disturbing others with the music). Select music, note its effect on you, and make necessary changes in choices. Try listening to music about three times a day for 20–30 minutes. In some patients this makes pain more tolerable or reduces pain and the need for pain relievers.
   • **Physical exercise** at least once a day. At first this may be very limited, such as merely pointing toes and/or squeezing a ball with the hand. But some degree of physical activity tends to be a surprisingly important part of the daily plan.
   • **Conversation with a friend** at least once a day. Examples are telephone calls or arranging to stagger visitors from day to day.
   • Daily viewing of **specially selected videotapes or TV programmes**. Avoid having the TV on most of the time. If you like them, **books or magazines** are a good substitute for TV.

5. Consider a **written schedule** of daily activities. You may want to ask a friend or your nurse to help with this.

6. Plan for periods of rest. Don't "overdo" it. **Pace yourself**.

7. **Vary your activities at regular intervals**. Anything can become boring after a while. If in doubt, try changing to a different activity at least every hour.

8. **Change your daily routine**. Every day does not have to be the same. "Variety is the spice of life."

9. Consider a **special treat at the end of the day** as a reward for carrying through with your routine.

10. It may be **difficult to get started** with your daily plans. But you may find that after you make the initial effort, it gets easier.

From: _____   Contact: _____

■ May be duplicated for use in clinical practice. From McCaffery, M., Beebe, A., and Latham, J (ed.): *Pain: Clinical Manual for Nursing Practice*, Mosby, an imprint of Times Mirror International Publishers Ltd, London, 1994.

Learning and Using Relaxation Techniques

TO: _____ (patient's name) DATE: _____

1. Find a technique that works for you. Your nurse or therapist may be able to describe some alternatives. Also, you may wish to listen to some tape-recorded ones.

2. Stick with the same technique once you have selected one. You may combine several, but keep your relaxation exercise essentially the same each time. This helps you become conditioned to it, that is, you learn the skill faster and relax faster and better each time.

3. Be patient. It may take several practise sessions before you experience much benefit.

4. Practise at least once a day; twice a day is probably better. Relaxation is considered a skill that can be learned with repeated practise. Even if your pain subsides, continue to practise relaxation daily so you will remember how when you need to use it again.

5. When you are beginning to learn relaxation, practise when you feel fairly free of pain and tension. It's hard to learn anything when you're upset or in pain. Later, when you have learned the skill of relaxation, you will be able to use it more successfully during periods of distress or pain. However, try not to let things get that bad.

6. Use relaxation preventively, before pain and tension increase. Keep pain and distress under control.

7. During any given day, you may practise relaxation and then use it whenever needed to deal with pain and tension. If you find that your total time spent in relaxation is 1 hour or more, talk with your nurse. Other measures may be needed.

8. Do not expect success every time. Measure success by the fact that you tried. Your ability will vary. You cannot force relaxation to happen. You can only give it an opportunity to do so. Everybody who practises anything, such as tennis or piano, knows that some days they perform well and some days they do not.

9. When you need to use something brief, select some small, helpful portion of the longer technique. Once you have learned a relaxation technique, note which parts are most helpful to you.

10. Check for tension at intervals throughout the day. For example, about every hour, quickly note your body from head to toe and use a brief technique to help decrease any tension you find.

11. Get ready to relax if you are using a relaxation technique lasting 5 minutes or longer. To obtain the maximal benefit from a relaxation technique, prepare for it in the following ways:

    • Get into a comfortable, well-supported position. Lying down or using a reclining chair may be best.

    • If you lie down, try elevating your legs and putting a small pillow under your neck as shown in the figure on the right. This gives you a head start on relaxing, since elevating your legs in this manner relieves a lot of tension in the muscles of the lower back and the neck.

    • If you sit up, support your arms, e.g. place them in your lap, on a table in front of you, or on the chair's armrests. Do not dangle your arms.

    • Do not cross your legs or arms. They become heavy and may begin to cut off circulation, causing prickling sensations.

    • Try to create a quiet environment. Take the telephone off the hook, and consider placing a "Do not Disturb" sign on your door. If there are noises that cannot be eliminated, listen to them before you begin your relaxation technique. This allows you to identify and, if necessary, respond to sounds so you may more easily ignore them later. Sometimes the steady noise of a fan, air conditioner, or "easy-listening" radio music will help override other distracting sounds. If your technique is taped, listen to it with a headset to minimize environmental noises.

    • Empty your bladder.

continued

Learning and Using Relaxation Techniques (cont'd.)

• Loosen tight clothing, and take off any uncomfortable items, e.g. eye glasses.
• Put down anything you are holding so you don't have to worry about dropping it as you relax.
• If you are "cold natured", cover yourself.
• If you wish to evaluate how well relaxation is working for you, try one of the following:

Before and after relaxation, take your pulse rate. Sometimes you will notice a decrease in your heart rate after relaxation.

Before and after relaxation, rate your pain and distress. Use a 0–10 scale for each. For distress, 0 equals no distress,and 10 equals worst distress can be. For pain, 0 equals no pain, and 10 equals worst pain can be. Sometimes you may note a decrease in both; other times, pain may remain the same, but your distress will decrease.

Ask someone to gently move a body part, e.g. bend your arm for you, to test for any feelings of tension.

Your nurse or therapist can show you pain and distress scales and help you learn to count your pulse.

From: _____   Contact: _____

Deep Breath/Tense, Exhale/Relax, Yawn for Quick Relaxation

TO: _____   (patient's name)   DATE: _____

1. Clench your fists; breathe in deeply and hold it a moment.

2. Breathe out slowly and go limp as a rag doll.

3. Start yawning.

Additional points: Yawning becomes spontaneous. It is also contagious, so others may begin yawning and relaxing too.

From: _____   Contact: _____

Humour for Relaxation

TO: _____ (patient's name)   DATE: _____

Laugh when you hurt? Hurting is rarely funny, but people who hurt sometimes find that occasional humour is one of the most effective ways to deal with pain. Why not try some of the following?

1. Watch television programmes that are really funny to you.

2. Listen to recordings by comedians that you find very funny.

3. Read books that make you laugh.

Something funny can certainly be distracting, but its value seems to go beyond a momentary redirection of thoughts. Humour may produce relaxation.

For example, when you laugh, it is almost impossible to maintain muscle contraction. A simple example of this is when two or more people attempt to lift a heavy object in unison. One of them may be in charge of coordinating the efforts. That person counts or gives some cue to signal everyone to lift at the same time. But if they laugh, they fail. The result is familiar: the lifters become limp, drop the object, and sometimes actually fall to the floor. Laughter causes skeletal muscle relaxation; the skeletal muscles become too limp to hold or lift an object.

From: _____   Contact: _____

Heartbeat Breathing for Relaxation

TO: _____ (patient's name)   DATE: _____

Before you do this, if you are unsure about how to find and count your pulse rate (usually radial pulse at the wrist), ask your nurse or therapist to help you.

1. Take a deep, comfortable breath.

2. Close your eyes or focus on your hands.

3. Count your radial pulse (at the wrist) for two beats.

4. Inhale while you count the next two beats.

5. Exhale while you count the next three beats.

6. Inhale and exhale in this manner several times.

Additional points: You can do this quickly if you are suddenly anxious or fearful. You can do this without drawing attention to yourself. The pulse (heart) rate usually slows noticeably.

From: _____   Contact: _____

■ May be duplicated for use in clinical practice. From McCaffery, M., Beebe, A., and Latham, J. (ed.): *Pain: Clinical Manual for Nursing Practice*, Mosby, an imprint of Times Mirror International Publishers Ltd, London, 1994.

> ## Progressive Relaxation Instructions

TO: _____ (patient's name) DATE: _____

This technique consists of:
1. Tense (or contract) and then relax specific muscle groups.
2. Usually tense/relax is done twice with each muscle group.
3. In the following script, 14 muscle groups are used, but many different groups may be used.

You may perform this technique from memory or by referring to the written directions. However, most people prefer to have it tape-recorded. Listening to the tape with a headset helps decrease distracting noises in the environment. You may choose your nurse or someone else to do the record.

Before recording, follow the directions for at least one or two sets of tense/relax. Have your recorder note approximately how many seconds you prefer to contract your muscles for and for how many seconds you prefer to remain relaxed between muscle contractions.

You may do this relaxation technique in any comfortable, well-supported position, sitting or lying down. To get the most out of relaxation, prepare yourself and the environment. Your nurse can give you a list of suggestions.

Changing the script. The script may be changed in several ways. In the script, each muscle group is noted with a bullet (•). Go over each of these. If you do not understand the directions for the muscle contraction, ask for an explanation or change the directions. If you want a longer technique (up to 20 minutes), divide the muscle groups into smaller groups; if you want a shorter technique, combine some muscle groups into one group or perform each muscle contraction only once with each muscle group. Determine if any muscle groups should be omitted. Some muscle contractions may increase your pain. If you are prone to leg cramps, you may wish to omit all muscle contractions involving the legs and feet. Also, the sequence may be changed, e.g. you may begin at the toes and progress to the upper body.

Following are the exact words, designed for tape-recording, that may be used in the instructions:

(*Name of patient*), this is (*name of person speaking*). You have probably chosen to listen to this because you want to give yourself a chance to experience and benefit from relaxation. Together we will do what we can at this moment. We cannot make it happen. Sometimes you will feel relaxed, sometimes you won't. All we can do is go through the technique and give it a chance to work.

You may close your eyes now or find something to focus on. Breathe in deeply, hold your breath a moment, and breathe out slowly. Now you may breathe in your usual way, just slowly and regularly.
• Clench your right fist and hold it.
  Feel the tension. Now let it relax. Feel the difference. Notice the feelings of relaxation.
  Now, with less tension, clench your right fist again and hold it.
  Feel this level of tension. Now let it relax. Notice the feelings of relaxation in your hand.
• Clench your left fist and hold it.
  Feel the tension. Now let it relax. Feel the difference. Notice the feelings of relaxation.
  Now, with less tension, clench your left fist again and hold it.
  Feel this level of tension. Now let it relax. Notice the feelings of relaxation in your hand.
• Press your upper right arm toward your ribs and press the elbow back. Hold it.
  Feel the tension. Now let it relax. Feel the difference. Notice the feelings of relaxation.

continued

Progressive Relaxation Instructions (cont'd.)

Now, with less tension, once again press your upper right arm toward your ribs and press the elbow back. Hold it. Feel this level of tension. Now let it relax. Notice the feelings of relaxation in your arm.
- Press your upper left arm toward your ribs and press the elbow back.
  Hold it. Feel the tension. Now let it relax. Feel the difference. Notice the feelings of relaxation.
  Now, with less tension, once again press your upper left arm toward your ribs and press the elbow back. Hold it. Feel this level of tension. Now let it relax. Notice the feelings of relaxation in your arm.
- Wrinkle your forehead and hold it.
  Feel the tension. Now let it relax. Feel the difference. Notice the feelings of relaxation.
  Now, with less tension, once again wrinkle your forehead and hold it.
  Feel this level of tension. Now let it relax. Notice the feelings of relaxation in your forehead.
- Wrinkle your nose and shut your eyes tightly. Hold it.
  Feel the tension. Now let it relax. Feel the difference. Notice the feelings of relaxation.
  Now, with less tension, again wrinkle your nose and shut your eyes. Hold it.
  Feel this level of tension. Now let it relax. Notice the feelings of relaxation in your nose and eyes.
- Clench your teeth, pull back the corners of your mouth, and press your tongue against the roof of your mouth.
  Hold it. Feel the tension. Now let it relax. Feel the difference. Notice the feelings of relaxation.
  Now, with less tension, again clench your teeth, pull back the corners of your mouth and press your tongue against the roof of your mouth. Hold it. Feel this level of tension. Now let it relax. Notice the feelings of relaxation in your mouth and jaw.
- Press your head backwards and hold it. Feel the tension. Now let it relax. Feel the difference. Notice the feelings of relaxation.
  Now, with less tension, again press your head backwards and hold it.
  Feel this level of tension. Now let it relax. Notice the feelings of relaxation in your neck.
- Bring both shoulders upward toward your ears and hold it.
  Feel the tension. Now let it relax. Feel the difference. Notice the feelings of relaxation.
  Now, with less tension, bring both shoulders upward toward your ears and hold it.
  Feel this level of tension. Now let it relax. Notice the feelings of relaxation in your shoulders.
- Make your stomach hard, pull it inward, and hold it.
  Feel the tension. Now let it relax. Feel the difference. Notice the feelings of relaxation.
  Now, with less tension, again make your stomach hard, pull it inward, and hold it.
  Feel this level of tension. Now let it relax. Notice the feelings of relaxation in your stomach.
- Press your right leg backwards and hold it.
  Feel the tension. Now let it relax. Feel the difference. Notice the feelings of relaxation.
  Now, with less tension, again press your right leg backwards and hold it.
  Feel this level of tension. Now let it relax. Notice the feelings of relaxation in your leg.
- Press your left leg backwards and hold it.
  Feel the tension. Now let it relax. Feel the difference. Notice the feelings of relaxation.
  Now, with less tension, again press your left leg backwards and hold it.
  Feel this level of tension. Now let it relax. Notice the feelings of relaxation in your leg.
- Point your right toes, stretch, and hold it.

continued

■ May be duplicated for use in clinical practice. From McCaffery, M; Beebe, A; and Latham , J (ed.): *Pain: Clinical Manual for Nursing Practice*, London, 1994, Mosby, an imprint of Times Mirror International Publishers Ltd.

Progressive Relaxation Instructions (cont'd.)

Feel the tension. Now let it relax. Feel the difference. Notice the feelings of relaxation.

Now, with less tension, again point your right toes, stretch, and hold it.

Feel this level of tension. Now let it relax. Notice the feelings of relaxation in your leg and foot.

Point your left toes, stretch, and hold it.

Feel the tension. Now let it relax. Feel the difference. Notice the feelings of relaxation.

Now, with less tension, again point your left toes, stretch, and hold it.

Feel this level of tension. Now let it relax. Notice the feelings of relaxation in your leg and foot. (End of instructions.)

Additional points: Once you have gained skill in using this technique to produce relaxation, you may find that when your time is limited you can benefit from using one small part of it, e.g. briefly clenching and relaxing your fists. This can be a practical way of integrating relaxation into your daily life. To prevent tension from building up, at intervals throughout the day you might clench your fists, note the tension, and then relax, noting the feelings of relaxation. Relaxation in one part of the body may spread throughout the body.

From: _____   Contact: _____

| **Using Imagery for Pain Relief** |

TO: _____ (patient's name)   DATE: _____

'Imagery for pain relief' means using of your imagination to help reduce your pain.

Your pain is certainly real, but you may be able to use your imagination in some way that helps relieve the pain. If you decide to try this, consider the following:

1. Find a technique that you like, one that makes sense to you. You may want to develop your own. The trick, of course, and it is admittedly a big trick, is to find the image that will relieve your particular pain.

2. Use your own image or representation of your pain and what relieves it. Although some imagery techniques suggest certain images for pain relief, these images are fairly vague because it is important for you to substitute your own personal images. Also, some techniques simply refer to areas of discomfort without much description. Again, use your own personal image of your pain.

3. If you feel you do not know enough about the cause of your pain or how it might be relieved, ask your nurse or doctor for information.

4. You need not use "medically correct" images. For example, some people have achieved pain relief by imagining their pain as a sound that gets quieter, a shape that becomes smaller, or a vicious animal that becomes friendly or eventually disappears.

5. Include your religious, spiritual, or "good luck" charms or rituals. For example, you may want to recite a passage of scripture, hold a rosary or rabbit's foot, or visualize a white light surrounding your body.

6. You may imagine how your pain is relieved and/or imagine the final result of being comfortable. If you prefer, you need not focus on your pain or imagine how it is relieved—just that it is relieved and you are comfortable. You may remember how you felt before the pain occurred.

7. If you wish you may practise your imagery technique or develop it over time. You may practise it in the absence of pain. Especially at first, some people like to practise imagery so they feel more familiar with it when they need it. You may decide on an image that relieves a little bit of pain each day rather than one that relieves all of the pain at once, especially if your pain is prolonged and severe.

8. If you decide to use more than one image or technique, use only one at a time. Most people concentrate more intensely and get a better effect this way. Trying to concentrate on two different images may dilute the effect of both of them.

9. Consider using a relaxation technique first, right before you begin the imagery. The imagery for pain relief may work better if you are relaxed and ready to concentrate.

10. Get comfortable. Get into a position with good support, e.g. lying down or sitting in a reclining chair. Loosen clothing or take off anything uncomfortable, e.g. your shoes. Empty your bladder before you begin.

11. Try to prevent interruptions. If your technique is tape-recorded, using a headset will help eliminate some of the noises around you. Taking the phone off the hook and posting a "Do not disturb" sign may help.

technique.

continued

Using Imagery for Pain Relief (contd.)

12. You may keep your eyes closed or open during the imagery technique. You may concentrate better with your eyes closed.

13. If you cannot concentrate, try counting each breath you take, saying each number silently to yourself before or after you breathe in or out. If this doesn't work, try again later. Perhaps you are too tired and need to rest. Or, you may be in too much pain and need another type of pain relief now.

14. If you are using an imagery technique that lasts for several minutes or more than a few seconds, remember that you do not always have to use the entire technique. You may select part of the image and focus on it only momentarily, perhaps as you stare into space. When the total imagery technique is used and effectively relieves pain, sometimes this effect can be maintained by frequently but briefly recalling a portion of the technique. Also, brief recall of the image may be helpful when you are unable to concentrate on using a lengthy imagery 15. The amount of time spent using an imagery technique for pain relief probably should not be more than 20 minutes at a time, and total time spent each day should not exceed 1 hour. If you are spending more time than this, discuss it with your nurse. You may need additional pain-relief measures.

16. Expect the effect of imagery to vary. It may not work every time you use it, or it may work better at some times rather than others. Measure success by the fact that you gave it a try.

17. Use other methods of pain relief, too. Rarely is imagery all that is needed for acceptable pain relief.

18. Use your imagery technique preventively, if possible. If you can predict when pain will return, use imagery before pain returns to try to prevent it from returning. At the very least, use imagery before pain increases to an intense level.

19. Be selective about the people you talk to about your use of imagery. Not everyone is open-minded about its possible value. Find out how others feel about imagery before you tell them what you do. If you want to close your eyes and prevent interruptions while you use imagery, you may simply tell others that you would like a few moments to rest your eyes. In preparation for a painful procedure, you could explain that you will be trying to concentrate on something else while the procedure is performed.

20. If you have any concerns about imagery or if you experience any unwanted side effects from using it, let your nurse know at once.

From: _____   Contact: _____

Emptying the Sandbag

TO: _____ (patient's name)   DATE: _____

1. This imagery technique is usually used to relieve pain in one area at a time. If you have pain in several areas of your body, decide which area of discomfort you want to relieve first.
2. Get into a well-supported, comfortable position. You may want to use a reclining chair or lie down.
3. Close your eyes, unless you feel better with them open. Most people can concentrate and imagine better with their eyes closed.
4. A brief relaxation technique at the beginning may be helpful, especially if you feel tense or find it hard to concentrate. Use whatever relaxes you, e.g. music. Or, ask your nurse about a brief technique such as slow, rhythmic breathing.
5. Breathe in slowly, deeply; breathe out slowly. Then continue to breathe slowly and evenly in whatever way is comfortable. This may be all that is needed to help you feel reasonably calm and comfortable.
6. Concentrate on your body being an empty sack or bag.
7. Gradually, at your own pace, focus on or imagine filling the bag slowly with sand. Feel your body get heavier and heavier as this happens. You may begin anywhere. For example, you may imagine filling your body from your toes up to your head. You may want to think of each area of your body as it fills with sand and gets heavier.
8. Continue filling the sandbag, your body, until it is completely full of sand; until the skin or covering has no more room, and until the bag, or your body, feels very heavy.
9. If a second person is available, indicate when you are ready to have help with this part. When the sandbag is completely full, you might raise your hand as a signal that you are ready for the following assistance: placing one hand on top of the area of pain and the other hand underneath. If this is impossible or uncomfortable, place the hands near the pain. The use of someone's hands is merely to help you focus on where the pain is. Another person is not essential. If a second person is not available, simply think about or focus on where the pain is.
10. Imagine making a small slit in the sandbag, usually in the back.
11. Imagine the sand slowly trickling out.
12. Begin to imagine the pain also trickling out slowly with the sand.
13. Continue thinking about, imagining, or visualizing the sand and pain slowly trickling out until the sandbag empties completely, is flat, depleted, and weightless.
14. Repeat the above steps 6 through to 13 for each area of pain.

Additional points: This technique can be done from memory. But, you may concentrate better if you tape-record the above steps or ask someone to read them to you each time you want to use the technique. Beginning with step number 2, each step may be read in a slow monotone voice with pauses between each step. You may want to omit number 4 or add a brief relaxation technique. Except for number 4, each step may be read almost exactly as it is written.

You may wish to develop your own image of your pain, e.g. colour, size, weight, temperature, sound, texture (e.g. feeling sharp or jagged around the edges), and smell of the pain. You may then imagine these sensory images changing or leaving the body as the sandbag empties.

From: _____   Contact: _____

Breathing Out Pain

TO: _____ (patient's name)   DATE: _____

NOTE: In these instructions for pain relief imagery, a blank is left (i.e._____) for you to fill in your own area(s) of discomfort. Before using these instructions, decide what words you will use for the blanks.

Instructions: You may close your eyes, if you wish, and take a slow, deep breath. You may feel yourself relax as you breathe out. Continue breathing comfortably and slowly, at whatever depth is natural for you, feeling your body relax each time you breathe out.

If you wish, the next time you breathe in you may imagine that your breath goes to your _____, bringing nutrients, comfort, and calm. As you breathe out, you imagine that the air goes out through your _____, taking with it the discomfort, leaving behind relaxed, healthy, comfortable tissues.

Each time you breathe in you may picture the air flowing through to your _____, bringing health and comfort. As you breathe out, the air once again flows out through your _____, leaving calm, relaxation, health, and comfort behind.

I will pause now and you may continue to breathe slowly and imagine more and more comfort with each breath that flows through your _____

When you are ready, you may end this image by counting silently to yourself from one to three. At the count of three breathe in, open your eyes, and say to yourself that you feel alert and relaxed.
I will wait now until you are ready to end this for yourself. Take your time. Enjoy the experience.

Additional points: If you already have a mental image of your pain, you may try to work with your image by breathing through it, gradually changing it to a more comfortable image. For example, if you see your pain as red and hard you may try to use your breaths to change the image to soft and white, or whatever you think of as a comfortable image.
Another variation is to imagine that there is a hole in your body near the painful area. As you breathe out, you may imagine the pain going out of your body through the hole.

From: _____   Contact: _____

Ball of Healing Energy

TO: _____ (patient's name)   DATE: _____

NOTE: These instructions for pain-relief imagery use the phrase "area that hurts", but you may substitute the name of your area of discomfort, e.g. "lower back".

Instructions: Now, if you wish, you may close your eyes. Take a slow, deep breath. You may feel yourself relax as you breathe out. Continue to breathe comfortably and slowly, at whatever depth is natural for you. Perhaps you can feel yourself relax each time you breathe out.

Now if you wish, you may begin to imagine a ball of white light, or healing energy, forming on your chest or in your lungs. This ball of white light or healing energy need not be terribly clear or vivid. Anything you want to imagine is suitable. It may be dim or abstract or very clear. Anything may be effective as long as you understand it as being positive, helpful, or healing.

When you are ready you may circulate this ball of white light and healing energy to the area that hurts. The next time you breathe in you may use that air to send the ball of healing energy to the area that hurts. When you breathe out you may use that air to send the ball away from your body, letting it take with it the hurt and tension, leaving behind feelings of comfort and healthy tissue.

You may, if you wish, continue to circulate the ball of healing energy with every breath you take. The ball of healing energy enters your body again, purified, and as you breathe in you may send the ball of healing energy to the area that hurts. As you breathe out you may send the ball of healing energy away from your body, letting it leave behind comfort and health.

Each time the ball of healing energy leaves your body it may take away twice as much of the hurt and leave behind twice as much comfort and health. The ball may get larger and larger as it does this.

I will pause now to allow you time to circulate the ball of healing energy or white light. When you are ready to end this, you may signal to me by raising your hand. . . . Take your time. . . .

Now that you are ready to end this technique, count silently to yourself from one to three. At the count of three breathe in deeply, open your eyes, and as you breathe out, say to yourself "I feel relaxed and alert."

Additional points: Healing energy is an ancient concept, and visualizing the sun or a white light is considered by many to be a powerful image for healing and pain relief. However, you may wish to substitute something else for this ball of energy. For example, you may prefer to use "God's healing power". You may wish to begin or end with scripture you find comforting.

Or, you may want to decrease or change certain specific qualities of the pain sensation. If you have burning pain, you may want to substitute something cool or cold, e.g. cold water, for the ball of energy.

Another variation is to have the ball of energy take away specific items, such as swelling, toxins, tension, or bacteria.

Obviously, you need not have someone read these instructions to you. You may be able to do it well from memory.

From: _____   Contact: _____

Planning for the Future—Review of Pain Relief Measures

TO: _____ (patient's name)   DATE: _____

Purpose: To use the information available from a recent episode of pain to plan the best possible pain relief for any future occurrence of similar pain. This is accomplished by identifying the effect of pain relief measures used for a recent episode of pain.

Nature of pain: _____

From (date): _____   to: _____

Medications used in relation to problem of pain (e.g. narcotic and non-narcotic analgesics, tranquillizers, antidepressants, sleeping pills, muscle relaxants):
Medication name, dose, frequency:

Helpful?   Other comments:

Non-pharmacological (non-drug) pain-relief measures (e.g. relaxation, distraction, TENS, exercise):
Method, frequency:

Helpful?   Other comments:

Summary of what did help: **Summary of what did not help:**

Plans for pain relief if situation occurs again (e.g. at home, or if readmit to hospital, return to accident and emergency):

Plans for pain relief at home or in immediate future, if applicable:

From: _____   Contact: _____

Pace Yourself

TO: _____ (patient's name)   DATE: _____

What is pacing? It's doing things throughout the day for periods of time that do not make your pain worse. Many people with chronic pain push or force themselves for a day or so, and then end up with much worse pain and are unable to do much for several days. Pacing is the opposite of this. The purpose of pacing is to make it possible for you to be active every day. Pacing and the big push are compared below.

Pacing

Take a break before you need it.

Benefits:

1. Pain stays manageable.

2. Able to maintain a certain level of activity day after day. No need to take time off.

3. Every day you are able to accomplish something you want or need to do.

Big Push

Force yourself.

Results:

1. Pain increases significantly. Medication intake increases. Irritability increases.

2. Must take time off to recover. Recovery may be slow and depressing.

3. You accomplish your goal but while you are recovering you can't do much at all.

By trial and error you can find out what you can do and for how long without your pain increasing or returning. For example, you may find that you can work at a certain activity for 30-minute periods, taking a 5-minute break every half hour. Setting a timer helps you remember. At the end of the day you may discover that you have worked productively for a total of 5 hours without increasing your pain. However, if you had pushed yourself to work 3 hours straight without a break, you might have increased pain and achieved less.

From: _____   Contact: _____

Overall Daily Plan

TO: _____ (patient's name)   DATE: _____

As a general rule, keep your pain under control by using your approaches to coping with pain before you really need them. Work out a daily schedule that includes each of the following to some extent in some way. Keep your pain under control. Don't wait until your pain is severe before you use something like relaxation, rest periods, or medication.

1. Pacing. Plan to rest before your pain increases and before you get tired.

2. Exercises. At least once a day, perform exercises that are appropriate for you. You may need to be advised by a physiotherapist. The main purposes of the exercises are to:
   • Stretch muscles to reduce soreness and muscle spasm.
   • Strengthen muscles.
   • Improve general physical fitness (this helps avoid further injury).
   • Increase ability to perform other activities.

3. Relaxation. Allow yourself to relax completely for at least 10 minutes once a day. You may use a relaxation tape, prayer, listening to music, or anything else that brings you peace of mind and contentment. Pain is stressful and frustrating, so you need to give yourself a real break from stress by truly relaxing. Just sitting down watching TV is not really profound relaxation. You may want to ask your nurse about relaxation techniques. Relaxation is a way to recharge yourself. Afterwards you'll feel more energetic and able to think clearly.

4. Medications for pain. These should be taken regularly by the clock, or at least before pain begins or increases.

5. Things to do every day. Do something every day that involves these three things:
   • Work (for wages, volunteer work, or study). Be sure you feel capable.
   • Family or close friend. Be sure you hug somebody.
   • Fun. Be sure you laugh.

From: _____ Contact: _____

Index